PATHOLOGIC BASIS OF DISEASE

SELF ASSESSMENT AND REVIEW

PATHOLOGIC BASIS OF DISEASE

SELF ASSESSMENT AND REVIEW

CAROLYN C. COMPTON, M.D., Ph.D.

Associate Professor of Pathology,
Harvard Medical School
Associate Pathologist,
Massachusetts General Hospital, Boston

3rd Edition

W.B. SAUNDERS COMPANY
Harcourt Brace Jovanovich, Inc.

Philadelphia   London   Toronto
Montreal   Sydney   Tokyo

W. B. SAUNDERS COMPANY
Harcourt Brace Jovanovich, Inc.

The Curtis Center
Independence Square West
Philadelphia, PA 19106

Library of Congress Cataloging-in-Publication Data

Compton, Carolyn C.

Pathologic basis of disease : self assessment and review /
Carolyn C. Compton.—3rd ed.

p.   cm.

1. Pathology—Examinations, questions, etc.
   I. Title.   [DNLM: 1. Pathology—examination
   questions.   QZ 18 C738p]

RB119.C65   1990

616.07—dc20
DNLM/DLC

for Library of Congress   89–70335
                                                        CIP

ISBN 0–7216–2974–1

Editor: Richard Zorab
Designer: Terri Siegel
Production Manager: Ken Neimeister
Manuscript Editor: Wendy Andresen

PATHOLOGIC BASIS OF DISEASE: Self Assessment and Review, Third Edition   ISBN   0–7216–2974–1

Printed in the United States of America.

Last digit is the print number: 9   8   7   6   5   4   3

Our delight in any particular study . . .
improves in proportion to the application which we bestow upon it.
Thus, what was at first an exercise
becomes at length an entertainment.

Addison

Many of those who can teach, can do, and do do.

David Seegal
The Pharos of Alpha Omega Alpha (1963)

Preface

This book was written for students of pathology. I intended it to serve as a working tool for studying and synthesizing information contained in the companion textbook, *Robbins Pathologic Basis of Disease*, 4/E. The questions are formulated in the traditional style of standardized examinations, which may help in preparation for quizzes, finals, or boards, but they are not meant to be examples of actual test questions. Actually, I was not expecting anyone who used this book to be able to answer all the questions correctly. Anyone who can does not really need this book. It is hoped that the mix of questions will help both to reinforce knowledge already acquired and to focus on new material for further study.

I have tried to design the questions to cover major issues and important details. The short explanations at the end of each chapter give concise answers to each question and expand on each answer choice. For more information about the topic of the question or the answer choices, you may want to consult the referenced pages of the textbook shown in parentheses after each answer or set of answers.

Acknowledgments

The author thanks

1. My students and residents, from whom I am always learning

2. My friends, who provided both moral and editorial support

3. My parents, who encouraged all my academic efforts, including this one

4. Dr. Stan Robbins and Dr. Ramzi Cotran, my much admired mentors

Answer: All of the above

Contents

1 General Pathology 1

    ANSWERS 13

2 Pediatric and Genetic Diseases 36

    ANSWERS 41

3 Nutritional Diseases 48

    ANSWERS 53

4 Infectious Diseases 61

    ANSWERS 66

5 The Cardiovascular System 74

    ANSWERS 81

6 The Respiratory System 91

    ANSWERS 96

7 The Hematopoietic and Lymphoid Systems 104

    ANSWERS 109

8 The Gastrointestinal Tract 117

    ANSWERS 126

9 The Liver, Biliary Tree, and Pancreas 139

    ANSWERS 145

10 The Kidneys and Urinary Tract 154
       ANSWERS 158

11 The Reproductive System 164
       ANSWERS 168

12 The Breast 174
       ANSWERS 177

13 The Skin 182
       ANSWERS 186

14 The Endocrine System 192
       ANSWERS 197

15 The Musculoskeletal System 204
       ANSWERS 209

16 The Nervous System 215
       ANSWERS 220

General Pathology

DIRECTIONS: For Questions 1 to 17, choose the ONE BEST answer to each question.

1. Generalized edema results from all of the following disorders EXCEPT:

A. Systemic hypertension
B. Congestive heart failure
C. Cirrhosis
D. Nephrotic syndrome
E. Hyperaldosteronism

2. Disorders that predispose to thrombosis include all of the following EXCEPT:

A. Pancreatic carcinoma
B. Pregnancy
C. Vitamin K deficiency
D. Sickle cell anemia
E. Severe burns

3. Chemical agents known to be carcinogenic in human beings include all of the following EXCEPT:

A. Cyclophosphamide (Cytoxan)
B. Asbestos
C. Arsenic
D. Saccharin
E. Vinyl chloride

4. Markedly increased susceptibility to pyogenic infections occurs in all of the following conditions EXCEPT:

A. Deficiency of the third component of complement (C3)
B. Common variable immunodeficiency
C. Chronic granulomatous disease of childhood
D. DiGeorge's syndrome
E. Chédiak-Higashi syndrome

5. The feature most important in differentiating a malignant from a benign tumor is:

A. Lack of encapsulation
B. High mitotic rate

C. Presence of necrosis
D. Presence of metastases
E. Nuclear pleomorphism (anaplasia)

6. In hypoxic cell injury, swelling of the cells occurs because:

A. Intracytoplasmic lipids accumulate
B. Intracytoplasmic proteins accumulate
C. Intracytoplasmic glycogen increases
D. Intracytoplasmic lipofuscin accumulates
E. Water enters the cell

7. Cell injury from chemically unstable molecules known as free radicals is a major feature of all of the following pathologic processes EXCEPT:

A. Mercury poisoning
B. Irradiation damage
C. Oxygen toxicity
D. Carbon tetrachloride poisoning
E. Bacterial infection

8. In an inflammatory response, neutrophils release molecules that have all of the following effects EXCEPT:

A. Chemotaxis of monocytes
B. Chemotaxis of lymphocytes
C. Degranulation of mast cells
D. Increased vascular permeability independent of histamine release
E. Connective tissue digestion

9. In immunologic reactions, lymphocytes make substances (cytokines) that are chemotactic for all of the following cells EXCEPT:

A. Neutrophils
B. Platelets
C. Eosinophils
D. Macrophages
E. Basophils

10. Mediators of increased vascular permeability in acute inflammatory responses include all of the following EXCEPT:

    A. Leukotriene E_4
    B. Complement complex C5b67
    C. Leukotriene C_4
    D. Bradykinin
    E. Platelet activating factor (PAF)

11. The most reliable evidence of chronicity in an inflammatory process in the liver (hepatitis) is the presence of:

    A. Lymphocytes
    B. Bile duct destruction
    C. Councilman bodies
    D. Fibrosis
    E. Plasmacytic infiltrates

12. A large aggregate of epithelioid histiocytes is seen in a microscopic section of an ovary removed at surgery. Your diagnosis is:

    A. Granulation tissue
    B. Granular cell tumor
    C. Granulosa cell tumor
    D. Granuloma
    E. Granulocytosis

13. All of the following neoplasms are malignant EXCEPT:

    A. Glomus tumor
    B. Ewing's tumor
    C. Wilms' tumor
    D. Seminoma
    E. Histiocytosis X

14. Hereditary conditions that are associated with a high risk of malignancy include all of the following EXCEPT:

    A. Von Hippel-Lindau disease
    B. Turcot's syndrome
    C. Patau's syndrome
    D. Fanconi's anemia
    E. Ataxia-telangiectasia

15. The diagnosis on a cervical cytology specimen is Class II. You would tell the patient that:

    A. Her Pap smear was perfectly normal
    B. Atypical cells were found, and the examination will need to be repeated
    C. A high-grade cervical dysplasia is present, and biopsy confirmation will be required
    D. Carcinoma in situ was found, and surgical excision of the lesion will be necessary
    E. Invasive carcinoma is present, and hysterectomy will be required

16. The cell surface antigen detected by monoclonal antibodies and known as CD5 is a marker for:

    A. T cells
    B. B cells
    C. Monocytes and granulocytes
    D. Myeloid stem cells
    E. NK cells

17. Stimuli to mast cell degranulation include all of the following EXCEPT:

    A. Antigen-IgE complexes
    B. Cold
    C. Interleukin-1
    D. Sunlight
    E. Bee venom

DIRECTIONS: For Questions 18 to 45, ONE or MORE of the completions given correctly finishes the incomplete statement. Choose:
    A—if only 1, 2, and 3 are correct
    B—if only 1 and 3 are correct
    C—if only 2 and 4 are correct
    D—if only 4 is correct
    E—if all are correct

18. In myocardial ischemia, irreversibly injured myofibers are distinguishable by which of the following light microscopic features?

    1. Cytoplasmic fatty change
    2. Cytoplasmic eosinophilia
    3. Cellular swelling
    4. Nuclear shrinkage

    A. 1, 2, 3   B. 1, 3   C. 2, 4   D. 4 only   E. All

19. Generation of free radicals is the major mechanism of cell injury in:

    1. Oxygen toxicity
    2. Radiation injury
    3. Carbon tetrachloride poisoning
    4. Ischemia

    A. 1, 2, 3   B. 1, 3   C. 2, 4   D. 4 only   E. All

20. Which of the following conditions are usually associated with delayed wound healing?

1. Severe granulocytopenia
2. Cushing's syndrome
3. Severe thrombocytopenia
4. Scurvy

    A. 1, 2, 3   B. 1, 3   C. 2, 4   D. 4 only   E. All

21. Cytotoxic lymphocytes are the major mediators of the pathogenesis of:

1. Renal transplant rejection
2. Arthus reaction
3. Graft-versus-host disease
4. Tuberculin reaction

    A. 1, 2, 3   B. 1, 3   C. 2, 4   D. 4 only   E. All

22. Secondary amyloidosis is associated with:

1. Ulcerative colitis
2. Rheumatoid arthritis
3. Renal cell carcinoma
4. Waldenström's macroglobulinemia

    A. 1, 2, 3   B. 1, 3   C. 2, 4   D. 4 only   E. All

23. Amyloid is:

1. Digested by amylase
2. Stained by oil red O
3. Sometimes generated from immunoglobulin heavy chains
4. Sometimes generated from transthyretin

    A. 1, 2, 3   B. 1, 3   C. 2, 4   D. 4 only   E. All

24. Hageman factor activates the:

1. Complement system
2. Kinin system
3. Fibrinolytic system
4. Coagulation system

    A. 1, 2, 3   B. 1, 3   C. 2, 4   D. 4 only   E. All

25. Red infarcts are usually encountered in:

1. Pulmonary embolism
2. Torsion of the testis
3. Superior mesenteric artery atheroembolism
4. Coronary artery thrombosis

    A. 1, 2, 3   B. 1, 3   C. 2, 4   D. 4 only   E. All

26. Shock is commonly associated with which of the following conditions?

1. *Escherichia coli* sepsis
2. Myocardial infarction
3. Cholera
4. Acute pancreatitis

    A. 1, 2, 3   B. 1, 3   C. 2, 4   D. 4 only   E. All

27. Human malignancies known to be caused by exposure to radiation include:

1. Acute leukemia
2. Thyroid carcinoma
3. Lung cancer
4. Osteosarcoma

    A. 1, 2, 3   B. 1, 3   C. 2, 4   D. 4 only   E. All

28. Neoplasms that are known to be associated with a defect of chromosome 22 include:

1. Adenocarcinoma of the lung
2. Meningioma
3. Malignant melanoma
4. Chronic myelogenous leukemia

    A. 1, 2, 3   B. 1, 3   C. 2, 4   D. 4 only   E. All

29. Factors that are assessed in the grading of a malignant tumor include:

1. Numbers of lymph nodes containing metastases
2. Size of the primary lesion
3. Degree of local invasion of the primary tumor
4. Number of mitoses in the primary tumor

    A. 1, 2, 3   B. 1, 3   C. 2, 4   D. 4 only   E. All

30. Shock is a frequent complication of large burn injuries that is commonly produced by:

1. Disseminated intravascular coagulation
2. *Pseudomonas* endotoxemia
3. Transudation of fluid from the wound
4. Anaphylaxis from smoke inhalation

    A. 1, 2, 3   B. 1, 3   C. 2, 4   D. 4 only   E. All

31. In a myocardial biopsy taken 2 hours after coronary occlusion and reperfusion, which of the following ultrastructural features would indicate that the myocytes had sustained irreversible ischemic injury?

1. Ribosomal detachment from the rough endoplasmic reticulum
2. Appearance of dense deposits in the mitochondria
3. Loss of intracellular glycogen
4. Loss of intracellular RNA

    A. 1, 2, 3   B. 1, 3   C. 2, 4   D. 4 only   E. All

32. An immunoperoxidase stain of an anaplastic tumor demonstrates the presence of desmin in the tumor cell cytoplasm. This finding is compatible with a diagnosis of:

1. Malignant schwannoma
2. Squamous cell carcinoma
3. Lymphoma
4. Rhabdosarcoma

    A. 1, 2, 3   B. 1, 3   C. 2, 4   D. 4 only   E. All

33. Contractile and cytoskeletal elements common to all cells include:

1. Spectrin
2. Actin
3. Myosin
4. Tubulin

   A. 1, 2, 3   B. 1, 3   C. 2, 4   D. 4 only   E. All

34. Pathologic forms of hyperplasia that are associated with an increased risk of malignancy in the tissue of origin and are therefore considered to be premalignant conditions include:

1. Adenomatous hyperplasia of endometrium
2. Follicular hyperplasia of lymph nodes
3. Hyperplasia of gastric mucosa (Ménétrier's disease)
4. Prostatic gland hyperplasia

   A. 1, 2, 3   B. 1, 3   C. 2, 4   D. 4 only   E. All

35. Cancers that commonly occur in tissues that have first undergone metaplasia, then become dysplastic, and finally become malignant include:

1. Squamous cell carcinoma of the endocervix
2. Squamous cell carcinoma of the bladder
3. Bronchogenic squamous cell carcinoma
4. Adenocarcinoma of the esophagus

   A. 1, 2, 3   B. 1, 3   C. 2, 4   D. 4 only   E. All

36. In which of the following diseases do calcium deposits commonly occur in *normal* tissues?

1. Wilson's disease
2. Multiple myeloma
3. Papillary carcinoma of the thyroid
4. Parathyroid carcinoma

   A. 1, 2, 3   B. 1, 3   C. 2, 4   D. 4 only   E. All

37. Factors that promote neutrophil adherence to the endothelium of blood vessels (a prerequisite for leukocyte emigration into tissues in an acute inflammatory response) include:

1. Leukotriene B_4
2. Endotoxin
3. Complement fragment C5a
4. Interleukin-1

   A. 1, 2, 3   B. 1, 3   C. 2, 4   D. 4 only   E. All

38. Predisposition to bacterial infection in diabetes mellitus is caused by basic defects in leukocyte function that include:

1. Reduced ability of leukocytes to stick to vascular endothelium
2. Reduced numbers of circulating white cells

3. Defective phagocytic function
4. Deficiency of leukocyte glucose-6-phosphate dehydrogenase (G6PD)

   A. 1, 2, 3   B. 1, 3   C. 2, 4   D. 4 only   E. All

39. Factors that are important in protecting normal cells from potential injury from free radicals generated in the course of an inflammatory response include:

1. Glutathione peroxidase
2. Serum ceruloplasmin
3. Catalase
4. α_2-Macroglobulin

   A. 1, 2, 3   B. 1, 3   C. 2, 4   D. 4 only   E. All

40. Pathologic lesions produced by vascular congestion include:

1. Nutmeg liver
2. Brown induration of the lung
3. Splenic Gandy-Gamna bodies
4. Strawberry gallbladder

   A. 1, 2, 3   B. 1, 3   C. 2, 4   D. 4 only   E. All

41. Amyloid of the AA type, in which the fibrils are composed mostly of amyloid-associated (AA) protein, occurs in association with which of the following conditions?

1. Senile cardiac amyloidosis
2. Hereditary neuropathic amyoidosis
3. Medullary carcinoma of the thyroid
4. Ulcerative colitis

   A. 1, 2, 3   B. 1, 3   C. 2, 4   D. 4 only   E. All

42. Tumors that tend to spread over the surfaces of viscera or body cavities rather than metastasizing via blood vessels or lymphatics include:

1. Colon carcinoma
2. Ovarian carcinoma
3. Renal cell carcinoma
4. Mesothelioma

   A. 1, 2, 3   B. 1, 3   C. 2, 4   D. 4 only   E. All

43. In the United States, which of the following tumors occur(s) with greater frequency in males than in females?

1. Pancreatic carcinoma
2. Colon carcinoma
3. Bladder carcinoma
4. Hepatocellular carcinoma (hepatoma)

   A. 1, 2, 3   B. 1, 3   C. 2, 4   D. 4 only   E. All

44. Oncogenic retroviruses:

1. Are RNA viruses
2. Contain the enzyme reverse transcriptase
3. Cause transformation via oncogenes or proto-oncogenes
4. Cause more types of human malignancy than all other oncogenic viruses

    A. 1, 2, 3   B. 1, 3   C. 2, 4   D. 4 only   E. All

45. Proto-oncogenes are known to:

1. Be normal genes in animal cells
2. Give rise to viral oncogenes (*v-onc*)
3. Encode proteins serving vital cell functions
4. Give rise to cellular oncogenes (*c-onc*)

    A. 1, 2, 3   B. 1, 3   C. 2, 4   D. 4 only   E. All

DIRECTIONS: For Questions 46 to 71, you are to decide whether EACH choice is TRUE or FALSE.

For each of the following statements about histocompatibility (HLA) antigens, decide whether it is TRUE or FALSE.

46. Histocompatibility antigens are the antigens that evoke graft-versus-host disease

47. Class II HLA (HLA-D) antigens are found on the cell surface of all normal nucleated cells

48. Class II HLA (HLA-D) antigens evoke the formation of humoral antibody in genetically incompatible transplant recipients

49. The chance that two siblings will be HLA identical is 50%

50. The genes that determine the magnitude of immune responses are located within the HLA gene complex

51. Recognition of a virally infected cell by a T lymphocyte is dependent on the presence of class II HLA antigens on the infected cells

52. Individuals who possess HLA-B27 antigen are nearly 100 times more likely to get ankylosing spondylitis than those who do not

For each of the following statements about tissue atrophy, decide whether it is TRUE or FALSE.

53. Atrophic cells contain fewer than normal numbers of cytoplasmic organelles (mitochondria, endoplasmic reticulum, etc.)

54. Atrophy occurs in otherwise normal tissues if their workload is decreased

55. Atrophy begins to occur in most tissues immediately after death of the individual

56. Atrophy occurs in otherwise normal tissues if the blood supply is decreased

57. The appearance of autophagic vacuoles in cells undergoing atrophy signals irreversible cell injury and impending cell death

For each of the following statements about the acquired immunodeficiency syndrome (AIDS), decide whether it is TRUE or FALSE.

58. The disease is caused by a retrovirus infection

59. The AIDS virus can also cause neoplastic transformation of normal cells

60. The number of helper T cells in the peripheral blood is characteristically increased

61. Immunoglobulin levels are characteristically normal or elevated

62. Death from this disease is usually caused by metastatic Kaposi's sarcoma

63. Lymphomas of B cells are more common than T-cell lymphomas in AIDS

64. Hemophiliacs are at high risk of developing AIDS

For each of the following statements about general tumor biology, decide whether it is TRUE or FALSE.

65. The rate of cell proliferation in most solid tumors is less than that of normally renewing intestinal epithelium

66. Most malignant tumors grow more rapidly than benign tumors

67. Most tumors are clones derived from a single transformed cell

68. Tumor cells require greater amounts of growth factors in vitro than their normal counterparts

69. Tumor cells capable of metastasis secrete enzymes that digest basement membrane components

70. Nonrandom karyotype alterations are associated with malignant but not benign tumors

71. Hereditary predisposition exists for most cancers, including the most common forms

DIRECTIONS: For Questions 72 to 99, the set of lettered headings is followed by a list of numbered words or phrases. For each numbered word or phrase choose:

A—if the item is associated with (A) only
B—if the item is associated with (B) only
C—if the item is associated with *both* (A) and (B)
D—if the item is associated with *neither* (A) nor (B)

For each process or lesion listed below, choose whether it is primarily characterized by an inflammatory response, an immunologic response, both, or neither.

  A. Inflammatory response
  B. Immunologic response
  C. Both
  D. Neither

72. Suture granuloma

73. Marantic endocarditis

74. Streptococcal pneumonia

75. Sunburn

76. Hashimoto's thyroiditis

77. Lead poisoning

For each of the biologic properties described below, decide whether it is characteristic of epidermal cells, fibroblasts, both, or neither.

  A. Epidermal cells (keratinocytes)
  B. Fibroblasts
  C. Both
  D. Neither

78. Under physiologic conditions, undergo continuous proliferation throughout life

79. Respond so rapidly to surgical skin incisions that migration across the wound is complete within 24 to 48 hours

80. Produce type IV collagen

81. Produce type II collagen

82. Synthesize fibronectin

83. Are induced to migrate by fibronectin

84. Are induced to divide by a factor secreted by activated macrophages

85. Are induced to divide by transforming growth factor-α (TFG-α)

86. Are induced to divide by platelet-derived growth factor (PDGF)

87. Produce interleukin-1

For each of the conditions listed below, decide whether it is causally related to cigarette smoking, alcohol abuse, both, or neither.

  A. Cigarette smoking
  B. Alcohol abuse
  C. Both
  D. Neither

88. Esophageal carcinoma

89. Acute esophagitis

90. Pancreatic carcinoma

91. Acute pancreatitis

92. Gastric carcinoma

93. Acute gastritis

94. Renal cell carcinoma

95. Bladder carcinoma

96. Pharyngeal carcinoma

97. Hodgkin's disease

98. Breast carcinoma

99. Ovarian carcinoma

DIRECTIONS: Questions 100 to 282 are matching questions. For each numbered item, choose the most likely associated lettered item from those provided. Each numbered item has ONLY ONE answer. Within each group, each lettered item may be the answer to one, more than one, or none of the numbered items.

For each of the biologic properties of mast cell mediators of type I (anaphylactic type) hypersensitivity reactions listed below, decide whether it is produced by leukotriene C_4, histamine, prostaglandin D_2, all of these, or none of these.

    A. Leukotriene C_4
    B. Histamine
    C. Prostaglandin D_2
    D. All of the above
    E. None of the above

100. Stored in granules in mast cell cytoplasm

101. Causes smooth muscle spasm

102. Attracts eosinophils

103. Increases vascular permeability

104. Causes platelet aggregation

105. Attracts neutrophils

For each of the autoantibodies listed below, choose the autoimmune disease with which it is most strongly linked.

    A. Grave's disease
    B. Sjögren's syndrome
    C. Lupus
    D. Systemic sclerosis (scleroderma)
    E. Primary biliary cirrhosis
    F. Goodpasture's syndrome
    G. Myasthenia gravis
    H. Type A fundal gastritis

106. Anti-double-stranded DNA

107. Scl-70 (anti-DNA topoisomerase I)

108. Anti-basement membrane

109. SS-B(La) (antiribonucleoprotein)

110. Anticentromere (anticentromeric proteins)

111. Anti-intrinsic factor

112. Antimitochondria

113. Antihistone

114. Antiacetylcholine receptor

115. Anti-TSH receptor

For each of the causes of fatty liver listed below, decide whether it increases free fatty acid entry into liver cells, decreases fatty acid oxidation, increases triglyceride formation, decreases apoprotein synthesis, or does all of these.

    A. Increases free fatty acid entry into liver cells
    B. Decreases fatty acid oxidation
    C. Increases triglyceride formation
    D. Decreases apoprotein synthesis
    E. All of these

116. Alcohol ingestion

117. Phosphorus poisoning

118. Carbon tetrachloride poisoning

119. Corticosteroid therapy

120. Starvation

For each of the descriptions of intracellular pigment accumulation listed below, decide whether it refers to lipofuscin, melanin, hemosiderin, or none of these.

    A. Lipofuscin
    B. Melanin
    C. Hemosiderin
    D. None of these

121. Accumulates in cartilage of patients with ochronosis

122. Accumulates in lungs of patients with mitral stenosis

123. Accumulates in lungs of coal miners

124. Accumulates in synovium of patients with pigmented villonodular synovitis

125. Accumulates in colonic mucosa of some laxative abusers

For each of the situations listed below, decide whether the cellular response it typically engenders is hypertrophy, hyperplasia, metaplasia, dysplasia, or none of these.

    A. Hypertrophy
    B. Hyperplasia
    C. Metaplasia
    D. Dysplasia
    E. None of these

126. Response of cardiac muscle to systemic hypertension

127. Response of bronchiolar epithelium in chronic bronchitis

128. Response of adrenocortical cells to a pituitary adenoma producing ACTH

129. Response of prostatic stroma in benign prostatic hypertrophy

130. Response of colonic epithelium in long-standing ulcerative colitis

For each of the characteristics of autoimmune disease listed below, decide whether it describes systemic lupus erythematosus (SLE), Sjögren's syndrome, scleroderma, all of these, or none of these.

    A. Systemic lupus erythematosus (SLE)
    B. Sjögren's syndrome
    C. Scleroderma
    D. All of these
    E. None of these

131. The disease occurs with increased incidence in hereditary deficiency of the second component of complement (C2)

132. A 40-fold increased risk of lymphoid malignancy is incurred

133. An underlying epithelial malignancy is found in 10% of patients

134. Dermatomyositis is an associated disorder

135. Articular (joint) pain is a common symptom

136. Anticentromere antibodies are characteristic

137. Glomerular lesions are extremely rare

138. The most common cause of death is renal failure

139. Immunoglobulin deposition is found in normal-appearing skin

140. Response to corticosteroids is excellent

For each of the characteristics of immunodeficiency disease listed below, decide whether it describes X-linked agammaglobulinemia of Bruton, common variable immunodeficiency, DiGeorge's syndrome, or none of these.

    A. X-linked agammaglobulinemia of Bruton
    B. Common variable immunodeficiency
    C. DiGeorge's syndrome
    D. None of these

141. Characterized by a failure of pre-B cells to mature into B cells

142. Caused by a defect in lymphoid stem cells

143. Associated with tetany

144. Associated with a high incidence of systemic lupus erythematosus

145. Often accompanied by nontropical sprue (gluten-sensitive enteropathy)

146. Associated with an increased incidence of lymphoid malignancy

147. Associated with noncaseating granulomas in the liver

For each of the conditions listed below, decide whether the major pathogenetic mechanism of the associated tissue edema and/or ascites is related to:

    A. Decreased plasma oncotic pressure
    B. Increased hydrostatic pressure
    C. Increased endothelial permeability
    D. Lymphatic obstruction
    E. None of these

148. Nephrotic syndrome

149. Congestive heart failure

150. Cirrhosis

151. Thermal burn

152. Kwashiorkor

153. Bee sting

154. Pregnancy

155. Excessive salt intake

156. Hydrops fetalis

157. Constrictive pericarditis

158. Metastatic carcinoma

159. Ménétrier's disease

For each of the conditions listed below, decide whether it most commonly produces coagulation necrosis, liquefaction necrosis, enzymatic fat necrosis, caseous necrosis, or none of these.

    A. Coagulation necrosis
    B. Liquefaction necrosis
    C. Enzymatic fat necrosis
    D. Caseous necrosis
    E. None of these

160. Pulmonary nocardiosis

161. Myocardial infarction

162. Pott's disease

163. Tuberculoid leprosy of skin

164. Acute pancreatitis

165. Wet gangrene of the great toe

166. Giardiasis (small bowel)

167. Cerebral infarction

168. Acute tubular necrosis (kidney)

For each of the conditions listed below, decide whether it is an example of an immunologically mediated disorder of the anaphylactic type (type I), cytotoxic type (type II), immune complex type (type III), cell-mediated type (type IV), or whether it is not an immunologically mediated disorder at all.

   A. Type I, anaphylactic type immune response
   B. Type II, cytotoxic type immune response
   C. Type III, immune complex disorder
   D. Type IV, cell-mediated hypersensitivity response
   E. Not an immunologically mediated disorder

169. Erythroblastosis fetalis

170. Poison ivy dermatitis

171. Hay fever

172. Polyarteritis nodosa

173. Serum sickness

174. Graft-versus-host disease

175. Dopamine-induced hemolytic anemia

176. Penicillin-induced urticaria

177. Cyclosporine-induced renal injury

178. Chlorpromazine-induced cholestatic jaundice

179. Pulmonary asbestosis

180. Chronic berylliosis

For each of the biologic characteristics listed below, decide whether it describes B cells, T cells, macrophages/monocytes, all of these cell types, or none of these.

   A. T cells
   B. B cells

   C. Macrophages/monocytes
   D. All of the above
   E. None of the above

181. Found in the circulating blood

182. Found in the cortex of lymph nodes

183. Display IgG on their cell surface

184. Do not usually display HLA-DR antigens on their cell surface

185. Do not have cell surface receptors for complement

186. Are able to lyse antibody-coated target cells by means of a nonphagocytic mechanism

187. Function in the negative regulation (turning off) of the immune response

188. Are capable of lysing tumor cells without previous sensitization

189. Initiate delayed-type cell-mediated hypersensitivity responses

190. Produce leukotriene mediators of anaphylaxis

191. Respond chemotactically to leukotriene B_4

192. Arise from stem cells in the bone marrow

For each of the situations listed below, decide whether bilirubin, hematin, ceroid, lipofuscin, or none of these pigmentations would be expected to be seen.

   A. Bilirubin
   B. Hematin
   C. Ceroid
   D. Lipofuscin
   E. None of these

193. Myocytes of an elderly, malnourished individual

194. Hepatocytes in an elderly, malnourished individual

195. Kupffer's cells in a patient recovering from hepatitis

196. Sinus histiocytes in the peribronchial lymph nodes of a smoker

197. Skin keratinocytes in Addison's disease

198. Kupffer's cells in an individual with hereditary spherocytosis

199. Kupffer's cells in large bile duct obstruction

200. Splenic phagocytes in malaria

201. Splenic phagocytes after a hemolytic transfusion reaction

202. Dermal macrophages of tattooed skin

For each of the conditions listed below, decide whether the associated inflammatory cell infiltrate is composed predominantly of neutrophils, monocytes/macrophages, eosinophils, plasma cells, or lymphocytes.

    A. Neutrophils
    B. Monocytes/macrophages
    C. Eosinophils
    D. Plasma cells
    E. Lymphocytes

203. Acute myocardial infarction (2 to 3 days in age)

204. Acute B viral hepatitis

205. Sarcoidosis

206. Primary tuberculosis

207. Polyarteritis nodosa

208. Reflux esophagitis

209. Primary syphilis

210. Löffler's syndrome

211. Paragonimiasis (lung fluke infection)

212. Bronchial asthma

For each of the biologic effects listed below, decide whether it is produced by one of the following cytokines, all of these, or none of these:

    A. Interleukin-1 (IL-1)
    B. Interleukin-2 (IL-2)
    C. Tumor necrosis factor-α (TNF-α)
    D. γ-Interferon (IFN-γ)
    E. All of the above
    F. None of the above

213. Made by virtually any cell

214. Activates macrophages

215. Made only by activated T cells

216. Stimulates natural killer (NK) cell growth

217. Induces expression of HLA class II molecules in many cells

218. Directly kills bacteria

219. Stimulates mast cell growth

220. Has direct antiviral activity

For each of the properties listed below, decide whether it is characteristic of CD4+ helper T cells, natural killer (NK) cells, CD8+ cytotoxic T cells, all of these, or none of these.

    A. CD4+ helper T cells
    B. Natural killer (NK) cells
    C. CD8+ cytotoxic T cells
    D. All of the above
    E. None of the above

221. Lack the ability to destroy tumor cells

222. Are not phagocytic

223. Contain granules in their cytoplasm

224. Are capable of lysing only antibody-coated cells

225. Possess cell surface receptors for the Fc fragment of IgG

226. Recognize antigens only in association with class I HLA antigens

227. Recognize antigens only in association with class II HLA antigens

For each of the conditions listed below, decide whether it is characterized by inflammation of the serous, fibrinous, suppurative, granulomatous, or lymphoplasmacytic type.

    A. Serous inflammation
    B. Fibrinous inflammation
    C. Suppurative inflammation
    D. Granulomatous inflammation
    E. Mononuclear cell inflammation

228. Cat-scratch lymphadenitis

229. Acute viral pneumonia

230. Acute appendicitis

231. Rheumatic pericarditis

232. Chronic brucellosis

233. Adult hyaline membrane disease (diffuse alveolar damage)

234. Second-degree thermal burns

235. Friction blisters

236. Acute viral hepatitis

237. Acute ascending cholangitis

238. Initial stage of primary biliary cirrhosis

239. Uremic pericarditis

For each of the chemical carcinogens listed below, decide whether it is primarily associated with cancer of the lung, skin, stomach, bladder, or none of these malignancies.

    A. Lung cancer
    B. Skin cancer
    C. Stomach cancer
    D. Bladder cancer
    E. None of the above

240. Aflatoxin B_1

241. Beta-naphthylamine (an azo dye)

242. Busulfan

243. Vinyl chloride

244. Chromium compounds

245. Nitrosamines

246. Benzidine

For each of the tumor types listed below, decide which of the following substances would be expected to be found in the tumor cells by immunohistochemical stains and would help to identify the tumor.

    A. Alpha-fetoprotein
    B. Carcinoembryonic antigen
    C. Desmin
    D. Human chorionic gonadotropin
    E. None of the above

247. Lymphoma

248. Neuroblastoma

249. Hepatoma

250. Colonic carcinoma

251. Choriocarcinoma

252. Medullary carcinoma of the thyroid

253. Rhabdosarcoma

For each of the neoplasms listed below, decide if Epstein-Barr virus, papillomavirus, herpes simplex type 2, hepatitis B virus, or none of these viruses is thought to be causally related to at least some tumors of that type.

    A. Epstein-Barr virus
    B. Papillomavirus
    C. Adenovirus
    D. Hepatitis B virus
    E. None of these

254. Cervical carcinoma

255. Breast carcinoma

256. Nasopharyngeal carcinoma

257. Burkitt's lymphoma

258. Cutaneous squamous cell carcinoma

259. Adult T-cell leukemia

260. Fibrosarcoma

261. Cholangiocarcinoma

262. Hepatoma

263. Angiosarcoma of the liver

For each of the paraneoplastic syndromes listed below, decide whether bronchogenic carcinoma, pancreatic carcinoma, renal cell carcinoma, prostatic carcinoma, or none of these is a very strongly associated underlying malignancy.

    A. Bronchogenic carcinoma
    B. Pancreatic carcinoma
    C. Renal cell carcinoma
    D. Prostatic carcinoma
    E. None of these

264. Malignant form of acanthosis nigricans

265. Hypercalcemia

266. Cancer-associated dermatomyositis

267. Hypertrophic osteoarthropathy

268. Hyponatremia

269. Polycythemia

270. Nephrotic syndrome

271. Anemia (nonmyelophthisic)

272. Malignancy-associated myasthenia gravis

273. Peripheral neuropathy

For each of the descriptions of molecular complexes found on the surfaces of cells of the immune system listed below, decide whether it characterizes CD3, CD4, CD8, all of these, or none of these.

    A. CD3
    B. CD4
    C. CD8
    D. All of these

274. Receptor for class I histocompatibility molecules

275. Receptor for class II histocompatibility molecules

276. Receptor for interleukin-2

277. Receptor for complement

278. Receptor for the Fc portion of IgG

279. Part of the class I histocompatibility molecular complex

280. Part of the class II histocompatibility molecular complex

281. Part of the T-cell antigen receptor (TCR) complex

282. Part of the B-cell antigen receptor

1

General Pathology

1. (A) Generalized noninflammatory edema results from imbalances in the factors determining body fluid compartmentalization that favor the entry of fluid into the extravascular compartment. Thus, common primary causes include increased hydrostatic pressure (congestive heart failure or cirrhosis with portal hypertension) and reduced plasma oncotic pressure resulting from either inadequate synthesis (cirrhosis) or increased loss (nephrotic syndrome) of albumin. Increased osmotic tension in the interstitial fluid related to sodium retention is another primary cause of generalized noninflammatory edema, which occurs in the presence of increased circulating levels of aldosterone.

Generalized edema occurs only in the presence of increased hydrostatic pressure in the venous or lymphatic system, the sites of resorption of extravascular interstitial fluid. Systemic hypertension in the arterial system does not produce this effect (pp. 87–89).

2. (C) A number of clinical states are associated with an increased incidence of thrombosis. Included among these are pregnancy and pancreatic carcinoma. The mechanisms underlying the thrombotic tendency in pregnancy are poorly understood but in pancreatic carcinoma may be related to the release of tissue thromboplastin and procoagulant factors from the tumor.

Conditions that produce intravascular stasis also predispose to thrombosis. Sickle cell anemia is a prime example (see Chapter 7, Question 13).

Severe tissue injury, such as that incurred in severe burns or trauma, causes release of tissue factor and predisposes to thrombosis. Other factors contributing to hypercoagulability in burns and trauma include direct endothelial injury and immobilization with vascular stasis.

Vitamin K deficiency, in contrast, produces a bleeding tendency rather than a predisposition to thrombosis. Because vitamin K is essential to the biosynthesis of

prothrombin and clotting factors VII, IX, and X, vitamin K deficiency produces a coagulopathy on the basis of the depletion of these factors (see Chapter 3, Question 14, and pp. 97–100).

3. (D) It is now clear from both epidemiologic and experimental studies that a large number of chemical agents are capable of causing neoplastic transformation of cells, either by direct action or after metabolic transformation into a carcinogenic metabolite. Among the best studied chemical carcinogens are alkylating agents (e.g., cyclophosphamide), many of which are used for cancer chemotherapy and have resulted in the iatrogenic induction of second malignancies (particularly lymphoid neoplasms and leukemia). Asbestos is a well-known cause of mesothelioma, a tumor that rarely occurs in other than asbestos-exposed individuals. Arsenic exposure is a well-documented cause of cutaneous squamous cell carcinomas, and vinyl chloride is known to cause the otherwise rare hemangiosarcoma of liver. Saccharin, in contrast, has only been shown to promote bladder cancer in rats previously given marginal doses of carcinogens. There is no epidemiologic evidence that saccharin is carcinogenic in humans (pp. 271–273).

4. (D) The most important defense mechanisms against pyogenic infections are humoral immune responses and inflammatory reactions with neutrophilic phagocytosis. Thus, disorders that affect either of these processes are associated with increased susceptibility to pyogenic infection.

Because the third component of complement plays a critical role as an opsonin in inflammatory responses to pyogenic bacteria, C3 deficiencies increase susceptibility to infection by these organisms. Common variable immunodeficiency is associated with a defect in humoral immunity causing increased susceptibility to pyogenic infection. Chronic granulomatous disease of childhood and the Chédiak-Higashi syndrome are disorders in which the function of phagocytes is deranged and pyogenic infection is common. In chronic granulomatous disease of childhood, hydrogen peroxide (H_2O_2) production by neutrophils is deficient, leading to a defect in the myeloperoxidase-H_2O_2-halide bactericidal system and susceptibility to catalase-producing bacteria. In the Chédiak-Higashi syndrome, a number of defects in phagocyte function are present, including impaired chemotactic responses and deficient degranulation.

DiGeorge's syndrome, however, is a disorder of the cellular immune system only. Inflammatory mechanisms and humoral immunity are unimpaired in patients with DiGeorge's syndrome, and susceptibility to pyogenic infection is not increased (*pp. 51–52, 222*).

5. (D) Although a number of pathologic features, such as anaplasia with nuclear pleomorphism, high mitotic rate, lack of encapsulation, and presence of necrosis and hemorrhage, are typically associated with malignant tumors, benign tumors may occasionally display one or more of these features as well. Therefore, the only feature that is absolutely diagnostic of malignancy is metastasis. Although so-called benign tumors are capable of producing considerable morbidity and even mortality through local compressive effects or secretion of systemically active substances such as hormones, benign tumors never metastasize (*pp. 243–248*).

6. (E) Hypoxia is the most common cause of cell injury. It is usually caused by ischemia (decreased blood flow) to the tissue, but depletion of the oxygen-carrying capacity of the blood or toxic injury to intracellular oxidative enzymes can also cause hypoxic injury. One of the most common histologic hallmarks of hypoxic cell injury, especially in cells with a high rate of aerobic metabolism, is acute cellular swelling (cellular edema). It occurs as a result of an influx of sodium and an iso-osmotic quantity of water into the cell. Because the cell membrane pumps that normally keep the concentration of sodium inside the cell low compared with the extracellular fluid require ATP as their energy source, they will cease to function as oxygen tension within the cell decreases, in turn decreasing oxidative phosphorylation by mitochondria and generation of ATP. Glycogen supplies within the cell cytoplasm can serve as a temporary source of ATP generated from anaerobic glycolysis, but glycogen stores are quickly depleted. Very simply, loss of the biochemical means to produce ATP, the energy source that fuels the active transport enzyme systems of the cell membrane, leads to failure of these pumps to move ions (and fluid) out of the cell.

Although intracytoplasmic accumulations of abnormal amounts of lipid, protein, glycogen, or lipofuscin may occur in some forms of cell injury, they do not usually occur with hypoxia. Moreover, although accumulation of any of these substances may cause affected cells to increase in size, the process would not be known as cellular swelling. This term applies exclusively to intracellular edema (see Questions 18 and 116 and *pp. 4–5*).

7. (A) Free radicals are chemically unstable, highly reactive molecules that are generated in many types of chemical and toxic pathologic processes. They are capable of profound cellular injury, chiefly through their ability to damage unsaturated fatty acids in cell membranes. The initiation of free radicals requires either a powerful outside energy source (e.g., ionizing radiation) or oxidation-reduction reactions that add single extra electrons to molecules capable of accepting them (e.g., oxygen). Thus, molecules having an odd number of electrons are formed, and the unpaired electrons are free to participate in chemical bond formation, such as lipid peroxidation, causing cell membrane damage. Alternatively, free radicals may donate their extra electrons to yet another molecule, which in turn becomes a free radical.

In irradiation damage, free radical formation is usually mediated through the radiolysis of water, leading to the formation of hydroxyl radicals that are highly injurious to the cell. In oxygen toxicity, oxygen acts as an electron acceptor to form the highly reactive free radical superoxide. In carbon tetrachloride (CCl_4) poisoning, CCl_4 itself acts as an electron acceptor and becomes a free radical. In bacterial infection, reactive oxygen metabolites (superoxides) are elaborated within the lysosomes of neutrophils and macrophages after phagocytosis of bacterial organisms. Although free radicals constitute one of the major bactericidal mechanisms of phagocytes, they can also be released extracellularly and cause damage to the surrounding tissues.

Unlike the previously mentioned forms of injury, which are mediated by free radicals, mercury poisoning causes direct toxic damage to cells. Mercury binds to sulfhydryl groups of cell membrane and other proteins, causing increased membrane permeability and inhibition of ATPase-dependent membrane transport. Its toxic activity is not dependent on metabolic conversion or free radical formation (*pp. 9–13, 50, 57–58*).

8. (B) The azurophilic granules found in the cytoplasm of neutrophils are specialized lysosomes that contain myeloperoxidase, acid hydrolases, neutral proteases, and cationic proteins. The latter include a chemotactic factor for monocytes, factors that increase vascular permeability directly or by releasing histamine from mast cells, and factors that inhibit movement of other neutrophils and eosinophils. Among the neutral proteases are enzymes capable of digesting collagen, elastin, cartilage, and basement membrane material, resulting in connective tissue destruction.

Although activated lymphocytes release molecules (lymphokines) that are chemotactic for neutrophils, the reverse is not true. Neutrophils do not produce chemoattractants for lymphocytes (*p. 57*).

9. (B) Besides being able to initiate, carry out, and terminate immune responses, lymphocytes can also produce acute inflammatory responses through their ability to recruit various inflammatory cell types. Activated T cells manufacture and release various biologically active molecules called cytokines. A number of cytokines are chemotactic agents for neutrophils, eosinophils, macrophages, and basophils as well as other lymphocytes.

Platelets do not respond with chemotactic movement to any known substance. In fact, like the erythrocyte, the other blood-borne cell lacking a nucleus, the platelet appears incapable of directed cell movement toward a chemoattractant. Platelets can, however, be activated by molecules produced by other cells such as the platelet activating factor (PAF) derived from basophils, neutrophils, endothelial cells, and macrophages. "Activation" of platelets causes their aggregation and subsequent release of active constituents such as histamine and serotonin but does not involve chemotaxis (*pp. 47, 58, 168–169*).

10. (B) Increased permeability leading to tissue edema is one of the hallmarks of acute inflammation. Vascular leakiness is produced by a number of chemical mediators that act directly on blood vessels to increase permeability. Perhaps the best known among these mediators is histamine, an amine released from mast cells and sometimes platelets in response to various forms of tissue injury. Platelet activating factor (PAF), a mediator derived from basophils, can indirectly increase vascular permeability by causing platelets to release their cytoplasmic stores of histamine. In addition, PAF itself is a potent, direct mediator of vascular permeability. In extremely low concentrations, PAF induces vasodilatation and increases vascular permeability with a potency of 100 to 10,000 times greater than that of histamine.

Bradykinin, a potent vasoactive peptide generated during activation of the kinin system after tissue injury, not only increases vascular permeability but causes contraction of smooth muscle, blood vessel dilatation, and pain. Bradykinin is produced when the inactive factor XII of the coagulation system (Hageman factor) is activated through contact with collagen, basement membrane material, cartilage, or endotoxin. Activated factor XII converts the blood-borne factor prekallikrein to kallikrein, which in turn enzymatically mediates the conversion of kininogen to bradykinin.

The leukotrienes are arachidonic acid metabolites produced by leukocytes via the cyclooxygenase pathway. Leukotrienes C_4, D_4, and E_4 all cause intense vasoconstriction and bronchospasm and are at least 1000 times more potent than histamine in increasing vascular permeability.

The complement system consists of 18 component plasma proteases (together with their cleavage products) that are activated in inflammatory and immune responses. The end result of complement activation is production of the C5b-9 complex, which produces membrane lysis (hopefully of a microbial agent, although parenchymal cells may be injured). Cleavage products that have numerous biologic activities are produced during activation of the cascade. Among those that produce increased vascular permeability are C3A and C5A, the latter being the more potent. The C5b67

complex has no permeability effect but is a chemotactic agent (*pp. 53–58*).

11. (D) In general, tissue infiltration by mononuclear cells, principally lymphocytes, plasma cells, and macrophages, is considered one of the histologic hallmarks of chronic inflammation. However, in immunologically mediated forms of inflammation such as acute viral hepatitis, inflammatory infiltrates consist primarily of mononuclear cells regardless of the stage of the disease and, therefore, are not reliable indicators of the chronicity of the process. Both bile duct destruction and Councilman body formation (coagulative hepatocellular necrosis) can be seen in either acute or chronic phases of numerous inflammatory conditions of the liver. Bile duct proliferation or hepatocellular regeneration accompanied by ceroid pigment in Kupffer's cells (a sign of past hepatocellular destruction) would be indicative of an inflammatory process of longer duration.

Fibrosis is by far the most reliable indicator of chronicity in any inflammatory process, including that of the liver. Thus, a special stain for collagen is often routinely performed on liver biopsies to estimate the duration, degree of destruction, and subsequent scarring (indicative of irreversible damage) produced by inflammatory processes in the liver (*pp. 63–65, 923, 934–936, 941*).

12. (D) An aggregate of epithelioid histiocytes is known as a granuloma. Granulomas may occur either as nonspecific inflammatory responses to foreign bodies or as part of a type IV (cell-mediated) hypersensitivity response initiated by specifically sensitized T lymphocytes. Immunologic responses to various microorganisms including mycobacteria, viruses, fungi, protozoa, and parasites are often of the delayed hypersensitivity type and involve granuloma formation.

Granulation tissue is newly forming, immature connective tissue consisting of fibroblasts, watery extracellular matrix, and capillaries found at sites of tissue repair. It is the precursor of scar tissue. Granular cell tumors are histologically distinctive (usually benign) neoplasms of Schwann cell origin that may occur in almost any site in the body, although rarely in the ovary. Granulosa cell tumors, on the other hand, arise exclusively in the ovary and are derived from the granulosa cells of the ovarian follicle. Granulocytosis refers to the increased numbers of circulating neutrophils, a hallmark of acute inflammatory conditions such as infection. Although the names of these entities may bear certain etymologic similarities, they share no biologic similarities and are in no way related to granuloma (*pp. 65–69, 73–74, 182–183, 705, 1167–1168*).

13. (A) Unfortunately for oncologists, surgeons, and pathologists alike, names of tumors do not always correspond to the rules of nomenclature that are meant to indicate whether the tumor is benign or malignant. For example, a tumor name composed of the word root for the tissue of origin plus the suffix "oma" denotes a benign neoplasm of that tissue. Designations for malignant tumors are usually compound names: the tissue of origin plus "sarcoma" (if mesenchymal in origin) or "carcinoma" (if epithelial in origin). However, according to accepted nomenclature, it is impossible to know from the names of certain tumors whether they are benign or malignant. In these cases the information must simply be memorized (unpalatable a suggestion as this may be).

Glomus tumors are completely benign neoplasms that arise from the modified smooth muscle cells of glomus bodies in arterioles with arteriovenous anastomoses. They usually occur in the distal portions of the fingers and toes, where glomus bodies are most commonly found. Simple surgical excision is completely curative (both for the tumors and for the considerable pain they produce).

Ewing's tumor, Wilms' tumor, seminoma, and histiocytosis X all are examples of malignant neoplasms. Ewing's tumor, more correctly called Ewing's sarcoma, is a highly malignant type of primary bone tumor composed entirely of primitive mesenchymal cells. These tumors occur primarily in children and young adults, and when treated by the combined use of surgery, radiation, and chemotherapy, have a 5-year survival of 40 to 75%.

Wilms' tumor, another tumor that occurs predominantly in the pediatric age-group, is a malignant neoplasm of renal origin. It is composed of a number of different cell types, all derived from the mesonephric mesoderm. Like Ewing's sarcoma, the vastly improved long-term survival now associated with these neoplasms represents a triumph of aggressive combined-modality oncologic therapy. When treated with chemotherapy, radiation, and surgery, 95% of patients with Wilms' tumors survive at least 2 years.

Although they vary in their biologic behavior, all germ cell tumors of the testis are malignant neoplasms. Seminoma, the most common testicular germ cell tumor, is composed of uniform, undifferentiated cells thought to be derived from primary germ cells. Seminomas are extremely radiosensitive and tend to remain localized for a long time. Thus they have the best prognosis among the testicular germ cell neoplasms. More than 90% of seminomas that are confined to the testis (Stage I) or that have spread only to the lymph nodes below the diaphragm (Stage II) can be cured.

Histiocytosis X is a proliferative disorder of Langerhans cells or their bone marrow precursors. In its generalized form, histiocytosis X behaves like a malignant tumor. The focal form of this disease is a benign process, perhaps even nonneoplastic, and is known as eosinophilic granuloma. Diffuse histiocytosis, also known as the Letterer-Siwe disease, usually occurs in infants and children and is a rapidly progressive, lethal disease unless treated with intensive chemotherapy (this remarkably improves survival, at least in infants younger than 2 years) (*pp. 240–243, 539–540, 745–747, 1109–1110, 1115, 1342–1343*).

14. (C) For many types of cancer, it is now well established that heredity has a role, whether major or minor, in predisposing an individual to the development of malignancy. Some of the most striking and obvious associations between heredity and tumor risk are exemplified by hereditary disorders.

Von Hippel-Lindau disease is a rare autosomal dominant disorder that is characterized by a strong predisposition to the development of various benign and malignant tumors throughout the body. Among these, the most common and characteristic are retinal hemangioblastoma and hemangioblastoma of the cerebellum (*p. 140*).

Turcot's syndrome is an autosomal recessive disorder in which affected individuals develop brain tumors and polyps of the colon. These individuals are also at increased risk of colon carcinoma, but the magnitude of the risk is still uncertain and is not as great as in other familial intestinal polyposis syndromes (*p. 897*).

Fanconi's anemia is an autosomal recessive form of aplastic anemia. In addition to having profound marrow hypofunction, affected individuals are at increased risk of developing leukemia or lymphoma (*p. 689*).

Ataxia-telangiectasia is an autosomal recessive neurocutaneous disorder characterized by prominent vascular (capillary) dilatations of the head and neck along with cerebellar ataxia and nystagmus. There is neuronal loss in the cerebellum, medulla, spinal cord, and spinal ganglia. The thymus is either absent or poorly developed, and both cellular and humoral immune deficiencies result. This disorder is also associated with increased chromosomal breakage thought to result from decreased amounts of endonucleases needed for DNA repair. The immune defects and/or the susceptibility to chromosomal breakage predisposes to a high rate of leukemia and other neoplasms of the lymphoreticular system (*p. 267*).

Patau's syndrome is a cytogenetic disorder caused by trisomy of chromosome 13. The most severe malformations among all the chromosomal abnormalities occur in this syndrome, and few affected infants live longer than 1 year, most dying soon after birth. Neoplasms, however, are not a feature of this syndrome, perhaps because death occurs so prematurely (*p. 132*).

15. (B) Next to biopsy, cytologic diagnosis of cancer is the best histologic method. It is usually cheaper, quicker, and less traumatic for the patient because the specimen sample required is so small. Cytologic diagnosis has become the most widely used method of screening for carcinoma of the cervix and/or endometrium and is becoming more and more widely used in the diagnosis of cancers of the breast, gastrointestinal tract, tracheobronchial tree, and urinary tract.

At the present time, however, the most common cytologic examination performed is that on scrapings from the uterine cervical os, known as the Pap (Papanicolaou) smear. With this reliable and simple screening technique, preneoplastic and early, noninvasive lesions can be detected in time for curative therapy to be performed. By long-standing convention, the cytologic findings of Pap smear examinations are divided into five diagnostic categories or classes. Normal cytology is designated Class I. Cervical dysplasia is designated as

Class III, carcinoma in situ as Class IV, and invasive cancer as Class V. Class II cytology is an indeterminant category and refers to the presence of a few atypical cells in the smear. Atypical cells may occur in inflammatory and reparative processes in the cervix, but they may represent true dysplasia that cannot be definitively diagnosed from the cells present. A repeat cytologic examination is recommended when Class II cytology is obtained *(pp. 300, 1141)*.

16. (A) With the microscope alone, it is not possible to differentiate one kind of small lymphocyte from another. With the development of monoclonal antibodies to distinctive cell surface antigens and their use in immunohistochemistry, it has become possible to positively identify individual immune cells of any type and to further delineate functionally distinct subsets among cells of a given type. Tumors of these cell types can also be identified. These distinguishing antigens are cell surface glycoproteins, some of which have known receptor functions. The antigens recognized by well-defined monoclonal antibodies have been cataloged numerically by international convention and are now known by their CD (cluster designation) number. CD5, for example, is an antigen present on all T lymphocytes, both intrathymic and peripheral. Other specific markers for T cells include CD3 (associated with the T-cell antigen receptor) and CD7. Functional T-cell subsets such as helper/inducer cells and cytotoxic/suppressor cells can be recognized by their expression of CD4 and CD8, respectively.

B cells can be recognized by their specific CD19 and CD20 antigens. Blood monocytes and granulocytes express CD13; myeloid stem cells and mature monocytes express CD33. Natural killer (NK) cells have no unique antigens. Although all NK cells express CD16 (low-affinity receptor for Fc portion of IgG), the antigen is also present on granulocytes *(pp. 165–167)*.

17. (C) Mast cell degranulation is a key event in type I (hypersensitivity or anaphylactic type) immune reactions and is mediated by binding of antigen to IgE attached to mast cells via their Fc portion in a previously sensitized individual (i.e., someone in whom an earlier T-cell response to the antigen has occurred, inducing B-cell stimulation and IgE production). With degranulation, mast cells release numerous substances that cause the vascular leakage, smooth muscle spasm, and influx of granulocytes that characterize anaphylactic reactions (see Questions 100–105). Marked edema (if systemic, shock may ensue), watery nasal and/or conjunctival discharge, and bronchospasm are typical clinical manifestations.

Mast cell degranulation can also be induced by nonimmunologic stimuli, however. It can be triggered by chemical substances such as bee venom mellitin, complement fragments C3a and C5a (anaphylatoxins), or drugs (e.g., codeine, morphine). Physical stimuli such as sunlight, cold, heat, and trauma can also induce mast cell degranulation. It is important to remember that some forms of asthma, hay fever, and hives are not immunologically mediated.

Interleukin-1 is a powerful and ubiquitous cytokine that plays various roles in both immune responses and inflammatory reactions (see Questions 213–220), but it does not cause mast cell degranulation *(pp. 173–176)*.

18. (C) The morphologic changes associated with nonlethal (reversible) ischemic injury to cells typically include cellular swelling and cytoplasmic fatty change. Cellular swelling is the result of the loss of oxidative phosphorylation and generation of ATP in the hypoxic cell. Without ATP, membrane sodium pumps cannot be maintained, intracellular sodium accumulates, and water is osmotically drawn into the cell, causing the cell to swell (see Question 6). Fatty change results from alterations of lipid metabolism in the injured cell that cause lipids to accumulate in the cytoplasm.

In contrast to reversible injury, irreversible damage can be recognized only after it has produced the death of the cell and the morphologic features of necrosis develop, usually hours after the biologic death of the tissue. Cytoplasmic eosinophilia (a result of depletion of basophilic ribonucleic protein in the cytoplasm) and nuclear shrinkage are two of the light microscopic hallmarks of necrosis *(pp. 4–8, 16–17)*.

19. (A) Free radicals are chemically unstable, highly reactive molecules that are capable of profound biologic injury, usually through lipid peroxidation and consequent cell membrane damage. Generation of free radicals in cells is usually the result of oxidation-reduction reactions yielding a free electron. Molecules that absorb the free electron become unstable free radicals (see Question 7). Oxygen frequently acts as an acceptor of free electrons, yielding the highly reactive free radical superoxide; thus, free radical generation is a major pathogenetic mechanism in oxygen toxicity. Exogenous drugs or chemicals such as carbon tetrachloride can also act as electron-absorbing molecules productive of injurious free radicals.

Less commonly, ionizing radiation initiates free radical formation, usually through the radiolysis of water and the production of hydroxyl radicals, which are particularly damaging to cells.

In contrast to chemical and toxic types of cell injury, which often involve free radical formation, ischemic and hypoxic injuries have a different pathogenetic basis: namely, termination of aerobic metabolism. Loss of oxidative phosphorylation leads to depletion of cellular ATP. Concomitantly, lactic acid accumulates from anaerobic glycolysis, and cellular pH decreases. Depletion of ATP produces mitochondrial dysfunction, and oxygen deprivation with cellular acidosis produces both lysosomal and plasmalemmal membrane injury *(pp. 4–12)*.

20. (E) Repair of tissue injury is a complex process involving cell growth and collagen synthesis and remodeling. Numerous factors contribute to the well-orchestrated biologic events in wound healing, and the process may be delayed if any of these critical factors is altered. Because granulocyte collagenase is critical to collagen degradation in the remodeling of connective tissue essential to the repair process, granulocytopenia may be expected to delay wound healing. Granulocytopenia also predisposes to wound infection, which greatly slows the entire reparative process. Cushing's syndrome is the disease process caused by increased systemic levels of corticosteroids. It has long been known that corticosteroids have an inhibitory effect on the wound healing process, probably the result of both their anti-inflammatory action and their ability to directly suppress collagen synthesis. Thrombocytopenia may also interfere with wound healing because (1) excessive amounts of extravasated blood tend to accumulate in the wound site and serve as a medium for bacterial growth and (2) platelets are the source of a mitogen for fibroblasts and smooth muscle cells called platelet-derived growth factor (PDGF), which is believed to be important in the normal progression of fibroplasia at wound sites. Because vitamin C is critical to the hydroxylation of proline in the biosynthesis of collagen, deficiency of this vitamin, known as scurvy, produces profound defects in wound healing *(pp. 82–84)*.

21. (B) Renal transplant rejection and graft-versus-host disease are processes in which immunologically mediated cellular cytotoxicity plays a major part. In renal transplant rejection, cytotoxic lymphocytes of the host react against incompatible HLA antigens on the surface of the cells of the transplanted tissue. In graft-versus-host disease, in contrast, it is the immunocompetent lymphocytes of the transplanted tissue that react against the tissue antigens of the host.

The Arthus reaction is a localized immune complex–induced vasculitis resulting from the intracutaneous injection of antigen in a previously sensitized individual having circulating antibodies against that antigen. The immunologic process is humoral rather than cellular, and cytotoxic lymphocytes do not participate. Although a tuberculin reaction is a classic example of a delayed hypersensitivity response mediated by the cellular immune system, the reaction is not cytotoxic. Rather, memory T cells previously sensitized to the tuberculin antigen of *Mycobacterium tuberculosis* are stimulated to divide and secrete cytokines on reexposure to the antigen. The cytokines recruit inflammatory cells, especially monocytes and macrophages, to the site of antigen deposition. Cell-mediated cytotoxicity plays little if any role in this reaction *(pp. 181, 183–188)*.

22. (E) Amyloidosis occurring in association with an underlying predisposing condition is known as secondary amyloidosis. When occurring as a consequence of a chronic inflammatory condition, it is known as reactive systemic amyloidosis (secondary amyloidosis). Ulcerative colitis and rheumatoid arthritis are among the most frequent causes of this form of the disease. Reactive systemic amyloidosis may also occur in association with nonlymphoid tumors such as renal cell carcinoma. If the underlying disease is a plasma cell dyscrasia or B-lymphocyte malignancy, such as Waldenström's macroglobulinemia, the amyloidosis is categorized as immunocyte-derived or primary amyloidosis *(pp. 213–214)*.

23. (D) Despite its name, amyloid is not biochemically related to starch and is not digested by amylase. Rather, amyloid is a protein with a complex substructure and is commonly identified in histologic section by the Congo red stain. Oil red O is a stain used for neutral lipid. In immunocyte-derived amyloidosis, amyloid is generated from immunoglobulin light chains. In senile cardiac amyloidosis, as well as in familial amyloidotic neuropathies, the normal plasma protein transthyretin (previously known as "prealbumin"), which binds and transports thyroxine and retinol, is the major constituent of the amyloid *(pp. 213–216)*.

24. (E) Hageman factor is a critical agent in the complex series of events that follow vascular injury and are critical to hemostasis. The activated Hageman factor (factor XII), which is generated through the contact of serum with collagen or injured endothelium after vascular disruption, in turn activates several enzymatic cascades with diverse biologic effects. Hageman factor can activate the complement system, potentiating complement-mediated inflammatory responses. It also activates the kinin system, leading to the generation of the vasoactive inflammatory mediator bradykinin. Perhaps most important, Hageman factor plays the schizophrenic role of activating both the thrombogenic and anticlotting mechanisms. Plasminogen is proteolytically converted to plasmin by activated factor XII, which simultaneously initiates thrombosis through the intrinsic coagulation pathway *(pp. 53–54)*.

25. (A) Red infarcts are named for their hemorrhagic appearance. They are usually encountered in tissues with a double circulation such as the lungs and liver, in loose tissues, or in tissues previously congested. In most other tissues, they commonly occur with venous occlusion. Classic examples of red infarcts include pulmonary infarctions from pulmonary embolism and torsion of the testis, which causes venous occlusion and intense congestion before the development of infarction. Infarction of the small intestine with its submucosal loose connective tissue is typically hemorrhagic whether caused by arterial occlusion or venous thrombosis. Coronary artery thrombosis, in contrast, is an example of arterial occlusion in a solid tissue and typically produces a white infarct *(pp. 111–112)*.

26. (E) Shock is a state of inadequate perfusion of all body tissues. It first produces reversible hypoxic injury to cells but if sufficiently prolonged may cause irreversible organ damage or even death. A number of categories of disorders may produce hemodynamic or vascular collapse and shock (see Question 30). Among the most common are bacterial infections producing so-called septic shock, the result of pooling of blood in the peripheral circulation. Cardiogenic shock, the result of reduced cardiac output, is most commonly caused by myocardial infarction. The watery diarrhea of cholera leads to massive fluid losses and a reduction of the effective circulating blood volume, causing hypovolemic shock. Hypovolemic shock may also occur in acute pancreatitis, which causes excessive transudation and exudation of fluid from the site of inflammation into the peritoneal cavity (*pp. 114–115*).

27. (**E**) Radiant energy in the form of ultraviolet light, electromagnetic radiation (e.g., x-rays), or particulate radiation (e.g., alpha particles or beta particles of radioisotopes) is carcinogenic. Even therapeutic irradiation has been responsible for the induction of malignancies, especially leukemia. Head and neck irradiation in infants and children has resulted in the development of thyroid cancer later in life in 9% of those exposed. Osteogenic sarcoma has been a common consequence of exposure to radium among watch dial painters. Lung cancer occurs with a tenfold increased frequency among miners of ores containing radioactive elements (*pp. 273–275*).

28. (**C**) Although chromosomal changes are present in the cells of many types of human neoplasms, specific and consistent chromosomal defects have been identified in only about 20 different tumors. In about 90% of meningiomas, a partial deletion or monosomy of chromosome 22 is present. Similarly, 90% of adults with chronic myelogenous leukemia have myeloid cells that contain a specific chromosomal translocation, the distal segment of the long arm of chromosome 22 to chromosome 9 (the Philadelphia chromosome). To date, however, no nonrandom karyotypic changes have been discovered in many of the more common solid tumors such as adenocarcinoma of the lung or malignant melanoma (*pp. 260–261*).

29. (**D**) The grading of a malignant neoplasm is based on the degree of cytologic differentiation of tumor cells and the number of mitoses. In general, there is a positive correlation between the degree of anaplasia and the biologic aggressiveness of the tumor. In contrast to grading, staging of a tumor involves assessment of the size of the primary lesion, the extent of local infiltration, spread to regional lymph nodes, and the presence or absence of blood-borne metastases. Staging often affects the therapeutic approach to the tumor and almost always affects survival (statistically). In general, the greater the stage of the tumor, the worse the prognosis (*pp. 249–250*).

30. (**A**) Hemodynamic or vascular collapse causing inadequate perfusion of tissues is known as shock (see Question 26). Shock may be induced by a number of mechanisms and is a common clinical problem. The major categories of shock are delineated by hemodynamic mechanism rather than by specific cause and include (1) cardiogenic shock, encompassing all causes of reduced cardiac output; (2) hypovolemia, caused by hemorrhage or fluid loss of any kind; (3) pooling of blood in the peripheral vasculature, usually associated with neuropathic or infectious causes; (4) anaphylaxis, immunologically mediated systemic circulatory collapse; and (5) disseminated intravascular coagulation (DIC). DIC can be either a primary cause of shock or may complicate shock due to another cause.

Patients with severe thermal burns are at high risk of developing shock from at least three major complications of this devastating injury. With massive tissue injury, large amounts of tissue thromboplastin are released into the circulation and precipitate DIC by activating the extrinsic pathway of the coagulation system. Widespread vascular injury leads to progressive loss of fluid from burn wounds, producing hypovolemia and reduced circulating blood volume. Another common complication that not only produces shock but is the most common cause of death in severely burned patients is burn wound infection. The gram-negative bacillus *Pseudomonas aeruginosa* is now the most common cause of burn wound sepsis. This organism is the source of many powerful toxins, including endotoxin, which causes pooling of blood in peripheral vessels, producing what is known as endotoxic shock.

Although smoke inhalation may cause severe pulmonary complications including the acute respiratory distress syndrome, it is not known to cause anaphylaxis or shock (*pp. 105, 115, 698–701*).

31. (**C**) The sequence of morphologic events following acute hypoxic cellular injury is now known. The early changes are reversible if oxygen is restored, but if hypoxia continues, morphologic changes that correspond to irreversible cell injury develop. Among the early, reversible changes are ribosomal detachment from rough endoplasmic reticulum and loss of intracellular glycogen as the cell begins to generate ATP through anaerobic glycolysis. These changes are usually accompanied by acute cellular swelling as ATP concentration is reduced and the sodium ion pumps of the cell membrane cease to function.

Irreversible damage is associated with the appearance of dense deposits in the mitochondria and loss of intracellular RNA. In the heart, these changes can be seen as early as 30 to 40 minutes after ischemia. The loss of cytoplasmic RNA is the result of lysosomal membrane damage and leakage of enzymes into the cytoplasm. As a consequence, RNA, DNA, protein, and other cellular constituents undergo enzymatic digestion (*pp. 4–9*).

32. (**D**) The cytoskeletal intermediate filaments of different classes of cells can be separated biochemically and immunochemically into at least five distinctive types: keratin filaments, desmin, vimentin, glial filaments, and neurofilaments. Although vimentin is produced by a wide variety of cells, including all mesenchymal cells and many types of epithelial cells, the other intermediate filaments are more limited and specific in their distribution. Keratins are made only by epithelial cells. Glial filaments and neurofilaments are formed only by glial cells and neurons, respectively. Desmin is produced only by skeletal muscle cells.

Because of their cell-type specificity, intermediate filaments can be helpful in tumor diagnosis. The presence of desmin in an anaplastic tumor, for example, supports a diagnosis of rhabdosarcoma, because desmin is unique to skeletal muscle. Analogously, the intermediate filament that one would expect to be expressed in a squamous cell carcinoma is keratin. Lymphomas and malignant schwannomas may express vimentin, but the finding is nonspecific because vimentin is produced by a wide variety of cells. Lymphoma is best identified by surface markers that are specific for lymphocytes rather than by intermediate filament expression (see Question 16). Schwannomas can be recognized by their production of S100 protein (also made by melanomas) (*p. 301*).

33. (**C**) Although the fully differentiated, specialized cell types of the human body possess many unique structural and functional properties, they also share some features common to all human cells. Among these are the cytoplasmic proteins tubulin and actin. The latter is a ubiquitous contractile protein that plays a part in such cell functions as movement and cell shape changes. Tubulin is the major structural component of microtubules, which are essential to spindle formation in mitosis, cilia (epithelial cells) and flagellum (sperm) formation, phagocytosis, and intracellular transport of secretions.

Myosin is a contractile protein found in most but not all cells. It is found in higher concentration in cells specialized for contraction, smooth and striated muscle cells. Spectrin is an element of the filamentous meshwork of proteins lining the inner membrane surface of certain cells, particularly erythrocytes, but is not found in all cells (*pp. 29–30*).

34. (**B**) Hyperplasia refers to an increase in the number of cells in an organ or tissue that is capable of mitotic activity. In some circumstances, hyperplasia represents a normal physiologic response and is beneficial. Compensatory hyperplasia, such as occurs in the remaining kidney after unilateral nephrectomy, and hormonal hyperplasia, such as occurs in the endometrium during the proliferative phase of the menstrual cycle, are two common examples.

Postmenopausal endometrial gland hyperplasia, however, is distinctly abnormal and is considered a pathologic form of hyperplasia. It signifies an increase in the absolute or relative amount of estrogen present. When it continues unabated, the hyperplastic changes become excessive (complex or adenomatous hyperplasia) and may be associated with cytologic atypia. Atypical hyperplasia of the endometrium in postmenopausal women is considered a premalignant lesion. The greater the atypia present, the greater the risk of endometrial carcinoma.

Another form of pathologic hyperplasia that is associated with an increased risk of malignancy is diffuse hyperplasia of the gastric surface mucosal glands, a condition known as Ménétrier's disease. The transition from hyperplasia to neoplasia is less common in this setting than in the previously mentioned example of endometrial hyperplasia.

Follicular hyperplasia of lymph nodes and prostatic gland hyperplasia are not premalignant lesions. Follicular hyperplasia of lymph nodes is considered a physiologic form of hyperplasia, because it represents a normal immunologic response to an antigenic challenge.

Prostatic gland hyperplasia is so common in elderly men (it occurs in 95% of those over the age of 70) that it can be considered a normal aging process. Because it is extremely common, prostatic gland hyperplasia can often be found in a prostrate carcinoma, but the two conditions are not believed to be causally related (*pp. 32–33, 707, 847, 1118–1120, 1150*).

35. (**E**) Metaplasia is a reversible change in which the normal cell type of a tissue or tissue layer is replaced by another normal but inappropriate cell type. It represents a process of altered differentiation of stem cells as an adaptive response to chronic irritation. Metaplasia itself is a benign process, but malignant change can develop in metaplastic tissue that continues to be chronically irritated. Tissues in which these phenomena occur commonly include the endocervix and the lung. The normal endocervix and lung contain no squamous epithelium, and yet the most common type of carcinoma arising in these tissues is squamous cell carcinoma. These cancers arise from a glandular epithelium that first undergoes squamous metaplasia, becomes progressively more dysplastic, and finally becomes cancerous. Although less common than the above examples, squamous cell carcinoma of the bladder and adenocarcinoma of the esophagus are also examples of malignant transformation of metaplastic epithelium.

Squamous metaplasia of glandular epithelium is by far the most common type of metaplastic change. Adenomatous (glandular) metaplasia of squamous epithelium is comparatively unusual, and the only common example is Barrett's esophagus, which develops in response to chronic acid reflux from the stomach (*pp. 34–35, 833*).

36. (**C**) Calcium deposits in tissues are known as dystrophic calcifications when they occur in dead or dying tissue and metastatic calcifications when they occur in normal tissue. The cause of metastatic calcification is hypercalcemia. Any disorder that produces increased levels of serum calcium may be associated with metastatic calcification. Multiple myeloma with its characteristic lytic bone lesions commonly produces hypercalcemia. Myeloma cells are known to make an osteoclast activating factor that stimulates bone resorption, liberating calcium from the mineralized matrix. Parathyroid carcinoma is a rare cause of primary hyperparathyroidism that tends to cause greater elevations in serum calcium than any other form of hyperparathyroidism. In fact, death from this disease is more often caused by complications of hyperparathyroidism than by the tumor itself. Metastatic calcifications are usually numerous and widespread with this disease.

Wilson's disease is a disorder of copper metabolism and does not affect serum calcium levels at all.

Papillary carcinoma of the thyroid often produces dystrophic calcifications within the tumor itself. These laminated concretions of calcium and other mineral salts are known as psammoma bodies. Dead cells that slough off the tips of the papillary fronds formed by the tumor are thought to serve as nidi of calcium deposition (*pp. 35–36, 956–957, 1235*).

37. **(E)** One of the hallmarks of an acute inflammatory response is neutrophilic infiltration. Drawn to the site of inflammation by chemotactic substances, migrating neutrophils first marginate to the periphery of vessels in the region of inflammation, stick to the endothelium, and then emigrate through the vessel wall to invade the tissue where their phagocytic talents may be needed. Although small numbers of neutrophils may transiently marginate and stick to vascular endothelium under normal circumstances, these processes are markedly amplified in acute inflammation. Increased leukocyte adhesion is mainly the result of specific interactions between complementary "adhesion molecules" present on leukocyte and endothelial surfaces. Several factors are known to promote endothelial-leukocyte adhesion through the modulation of adhesion molecules. Factors produced in inflammatory responses that stimulate adhesion molecules on leukocytes (glycoproteins known as LFA-1, Mac-1, and p150,95) include complement fragment C5a and leukotriene B_4. Factors that stimulate adhesion molecules on endothelial cells include interleukin-1 and endotoxin. Some factors, such as the cytokine tumor necrosis factor (TNF), stimulate leukocyte and endothelial adhesion molecules (see Questions 213–220 and *pp. 45–48*).

38. **(B)** Normal leukocyte function is essential to the body's defense against bacterial organisms. Thus, disorders that are associated with defects in leukocyte function predispose affected individuals to bacterial infection. Diabetes mellitus is an example of a disorder that produces several basic defects in leukocyte function, including defective leukocyte adherence to vessel walls, impaired chemotaxis, and decreased phagocytosis.

The total number of circulating white cells and the leukocyte content of glucose-6-phosphate dehydrogenase are usually normal in diabetes mellitus (*pp. 51–52*).

39. **(A)** To protect themselves from the harmful effects of free radicals generated in inflammatory responses, normal tissues possess several antioxidant protective mechanisms. Serum proteins such as the copper-containing compound ceruloplasmin and the iron-free fraction of serum transferrin are important endogenous antioxidants that serve to inactivate free radicals. Cellular enzymes such as catalase and glutathione peroxidase are capable of detoxifying hydrogen peroxide, and the enzyme superoxide dismutase can inactivate superoxide. Ultimately, the prevention of tissue destruction by an acute inflammatory process depends on these mechanisms and the balance between production and inactivation of free radicals.

α_2-Macroglobulin is an antiprotease found in serum and various secretions. Although it is important in protecting normal tissues from the harmful effects of lysosomal proteases released from leukocytes during inflammatory reactions, it has no effect on free radicals (*pp. 12, 58*).

40. **(A)** "Congestion" is a general term referring to increased blood volume in tissue caused by reduced venous drainage. Congestion may occur as a systemic phenomenon (e.g., congestive heart failure) or a local process (e.g., involving one organ or part of an organ). Passive congestion of the liver produces a mottled pattern of tissue discoloration known as nutmeg liver because it resembles the cut surface of a nutmeg. The appearance is created by deeply reddened centrilobular zones surrounded by pale, yellow-brown zones of uncongested liver at the lobule periphery. Hypoperfusion of the centrilobular zone with ischemic necrosis also contributes to this disorder. Chronic passive congestion of the lungs produces a lesion known as brown induration—brown from hemosiderin deposition and indurated from collagen deposition in the chronically edematous alveolar septae. In the spleen, chronic passive congestion produces small fibrous nodules with hemosiderin deposition known as Gandy-Gamna bodies. They occur with increased portal pressure, which causes deposition of collagen in the basement membrane of the splenic sinusoids.

Strawberry gallbladder refers to the gross appearance of cholesterolosis of the gallbladder mucosa. The focal accumulations of lipid-laden macrophages are said to resemble the yellow flecks on the surface of a strawberry (*pp. 91–93, 751, 921, 973*).

41. **(D)** In contrast to amyloid of the AL type in which the fibrils are composed of immunoglobulin light chains, amyloid of the AA type is composed mostly of amyloid-associated (AA) protein. This type of amyloid characteristically occurs in two basic categories of disease: reactive systemic amyloidosis occurring in association with malignant tumors or chronic inflammatory conditions (e.g., ulcerative colitis) and the form of hereditary amyloidosis known as familial Mediterranean fever.

In senile cardiac amyloidosis and the hereditary neuropathic forms of amyloidosis, the amyloid is derived from transthyretin, a normal serum protein that binds and transports thyroxine and retinol (see Question 23). In the localized form of amyloidosis that occurs in association with medullary carcinoma of the thyroid, the amyloid is derived from thyrocalcitonin produced by the neoplastic cells (*p. 212*).

42. **(C)** Most malignant tumors tend to metastasize via the lymphatic or blood vessels. Only a few tumor types, such as ovarian carcinomas and mesotheliomas, deviate from these patterns and tend to spread over the surfaces of viscera or body cavities. This pattern of spread is so distinctive that mesothelioma can often be diagnosed radiologically by the thick rind of tumor tissue it produces over the surface of an involved lung. Similarly, the studying of the surfaces of the peritoneal cavity and the abdominal viscera by ovarian carcinoma is easily recognized at surgery.

Colon carcinoma is a classic example of a malignant tumor that metastasizes primarily via the lymphatic system. Renal cell carcinoma, on the other hand, is a common example of a tumor that typically spreads by a hematogenous route. Neither of these tumors characteristically spreads over body cavities or organ surfaces (*pp. 248, 807*).

43. (E) In the United States, with the exception of tumors of the female reproductive organs, every major type of malignancy occurs with greater frequency in males than in females. Moreover, the disparity between cancer death rates between men and women appears to be increasing. During the past 30 years, the cancer death rates among males has increased significantly, whereas among females, it has decreased slightly. The steady increase in the death rate among males has been ascribed mainly to lung cancer *(pp. 262–263)*.

44. (A) Although several different types of DNA viruses are known to be capable of causing neoplastic transformation of animal cells (e.g., papovaviruses, adenoviruses), the only oncogenic RNA viruses are retroviruses. All retroviruses contain the unique enzyme reverse transcriptase (a special RNA-dependent DNA polymerase). During infection of an animal cell, this enzyme catalyzes the transcription of their RNA genome into a DNA intermediate (called a provirus) from which more viral RNA is replicated. Acute transforming retroviruses contain genetic sequences (viral oncogenes) that confer transforming capacity. Slow transforming retroviruses lack oncogenes but cause transformation by inserting their proviral DNA near a proto-oncogene in the genome of the infected cell. The strong viral promotor sequences in the vicinity cause increased transcription of the proto-oncogene and conversion to a cellular oncogene *(c-onc)*. In humans, several different types of malignancies are causally related to infection by DNA viruses (e.g., cervical carcinoma and papillomaviruses; Burkitt's lymphoma and Epstein-Barr virus; hepatoma and hepatitis B virus). The only human malignancy presently known to be caused by a retrovirus is a form of T-cell leukemia/lymphoma caused by human T-cell lymphotrophic virus type 1 *(pp. 276–281)*.

45. (E) Proto-oncogenes are normal cellular DNA sequences. These genes are highly conserved throughout the biologic kingdom from yeasts to humans, suggesting that they play key roles in essential cell functions such as differentiation and growth regulation. Proto-oncogenes are the precursors of both viral *(v-onc)* and cellular oncogenes *(c-onc)*. Viral oncogenes are altered copies of proto-oncogenes that have become incorporated (transduced) into the viral genome during the process of viral replication in normal cells. Cellular oncogenes are proto-oncogenes that have been altered in situ to acquire transforming properties. This may happen when a viral promoter is inserted upstream from a proto-oncogene, leading to sustained and abundant (uncontrolled) expression *(pp. 279–282)*.

46. (True); 47. (False); 48. (False); 49. (False); 50. (True); 51. (False); 52. (True)

(46) Histocompatibility antigens are cell surface antigens encoded by a set of closely linked genes on chromosome 6 which are usually inherited en bloc. They are the antigens that evoke rejection of transplanted organs in an immunocompetent host or immune attack by immunocompetent cells from transplanted tissue on the tissues of an immunoincompetent recipient. Simply put, histocompatibility (HLA) antigens constitute the immunologic basis of "self," because they are the means by which lymphocytes from one individual can recognize "foreign" cells or tissues from a genetically nonidentical individual.

(47 and 48) Two major classes of HLA antigens have been defined. Class I antigens are glycoproteins coded by HLA-A, -B, and -C loci, each representing a separate gene within the major histocompatibility complex on chromosome 6. Class I antigens are present on virtually all nucleated cells and evoke the formation of humoral antibody in genetically nonidentical transplant recipients. Class II antigens are those encoded by the HLA-D locus (containing three subregions: DP, DQ, and DR) of the major histocompatibility complex. Although HLA stands for "human leukocyte antigens," it is only the class II HLA antigens that are distributed almost exclusively on leukocytes—specifically cells of the immune system (macrophages, most B cells, and a small percentage of T cells). Other cell types such as fibroblasts, endothelial cells, renal tubular cells, and epidermal keratinocytes can be induced to express class II HLA antigens by γ-interferon. In contradistinction to class I antigens, class II antigens evoke cellular rather than humoral immune responses to genetically nonidentical cells. Class II antigens are important in cell-to-cell interactions in antigen presentation.

(49) As mentioned earlier, the genes that code for both classes of HLA antigens are closely linked and inherited as a set that constitutes a haplotype. One set or haplotype is inherited from each parent. According to the laws of mendelian genetics, siblings can have only four possible combinations of haplotypes. There is only a 25% chance that two siblings will be HLA identical. The odds are 50% that two siblings will share one haplotype and 25% that they will not share any haplotype. The concept of haplotype sharing becomes important when genetically related or genetically identical organ transplant donors are sought.

(50 and 51) In both mice and humans, the genes controlling the magnitude of both cellular and humeral immune responses are located within the major histocompatibility complex. In humans, immune response (Ir) genes map within the HLA-D region, and HLA-D antigens function as Ir genes. T-cell-mediated cell-to-cell interactions in immune responses are critically dependent on cell surface HLA antigens. For example, recognition of a virally infected cell by a T lymphocyte is dependent on the coincident presence of class I HLA molecules on the infected cell. Viral infection alters class I molecules specifically, and the altered antigens become targets for (CD8+) cytotoxic T cells. Class II HLA antigens do not appear to play a part in this response.

(52) Various diseases are strongly associated with certain HLA types. Perhaps the best-known and strongest association is that between ankylosing spondylitis and HLA-B27. Individuals who possess the HLA-B27 antigen have a 90-fold greater chance of developing this disease than those who lack this antigen *(pp. 169–172)*.

53. (True); **54.** (True); **55.** (False); **56.** (True); **57.** (False)

(53, 54, 56) Atrophy refers to diminished size, either individual cells of diminished size or an entire tissue or organ composed of shrunken cells. On a cellular level, atrophy is due to a reduction in the structural components of the cell, including cytoplasmic organelles and cytostructural elements. Although atrophy may be accompanied by decreased cell function, it does not imply that the cells are dead or even moribund. Atrophy may occur in otherwise normal tissues in which the workload or blood supply has decreased. Other causes of atrophy are loss of innervation, inadequate nutrition, and loss of endocrine stimulation.

(55 and 57) Although autophagic vacuoles may be seen in cells undergoing atrophy, this is not a sign of irreversible cell injury. Autophagy is a mechanism by which injured or effete organelles are eliminated from the living cell. Autophagy is to be distinguished from autolysis, the process by which dead tissues are enzymatically digested by lysosomal enzymes released from necrotic cells *(pp. 30–31)*.

58. (True); **59.** (False); **60.** (False); **61.** (True); **62.** (False); **63.** (True); **64.** (True)

(58 and 59) Since the first cases of acquired immunodeficiency syndrome (AIDS) were reported in 1981, this devastating and lethal disease has been the subject of intensive research and enormous public concern. AIDS is an infectious disease transmitted sexually (in the United States, primarily in homosexual males but increasing among heterosexuals) or parenterally (e.g., blood transfusions or intravenous drug use) and is now known to be caused by a retrovirus known as human immunodeficiency virus (HIV). There are two known types of HIV (HIV-1 and HIV-2), both of which cause AIDS, but it is HIV-1 that is the causative agent in the United States and Central Africa. HIV-2 causes AIDS in West Africa. Although HIV belongs to a family of retroviruses that includes human T-cell leukemia viruses (HTLV-I and HTLV-II), HIV does not cause leukemia or any other malignancy. HIV is considered a "cytopathic" rather than a "transforming" virus. Both HIV and HTLV target CD4+ T helper cells. However, HIV causes impairment of function and destruction of helper cells, whereas HTLV causes neoplastic transformation.

(60 and 61) Typically, AIDS presents clinically with fever, weight loss, and persistent generalized lymphadenopathy. Affected individuals characteristically have a lymphopenia and a selective impairment of T-cell function. In contrast to the circulating T-cell population of normal individuals in which the ratio of helper (CD4) to suppressor cells (CD8) is approximately 2:1, this ratio is inverted in AIDS patients owing to a severe deficiency of CD4+ helper/inducer cells because these cells are the main target of HIV attack (the gp120 envelope glycoprotein of the AIDS virus specifically binds to the CD4 molecule present in high density on the surface of T helper cells and in low density on monocytes). Immunoglobulin levels, on the other hand, are often elevated in AIDS patients owing to polyclonal B-cell activation caused by infectious agents such as Epstein-Barr virus or cytomegalovirus or by HIV envelope glycoproteins. Despite elevated immunoglobulins and spontaneously activated B cells, AIDS patients cannot mount an antibody response to a new antigen. With the onset of full-blown AIDS syndrome, B-cell proliferation subsides, and lymph nodes become depleted of B as well as T cells.

(62 and 63) Although a particularly aggressive form of Kaposi's sarcoma is a feature of the AIDS syndrome in about 25% of patients and usually occurs in male homosexual patients rather than those in other risk groups, death from overwhelming infection usually ensues before death from metastatic tumor can occur. Non-Hodgkin's lymphomas, primarily high-grade B-cell neoplasms, are second only to Kaposi's sarcoma in frequency in AIDS patients. The genesis of these tumors is thought to be related to the long-term polyclonal B-cell proliferation that occurs concomitantly with dwindling T-cell function.

(64) As mentioned earlier, AIDS can be transmitted by transfusion of whole blood or blood components such as platelets or plasma. Thus, hemophiliacs, especially those who received factor VIII concentrates before 1985, are at high risk of developing AIDS. Factor VIII concentrates are produced by pooling blood obtained from several thousand blood donors. Since 1985, the risks of developing transfusion-related AIDS have been substantially reduced by screening of donated blood for anti-HIV antibodies, viral-inactivating heat treatment of clotting factor concentrates, and more rigid exclusion criteria for donors. At present, the most common mode of parenteral transmission of AIDS by far is intravenous drug abuse *(pp. 224–234)*.

65. (True); **66.** (True); **67.** (True); **68.** (False); **69.** (True); **70.** (False); **71.** (True)

(65 and 66) In general, the rate of growth of tumors is inversely related to their degree of differentiation: the more differentiated, the slower the growth. Thus, most malignant tumors grow faster than their benign counterparts.

(67) Strong evidence now exists that most human tumors are clonal—that is, derived from the proliferation of a single neoplastically transformed cell. Nevertheless, cellular heterogeneity within given tumors usually exists and may result from new mutations in the genetically unstable evolving neoplasm or variable expression of genes in different subsets of tumor cells.

(68) Many of the altered growth properties of malignant cells can be studied in cell culture. For example, it appears that malignant cells are less fastidious than normal cells and can grow and divide under conditions that would not support optimal growth of normal cells. Lacking a requirement for attachment to a solid substrate, cancer cells can grow in a fluid or semisolid medium and require lower serum concentrations in the medium for optimal growth than normal cells. They are also less susceptible to what has been called density-dependent inhibition of growth.

(69) Tumor cells capable of metastasis must be able

to attach to, invade, degrade, and penetrate the extracellular matrix around them. Malignant cells elaborate a number of proteolytic enzymes capable of digesting extracellular matrix components including collagenases, glycosidases, elastase, and plasmin. It is believed that the secretion of such enzymes contributes to the invasive potential of cancer cells. Compelling evidence now exists that tumor cells with the ability to invade through basement membranes and metastasize secrete type IV collagenase (type IV collagen is the major structural component of all basement membranes).

(**70**) Although it is clear that chromosomal abnormalities are present in most types of human cancer, the karyotypic alterations most often appear to be desultory. With some types of cancer, however, predictable (nonrandom) karyotype abnormalities occur in virtually every case, indicating that the alteration is a primary event in tumorigenesis. Chronic myelogenous leukemia was the first malignancy discovered to have a nonrandom karyotypic change, a 9–22 chromosomal translocation (the Philadelphia chromosome). Many other malignancy-associated nonrandom genetic alterations have since been defined. More recently, however, nonrandom karyotypic changes have been discovered in several types of benign tumors as well, including lipomas, meningiomas, and colonic adenomas in familial polyposis coli.

(**71**) Although environmental influences (e.g., chemical carcinogens, radiation, oncogenic viruses) play key roles in carcinogenesis, hereditary predisposition has been shown to be a contributing factor in a large number of human cancers, including the most common types. Examples of malignancies with a strong hereditary predisposition include breast cancer, childhood retinoblastoma, and familial polyposis coli. Overall, the risk that a close relative of a cancer patient will develop the same tumor is increased threefold over control populations (*pp. 250–268*).

72. (A); 73. (D); 74. (C); 75. (A); 76. (B); 77. (D)

Inflammation and immunologic responses are complex reactions that have evolved because of their overall benefit to the organism. However, these same reactions can also cause injury to the organism and form the basis of disease processes. In general, inflammation is (1) a programmed response to injury in vascularized living tissue due to almost any cause (e.g., trauma, burns, infection), (2) closely related to repair of the injured tissue, and (3) mediated primarily by granulocytes and macrophages and chemical factors derived from plasma. Immune responses, in contrast, are the body's strategic defense system against invasion by pathogens. They are characterized by highly specific offensive attacks directed against specific molecular substances known as antigens (belonging to the potential "invader") and are mediated by lymphocytes with the help of antigen-presenting cells (e.g., macrophages, dendritic cells, and Langerhans' cells). Inflammatory and immune responses overlap in two fundamental ways: (1) All immune reactions produce tissue injury and thereby cause inflammation; and (2) some cytokines produced by activated immune cells are actually mediators of inflammation (e.g., interleukin-1 and tumor necrosis factor) (see Questions 213–220). Thus, immune reactions are one category of inflammation-provoking injury, but many inflammatory responses do not involve immune reactions.

(**72**) A granulomatous response to an inert foreign body such as surgical suture material is a type of inflammation and, in contrast to type IV hypersensitivity responses with granuloma formation, requires no participation of the immune system (*pp. 65–68*).

(**73**) In contrast to infectious endocarditis, which evokes an inflammatory response in the surrounding valvular tissue, nonbacterial thrombotic (marantic) endocarditis is characterized by the formation of bland fibrin thrombi on valve leaflets with no significant accompanying inflammatory reaction. Although its pathogenesis is uncertain, marantic endocarditis is thought to be related to hypercoagulability (*pp. 636–637*).

(**74**) Streptococcal infection produces both an exuberant inflammatory response and an immunologic reaction to the organism. Because both responses are important host defense mechanisms against pyogenic bacteria, disorders that produce defects in either lead to increased susceptibility to staphylococcal and other pyogenic infections (*pp. 339–342*).

(**75**) Sunburn is a classic example of inflammation induced by cutaneous injury from the radiant energy of ultraviolet light (*pp. 3, 40*).

(**76**) Although the name implies an inflammatory response in the thyroid, Hashimoto's thyroiditis is an autoimmune disorder mediated by both cellular and humoral immune responses to thyroid antigens (*pp. 1220–1222*).

(**77**) Lead poisoning is caused by the direct toxic effects of lead on the hematopoietic system, the nervous system, the gastrointestinal tract, and the kidneys. Neither an inflammatory nor an immunologic response is evoked by this toxic process. Because of the insidious nature of the injury, the disease often goes unrecognized for a long time (*pp. 492–494*).

78. (A); 79. (A); 80. (A); 81. (D); 82. (C); 83. (C); 84. (B); 85. (C); 86. (B); 87. (A)

During cutaneous wound healing two diverse cell types, keratinocytes and fibroblasts, synchronously proliferate and interact to repair the defect.

(**78, 79, 80, 81**) Unlike fibroblasts, which normally undergo proliferation only in response to tissue injury (a "stable" cell type), epidermal cells undergo continuous proliferation throughout life (a "labile" cell type). After a cutaneous wound such as a clean surgical incision, epidermal cells rapidly migrate across the wound, establishing epithelial continuity within 24 to 48 hours. This speedy response takes place long before the reparative response of the underlying connective tissue has begun to evolve. The basal cells of the newly reformed epithelium lay down new basement membrane, the primary component of which is type IV collagen, the only collagen type now known to be produced by epidermal cells. Fibroblasts are capable of producing both type I and type III collagen, but neither keratinocytes nor fibroblasts produce type II collagen, a type found only in cartilage, intervertebral disks, and the vitreous body.

(82, 83, 84) Fibroblasts are capable of abetting the process of epithelial cell migration referred to earlier through their production of fibronectin. This large glycoprotein promotes epithelial cell attachment and spreading on the extracellular matrix below, although the mechanisms by which this occurs are still unclear. Moreover, there is recent experimental evidence that keratinocytes themselves can synthesize fibronectin.

Fibronectin may also be involved in the induction of connective tissue cell migration across the healing wound, because fibronectin fragments are known to be chemotactic for fibroblasts. In addition, fibroblasts are activated and induced to divide by a factor secreted by activated macrophages (usually plentiful in healing wounds).

(85) The "transforming" growth factors, TGFα and TGFβ, are actually misnomers, labeled as such when they were originally discovered in virally transformed cells and thought to be involved in neoplasia. They are now known to be produced by many normal cell types, including macrophages, and are thought to participate in normal processes such as embryogenesis and wound healing by inducing cell growth and differentiation. TGFα is a polypeptide similar to epidermal growth factor (EGF), a factor that is named for its ability to enhance epidermal proliferation and keratinization but that causes fibroblast proliferation as well. TGFα binds to EGF receptors on cells and produces the same biologic responses. TGFβ is a growth inhibitor to most cell types in culture but stimulates fibroblast activity and angiogenesis in vivo.

(86 and 87) Other factors that stimulate fibroblast activity and proliferation during the wound healing process are platelet-derived growth factor (PDGF) and interleukin-1 (IL-1). PDGF is a polypeptide stored in the alpha granules of platelets and released on platelet activation. It is a powerful mitogen and chemotactic factor for fibroblasts. IL-1 is a polypeptide produced mainly by macrophages that, among many other activities, stimulates collagenase production in fibroblasts. Many cells (e.g., monocytes, macrophages, endothelial cells, glial cells, keratinocytes) produce IL-1 (*pp. 58, 72–81*).

88. (C); 89. (C); 90. (A); 91. (B); 92. (D); 93. (C); 94. (A); 95. (A); 96. (C); 97. (D); 98. (B); 99. (D)

Sadly, a very great number of debilitating inflammatory conditions and human cancers are self-inflicted via the chronic use of two highly injurious substances, cigarettes and alcohol.

(88, 89, 90, 91, 92, 94, 95, 96, and 98) Both the esophagus and stomach are highly susceptible to injury and neoplastic transformation by cigarettes and alcohol. Acute esophagitis, acute gastritis, and esophageal carcinoma all are causally related to both cigarettes and alcohol. Pharyngeal carcinoma is also closely linked with both cigarette smoking and alcohol abuse. The pancreas responds somewhat differently from the esophagus in that acute pancreatitis has been linked only to alcohol abuse, whereas pancreatic carcinoma is associated with cigarette smoking. Cancers of the gastrointestinal tract are not the only malignancies caused by cigarette smoking, however. Transitional cell carcinoma of the bladder and renal cell carcinoma also occur with significantly greater frequency in cigarette smokers. Moderate alcohol consumption has been recently identified as a risk factor for breast cancer, but the associated increased risk is slight compared with genetic and hormonal risk factors (see Chapter 12, Question 7, and *pp. 469–471, 1193*).

(92, 97, 99) There is no known association between either cigarette smoking or alcohol abuse and Hodgkin's disease, gastric carcinoma, or ovarian carcinoma, but this is small consolation.

100. (B); 101. (D); 102. (E); 103. (D); 104. (E); 105. (E)

(100) Mast cell mediators of anaphylaxis are of two types: (1) primary mediators that are preformed and stored in cytoplasmic granules and (2) secondary mediators derived from cell membrane phospholipids that are synthesized de novo when mast cell degranulation is triggered. Primary mediators include histamine, chemotactic factors for eosinophils and neutrophils, heparin, neutral proteases (e.g., trypsin), and other inflammatory factors. Secondary mediators include platelet activating factor (PAF) and products of arachidonic acid metabolism, leukotrienes (B_4, C_4, D_4, and E_4), and prostaglandins (principally D_4).

(101 and 103) Vascular permeability is increased by histamine, leukotrienes C_4, D_4, and E_4, prostaglandin D_2, PAF, and complement-activating neutral proteases. Smooth muscle contraction is caused by all of the same substances except the neutral proteases. The leukotrienes and prostaglandin D_2 are far more powerful than histamine in inducing both these reactions, however.

(102 and 105) Several eosinophil chemotactic factors, neutrophil chemotactic factors, and inflammatory factors of anaphylaxis that are chemotactic for granulocytes are contained in mast cell granules. Leukotriene B_4 is also highly chemotactic for neutrophils, eosinophils, and monocytes. However, histamine, prostaglandin D_2, and leukotrienes C_4, D_4, and E_4 are not chemotactic.

(104) Of all the mast cell mediators, only PAF causes platelet aggregation. It also causes platelets to degranulate and release histamine. However, PAF itself is a potent direct-acting effector of both bronchospasm and increased vascular permeability (*pp. 173–176*).

106. (C); 107. (D); 108. (F); 109. (B); 110. (D); 111. (H); 112. (E); 113. (C); 114. (G); 115. (A)

In many systemic and organ-specific autoimmune diseases, distinctive autoantibodies are produced. Such antibodies may or may not be clearly related to the pathogenesis of the disease, do not occur in every case, and are almost never pathognomonic. Nevertheless, they are diagnostically useful markers and are frequently part of the clinical evaluation of patients with suspected autoimmune diseases.

(**106 and 113**) Antibodies to native double-stranded DNA and to histones are typical of systemic lupus erythematosus (SLE). Antihistone antibodies are also highly characteristic of drug-induced lupus, occurring in 95% of cases as compared with 70% of cases of SLE (*pp. 193–196*).

(**107 and 110**) Two antinuclear antibodies that are more or less unique to systemic sclerosis (scleroderma) have been identified: Scl-70 and an anticentromere antibody. Scl-70 is directed at DNA topoisomerase I and is present in about 70% of patients with the diffuse variant of the disease. The anticentromere antibody is present in only about 10% of those with diffuse scleroderma but occurs in 80 to 90% of those with the more limited form of the disease known as the CREST syndrome (an acronym for calcinosis, Raynaud's phenomenon, esophageal dysmotility, sclerodactyly, and telangiectasia) (*pp. 195, 204–205*).

(**108**) Anti-basement membrane antibodies are the diagnostic feature of Goodpasture's disease, the archetypal example of disease caused by autoantibodies. In fact, the once fatal disease is effectively treated by simultaneous immunosuppression to reduce further antibody production and plasma exchange to remove circulating antibodies and chemical mediators of immunologic injury (*p. 794*).

(**109**) Antibodies directed against ribonucleoprotein antigens designated as SS-A(Ro) and SS-B(La) are highly characteristic of Sjögren's syndrome and can be detected in as many as 90% of patients. SS-B(La) is considered more specific than SS-A(Ro), because the latter also occurs in 30 to 40% of patients with SLE. Remember, the "SS" stands for Sjögren's syndrome and not systemic sclerosis! A different antiribonucleoprotein (Smith antigen) antibody, anti-Sm, is highly specific for SLE and is not encountered in Sjögren's syndrome (*pp. 195, 202–203*).

(**111**) Antibodies to intrinsic factor (IF) and gastric parietal cells are distinctive features of type A fundal gastritis. The antibodies are thought to cause immunologic destruction of gastric parietal cells, the cells that make both HCl and IF. Thus, hypo- or achlorhydria is produced, and about 10% of patients develop an overt megaloblastic (pernicious) anemia as a result of their inability to absorb vitamin B_{12}, cofactor required for DNA synthesis (*pp. 843–844*).

(**112**) Antimitochondrial antibodies are encountered in 95% of patients with primary biliary cirrhosis (PBC), a chronic destructive inflammatory condition of intrahepatic bile ducts. Although PBC is characterized by a number of immunologic abnormalities, direct proof that the duct destruction is immunologically mediated is still lacking. Why antibodies to mitochondria develop is also unclear, but the phenomenon is virtually diagnostic of PBC (*pp. 953–954*).

(**114**) Myasthenia gravis is an autoimmune disease caused by antibodies to acetylcholinesterase receptors (AChR) of the postsynaptic membrane of the neuromuscular junction. Receptors are destroyed, and transmission of the nerve impulse across the neuromuscular junction is lost. About 85 to 90% of patients with myasthenia gravis have circulating anti-AChR, and its presence in the serum (but not its titer) correlates with severe or generalized disease (*pp. 1366–1367*).

(**115**) Grave's disease is autoimmune hyperthyroidism caused by antibodies to the TSH receptors on thyroid follicular cells that mimic the functions of TSH. Separate antibodies stimulate hyperfunction and growth, producing both goiter and hyperthyroidism (*pp. 1223–1224*).

116. (E); 117. (D); 118. (D); 119. (A); 120. (A)

(**116**) Fatty change refers to intracellular accumulation of neutral lipids within parenchymal cells produced by some imbalance in the cellular production, utilization, or mobilization of fat. It is usually the result of some form of nonlethal cell injury. Although it may occur in other organs, fatty change is most frequently observed in the liver, the major site of fat metabolism.

In the United States, alcohol is the most common cause of fatty liver. It has various lipogenic effects, including increased free fatty acid mobilization and entry into liver cells, decreased fatty acid oxidation, increased esterification of fatty acids to triglycerides, and decreased lipoprotein secretion.

(**117 and 118**) Toxic exposure to phosphorus or carbon tetrachloride produces lipid accumulation in liver cells principally by reducing apoprotein synthesis, which consequently decreases secretion of lipoprotein (the export form of lipid).

(**119 and 120**) Increased lipid mobilization from adipose tissue leading to excessive entry of free fatty acids into the liver is the major mechanism of hepatic fatty change caused by corticosteroids or starvation (*pp. 20–23*).

121. (D); 122. (C); 123. (D); 124. (C); 125. (A)

(**121**) Although pigment accumulation is usually not harmful to cells, it can be a reflection of certain distinctive pathologic processes. In patients with alkaptonuria, a rare inherited metabolic disease, accumulation of the brown-black pigment homogentisic acid occurs in the skin, connective tissue, and cartilage, where the pigmentation is known as ochronosis.

(**122**) Patients with mitral stenosis classically develop brown, indurated lungs. The color is due to hemosiderin accumulation, the result of pulmonary hypertensive vascular changes and chronic leakage of red blood cells.

(**123**) The color of the lungs in coal miner's disease, however, is due to a marked accumulation of an inhaled exogenous pigment, carbon.

(**124**) Pigmented villonodular synovitis is an unusual condition of unknown cause characterized by dramatic synovial overgrowth (probably neoplastic) usually involving the knee or hip. Typically, the proliferating mass of synovium is variably pigmented by hemosiderin, presumably of traumatic origin.

(125) In yet another bizarre condition called melanosis coli, the colonic mucosa becomes diffusely blackened by deposition of melanin-like pigment in mucosal macrophages. The pigment has recently been shown to be lipofuscin derived from apoptotic colonic epithelial cells that are injured by cathartics of the antracene (anthraquinone) type (Walket et al., Am J Pathol 131:465, 1988) (see Chapter 8, Question 20, and *pp. 24–26*).

126. (A); 127. (C); 128. (B); 129. (B); 130. (D)

Hypertrophy, hyperplasia, and metaplasia are adaptive changes that cells may undergo in response to alterations in their environment. In brief, hypertrophy refers to increase in cell size, hyperplasia to increase in cell numbers, and metaplasia to a change in cell type through altered cellular differentiation. Dysplasia, in contrast, is not considered to be an adaptive response. It refers to some derangement in normal cellular responses producing atypical development. In epithelial tissues, dysplasia is strongly associated with the development of malignancy and often precedes overt cancers.

(126) A classic example of hypertrophy is the response of cardiac muscle to systemic hypertension. Cardiac muscle cannot proliferate. Therefore, in response to an increased workload, each cell becomes larger by increasing its cytoplasmic content of contractile elements.

(127) One of the cardinal histopathologic features of chronic bronchitis is goblet cell metaplasia of the bronchiolar epithelium. In contrast to normal bronchioles, which are lined only by ciliated columnar cells and Clara cells, the bronchioles of patients with chronic bronchitis contain large numbers of mucin-producing goblet cells. They develop from the bronchiolar reserve cells as a result of chronic exposure to cigarette smoke. Early in the course of the disease, the metaplastic change is an adaptive one and appears to be reversible.

(128) Prolonged increased stimulation by ACTH typically induces adrenocortical hyperplasia. The hyperplasia may be nodular or diffuse, and its extent is a function of the duration and level of the ACTH excess.

(129) The "hypertrophy" referred to in the disorder known as benign prostatic hypertrophy is that of the entire gland, which diffusely enlarges. On microscopic examination, however, it becomes obvious that the glandular enlargement is due to hyperplasia of the stromal and glandular elements of this tissue.

(130) Perhaps the most important pathologic change associated with long-standing ulcerative colitis is dysplasia of the colonic epithelium. It has long been known that patients with ulcerative colitis are at greatly increased risk of developing colonic carcinoma. It is now clear that epithelial dysplasia precedes the development of malignancy in these patients, and it is therefore considered a premalignant change *(pp. 30–35)*.

131. (A); 132. (B); 133. (E); 134. (D); 135. (A); 136. (C); 137. (B); 138. (A); 139. (A); 140. (E)

As the name implies, autoimmune diseases are disorders caused by immunologic attack directed against constituents of the body's own tissues ("self antigens").

Both systemic lupus erythematosus (SLE) and scleroderma are primary disease processes involving multiple organ systems. Although Sjögren's syndrome may occur in primary form as an isolated disorder, it occurs more frequently as a secondary process in association with other autoimmune diseases.

(131, 135, 138, 139) SLE is believed to be caused by a fundamental defect in the immune system producing abnormalities of both B and T cells. The disease clearly has a genetic predisposition and a positive correlation with HLA-DR2 and -DR3 antigens. Furthermore, SLE is associated with inherited deficiency of the second component of complement (C2), the genes for which are located within the HLA region. Thus, the association of SLE and hereditary C2 deficiency may reflect genetic derangements in certain chromosomal regions governing the immune response. Although SLE involves virtually every organ system, joint involvement with articular pain is the single most common clinical manifestation and must be differentiated from other forms of arthritis. The most devastating manifestation, however, is kidney involvement with renal failure, the major cause of mortality. As in many other autoimmune disorders, skin involvement is common in SLE. In contrast to the skin involvement in dermatomyositis, scleroderma, and chronic discoid lupus erythematosus, however, immunoglobulin deposition is found along the dermoepidermal junction of normal-appearing as well as clinically involved skin in SLE.

(132 and 137) Sjögren's syndrome is an uncomfortable disorder characterized by dry eyes and dry mouth resulting from immunologically mediated destruction of lacrimal and salivary glands. It also has the unfortunate distinction of being associated with a 40-fold increased risk of developing a lymphoid malignancy. Another feature of Sjögren's syndrome that distinguishes it from SLE and scleroderma is the rarity of glomerular lesions, which are quite common in the latter two disorders. Instead of glomerular disease, renal involvement in Sjögren's syndrome takes the form of tubulointerstitial nephritis.

(133) Epithelial malignancy is most commonly associated with dermatomyositis, in which the incidence of underlying carcinoma is about 10%. SLE, Sjögren's syndrome, and scleroderma do not share this association.

(134) In another subset of patients without underlying malignancy, dermatomyositis is associated with other autoimmune connective tissue disorders including SLE, Sjögren's syndrome, and scleroderma.

(136) Scleroderma, a disorder characterized by altered collagen synthesis with systemic fibrosis, shares various serologic abnormalities with other autoimmune connective tissue disorders. Recently, however, two autoantibodies more or less unique to scleroderma and useful in establishing this diagnosis have been discovered: an anticentromere antibody and antibody against a nonhistone nuclear protein called Scl-70.

(140) Although immunosuppression with corticosteroids is of variable benefit in controlling the clinical

manifestations of most autoimmune connective tissue disorders, a consistently excellent response to this mode of therapy is associated only with mixed connective tissue disease *(pp. 195–209)*.

141. (A);   142. (D);   143. (C);   144. (A);   145. (B);   146. (B); 147. (B)

In contrast to immunodeficiencies that arise as a secondary consequence of infection, malnutrition, aging, autoimmune disease, or exposure to immunosuppressive agents, primary immunodeficiency disorders are almost always genetic in origin. Study of the specific defects inherent in each of these disorders has greatly broadened our understanding of the functions of individual components of the immune system.

(141 and 144) X-linked agammaglobulinemia of Bruton is a disease restricted to males and characterized by the virtual absence of immunoglobulin production. The disorder is a classic example of a primary B-cell deficiency in which the underlying defect is a failure in pre-B-cell maturation. Although patients with this disorder fail to mount humoral immune responses against infectious organisms, they are paradoxically at greatly increased risk of developing autoimmune diseases such as systemic lupus erythematosus, rheumatoid arthritis, and dermatomyositis. Although a high frequency of rheumatoid arthritis is also associated with common variable immunodeficiency, systemic lupus erythematosus is not particularly common in association with this disease as compared with X-linked agammaglobulinemia of Bruton.

(142) As in X-linked agammaglobulinemia of Bruton, common variable immunodeficiency and DiGeorge's syndrome are both characterized by derangements in immunocyte maturation rather than an underlying defect in lymphoid stem cells. Stem cell defects produce a much more serious disease known as severe combined immunodeficiency.

(143) DiGeorge's syndrome is a selective T-cell deficiency. It is caused by a failure of development of the third and fourth pharyngeal pouches, the embryologic origin of both the thymus and the parathyroids. Thus, the total absence of cell-mediated immunity is accompanied by deranged serum calcium regulation and tetany.

(145, 146, 147) Common variable immunodeficiency is the most common form of immunodeficiency with serious clinical impact. As its name implies, it represents a group of syndromes with variable functional defects of B cells or T cells or both. Disorders falling into this category have several unusual features in common, however. Patients with common variable immunodeficiency are often affected by a gluten-sensitive, sprue-like malabsorption syndrome. Furthermore, noncaseating granulomas without any consistent microbial cause are frequently found in the liver, lungs, spleen, and skin. Of graver significance is the association of this disorder with the development of lymphoid malignancy, which sometimes develops late in the course of this disease *(pp. 221–223)*.

148. (A);   149. (B);   150. (B);   151. (C);   152. (A);   153. (C);   154. (B);   155. (E);   156. (A);   157. (B): 158. (D); 159. (A)

Edema is the accumulation of an abnormal amount of fluid in the interstitial tissue spaces or body cavities. Ascites is a localized form of edema in which edema fluid collects in the peritoneal cavity. Edema is the result of a disturbance in the forces that normally keep about 75% of all the extracellular fluid in the body within the intravascular compartment. The remaining 25% is interstitial fluid that is separated from the intravascular fluid by a semipermeable endothelial barrier. Maintenance of this balance between the interstitial and intravascular fluid compartments depends on several factors: (1) the intravascular hydrostatic pressure, (2) the oncotic pressure exerted by the plasma proteins, (3) the hydrostatic pressure of the interstitial fluid, (4) the lymphatic drainage of the interstitial tissue spaces, and (5) the integrity of the vascular endothelium. Disorders that either decrease the plasma oncotic pressure, lymphatic drainage, or endothelial integrity or increase the intravascular hydrostatic pressure or the osmotic tension of the interstitial fluid (usually related to sodium retention) will promote edema.

(148, 152, 156, 159) Decreased plasma oncotic pressure is the major cause of edema in the nephrotic syndrome, kwashiorkor, hydrops fetalis, and Ménétrier's disease. In the nephrotic syndrome, excessive glomerular permeability results in the loss of large amounts of protein into the urine. Excessive protein loss is also the underlying problem in Ménétrier's disease, but in this condition, protein is secreted into the gut in the form of mucus produced by hyperplastic gastric mucosal cells. Underproduction (rather than excessive loss) of plasma proteins is the underlying defect in kwashiorkor and hydrops fetalis. In kwashiorkor, profound protein malnutrition produces severe protein deprivation in all tissues of the body, including the liver, severely limiting hepatic plasma protein production. In hydrops fetalis, the result of a hemolytic anemia produced by blood group incompatibility between mother and child, hypoxic injury to the liver leads to markedly reduced synthesis of albumin and other major plasma proteins.

(149, 150, 154, 157) Increased intravascular hydrostatic pressure is the major contributor to the edema associated with congestive heart failure and constrictive pericarditis. In congestive heart failure, the most common cause of edema, the failing heart is unable to generate a normal cardiac output. Consequently, blood is not adequately emptied from the venous system of the lungs (left heart failure) or the systemic venous system (right heart failure), and venous hydrostatic pressure increases, causing edema in the lungs or the periphery, respectively. In pregnancy and constrictive pericarditis, venous return to the heart is restricted by external compression, and hydrostatic pressure in the venous system proximal to the point of compression increases. Thus pregnancy-associated edema is primarily in the lower extremities, whereas the edema associated with constrictive pericarditis is characteristically systemic. In cirrhosis, hepatic scarring and obliteration of portal architecture greatly diminish portal flow through the liver and increase hydrostatic pressure in the portal system, producing ascites. In some cases of cirrhosis, decreased hepatic cell numbers and/or function may also lead to a decrease in albumin production and the resultant decrease in plasma oncotic pressure contributes to the ascites and edema. Unless accompanied by severe malnutrition, however, it is seldom severe enough to be a major factor. The major contribution to the edema and ascites in nearly all cases of cirrhosis is portal hypertension.

(151 and 153) Disruption of endothelial integrity with increased vascular permeability produces edema in thermal burns and bee stings. In thermal burns, direct tissue injury as well as mediators of vascular permeability generated in the accompanying inflammatory response lead to a massive outpouring of fluids into injured tissue. Bee stings most commonly produce a mild inflammatory response and localized edema. In sensitized individuals, however, IgE-mediated hypersensitivity responses lead to increased vascular permeability on a wider scale, producing hives or anaphylaxis.

(155) Excessive salt intake in normal individuals does not ordinarily cause edema. In those predisposed to sodium retention, however, edema may result from elevated osmotic pressure in interstitial fluid containing increased numbers of sodium ions *(pp. 87–90).*

(158) Edema associated with metastatic carcinoma is most often the result of lymphatic blockage by tumor. Other mechanisms, such as venous compression by tumor, protein wasting, and hepatic replacement by metastatic tumor, are possible but are less common.

160. (B); 161. (A); 162. (D); 163. (E); 164. (C); 165. (B); 166. (E); 167. (B); 168. (A)

Morphologic patterns of tissue necrosis depend on the balance between progressive enzymatic digestion of dead cells and coagulation of denatured proteins in the cytoplasm of dead cells. At least four distinctive morphologic patterns of necrosis can be recognized: coagulation necrosis, liquefaction necrosis, enzymatic fat necrosis, and caseous necrosis.

(161 and 168) Coagulation necrosis is the most common pattern of necrosis and is characterized by preservation of the basic cellular shape, permitting recognition of the cell outlines and tissue architecture despite the loss of nuclei from the dead cells. It is the result of coagulation of denatured proteins in dead cells and delayed proteolysis by lysosomal enzymes. This type of necrosis commonly occurs in myocardial infarction with ischemic necrosis of myocytes. Coagulation necrosis also predominates in acute tubular necrosis resulting from sudden severe ischemia to the kidney or after chemical injury such as mercuric chloride poisoning. In these injuries, entire renal tubules may undergo necrosis but the outlines of the tubular epithelial cells can still be recognized.

(160, 165, 167) Liquefaction necrosis is the result of enzymatic digestion of dead cells, resulting in oblitera-

tion of tissue architecture. This occurs when lysosomal enzymes within the dead and dying cells are activated (autolysis) or when the powerful hydrostatic enzymes of bacteria or leukocytes contribute to the digestion of dead cells (heterolysis). This pattern of necrosis characteristically occurs in pulmonary nocardiosis and wet gangrene of an extremity. In both these examples, the liquefactive action of bacteria and attracted leukocytes largely determines the pattern of necrosis. Liquefaction necrosis is also characteristic of ischemic destruction of brain tissue, but in this case it is primarily autolytic.

(164) Enzymatic fat necrosis is highly characteristic of acute pancreatitis. In this condition, powerful lipases and proteases are released into the surrounding peripancreatic fat and catalyze the decomposition of triglycerides that leak from the damaged adipose cells, producing free fatty acids. Indistinct outlines of necrotic adipose cells are seen in association with granular, basophilic deposits that represent calcium soaps formed by the reaction of calcium with the released free fatty acids.

(162) Pott's disease is the term by which tuberculous spondylitis is known. The granulomatous lesions of *Mycobacterium tuberculosis*, wherever they are found in the body, are characterized by a distinctive pattern of necrosis known as caseation. Caseous necrosis represents a combination of coagulative and liquefactive necrosis in which the outlines of the dead cells are neither totally destroyed nor well preserved. Grossly, caseous necrosis resembles clumped cheesy material, and microscopically, distinctive amorphous granular debris is seen. This pattern of necrosis is highly characteristic and virtually diagnostic of mycobacterial infection.

(163) Although tuberculoid granulomas are characteristic of the vigorous T-cell-mediated immune response mounted by individuals infected with *Mycobacterium leprae* in tuberculoid leprosy, the granulomatous lesions do not characteristically undergo necrosis and instead remain as hard tubercles.

(166) Infection with the intestinal flagellate *Giardia lamblia* usually produces dramatic symptoms such as copious watery diarrhea, cramps, and even malabsorption. Ironically, however, the organism often causes relatively few morphologic changes in the small bowel. Although the intestinal morphology may range from virtually normal to markedly abnormal with villous flattening, necrosis virtually never occurs *(pp. 16–19, 400).*

169. (B); 170. (D); 171. (A); 172. (C); 173. (C); 174. (D); 175. (B); 176. (A); 177. (E); 178. (E); 179. (E); 180. (D)

Although immune responses are essential for survival in a world filled with microbes, they can also cause debilitating and even fatal diseases. Disorders resulting from tissue-damaging immune reactions can be separated into four major categories based on the immunologic mechanism that mediates the disease.

(171 and 176) In type I disease, exposure to an antigen leads to the production of cytotropic IgE antibodies that become affixed to mast cells and basophils. On reexposure, antigen combines with the cell-bound antibody, causing release of vasoactive amines, increased vascular permeability, and edema within a few minutes of encountering the antigen. Depending on the allergen and the portal of entry, localized reactions may take the form of cutaneous swellings (hives, or urticaria), nasal and conjunctival discharge, hay fever, bronchial asthma, or allergic gastroenteritis. Systemic reactions, usually developing after an intravenous injection of the offending antigen, can produce a state of shock that is sometimes fatal. Hay fever and penicillin-induced urticaria are examples of localized type I (anaphylactic type) hypersensitivity response *(pp. 173–176)*.

(169 and 175) Type II (cytotoxic type) hypersensitivity responses are caused by the formation of antibodies directed toward antigens present on the surface of cells or other tissue components. The antigen may be one intrinsic to the cell membrane or an absorbed exogenous antigen. Antibody-coated cells are then susceptible to three separate modes of injury: (1) complement activation and direct complement-mediated membrane damage; (2) phagocytosis promoted by opsonization; or (3) antibody-dependent cell-mediated cytotoxicity by nonsensitized cells that have Fc receptors such as monocytes, neutrophils, eosinophils, and K cells. Erythroblastosis fetalis, a hemolytic anemia in neonates caused by blood group incompatibility between mother and child, is a prime example of a type II hypersensitivity reaction. In this disorder, the mother's immune system reacts to blood group antigens expressed by the fetal red blood cells. Another example is the hemolytic anemia induced by the antihypertensive agent alpha-methyldopa (dopamine). The drug initiates (in some unknown manner) the production of antibodies that are directed against intrinsic red blood cell antigens. As in erythroblastosis fetalis, the red cell antigens that are usually the target of the immunologic response in dopamine-induced hemolytic anemia are the Rh blood group antigens *(pp. 177–178)*.

(172 and 173) Immune complex disorders (type III hypersensitivity responses) are caused by antigen-antibody complexes that cause tissue damage through their ability to activate a variety of serum mediators, principally the complement system. Such a reaction usually requires at least two exposures to the antigen: a sensitizing exposure to induce circulating antibody followed by a second exposure sometime later. However, persistence of the antigen through the phase of the primary immune response when circulating antibody is present can also lead to immune complex formation. Polyarteritis nodosa is a necrotizing form of vasculitis thought to be produced by complement-fixing immune complexes that become localized to vessel walls, particularly the small or medium-sized muscular arteries. Although the inciting antigen is not known in most cases, about 30% of patients with polyarteritis nodosa have hepatitis B antigen in their serum and circulating HBsAg-anti-HBs immune complexes. Serum sickness is a systemic immune complex disorder caused by the formation of small, soluble antigen-antibody aggregates within the circulation. The inciting antigen in this disorder is usually a foreign protein contained in some therapeutic antiserum derived from an animal (e.g., horse tetanus antitoxin) or a drug *(pp. 178–182)*.

(170, 174, 180) Hypersensitivity responses mediated by specifically sensitized T lymphocytes are known as type IV (cell-mediated) reactions. Poison ivy dermatitis, graft-versus-host disease, and chronic berylliosis all are examples of cell-mediated hypersensitivity. Poison ivy causes a type of contact dermatitis in which a delayed hypersensitivity response is mounted against the plant-derived antigen affixed to epidermal cells. In graft-versus-host disease, the immunocompetent cells in the grafted tissue mount an immune response against the tissue of the immunocompromised recipient. In chronic berylliosis, T cells immunized against beryllium initiate granuloma formation, the hallmark of chronic berylliosis, through their production of lymphokines, which regulate macrophage activity *(pp. 182–183)*.

(177, 178, 179) In cyclosporine-induced renal injury, chlorpromazine-induced cholestatic jaundice, and pulmonary asbestosis, the tissue injury is caused by the direct toxic effects of the causative agent. Immunologic responses are not known to have any direct role in these disorders *(pp. 479–481, 486–489)*.

181. (D);   182. (D);   183. (B);   184. (A);   185. (A);   186. (E);   187. (A);   188. (E);   189. (A);   190. (C);   191. (C);   192. (D)

(181, 182, 192) The three major cell types that compose the immune system are T lymphocytes, B lymphocytes, and macrophages. In varying proportions, all of these cell types are found in the circulating blood (monocytes are the circulating form of macrophages) and in the peripheral lymphoid tissues, and all arise from stem cells in the bone marrow. In the cortex of lymph nodes, B cells are found primarily in the germinal centers, whereas T cells and macrophages are found predominantly in the paracortical zones *(pp. 165–167, 703–704)*.

(184, 185, 187, 189) T lymphocytes are the major effector cells in cellular immune reactions such as delayed hypersensitivity responses and in the regulation (both initiation and termination) of all immune responses. Unlike B cells and macrophages/monocytes, the great majority of T lymphocytes do not display HLA-DR antigens on their cell surface, nor do they have cell surface receptors for complement *(pp. 165–167, 170)*.

(183) B lymphocytes are the major effector cells in humoral immune responses. They express cell surface immunoglobulin (IgG) that is thought to be identical in specificity to the immunoglobulin secreted by that cell when it differentiates into a plasma cell *(p. 167)*.

(190 and 191) Macrophages have several key roles in the immune response. They function as antigen-presenting cells and also act as powerful effector cells in certain cell-mediated immune responses, usually under the direction of cytokines produced by activated T cells.

Along with mast cells and neutrophils, macrophages produce lipoxygenase derivatives of arachidonic acid, known as leukotrienes. Leukotrienes C_4, D_4, and E_4 are powerful mediators of anaphylaxis. In addition, macrophages respond chemotactically to another of these lipoxygenase derivatives, leukotriene B_4, a mediator of acute inflammation (*pp. 55–56, 60–62, 167*).

(186 and 188) Although macrophages are capable of phagocytizing and lysing antibody-coated target cells, only natural killer (NK) cells are capable of lysing antibody-coated target cells by means of a nonphagocytic mechanism. This process is called antibody-dependent cellular cytotoxicity (ADCC). Obviously, however, ADCC requires previous sensitization by the antigen and the production of cytophilic antibody. NK cells are also capable of lysing target cells, such as tumor cells or virus-infected cells, without previous sensitization. Although NK cells share some cell surface properties with T cells, B cells, and macrophages, they are thought to be distinct from any of these cell types. They are considered to be important as the first line of defense against tumors and viral infections (*pp. 167–168*).

193. (D); 194. (D); 195. (C); 196. (E); 197. (E); 198. (E); 199. (A); 200. (B); 201. (B); 202. (E)

Pigment accumulation in cells is most often the result of a pathologic process. Normal examples of pigment accumulation are few and include melanin in melanocytes and neighboring basal keratinocytes of the skin and iron stores in the form of hemosiderin in the bone marrow. Examples of pathologic accumulations of pigment in cells are much more numerous, however, and certain disorders characteristically produce accumulations of a specific pigment type.

(193 and 194) Lipofuscin, an insoluble brown pigment that is the product of cell membrane breakdown—often the result of lipid peroxidation by free radicals—is considered "wear-and-tear" or aging pigment. It is present in abundance in the heart and liver of elderly, malnourished individuals. In severe cases, when lipofuscin deposition is accompanied by organ shrinkage, the condition is known as brown atrophy. Lipofuscin is not injurious to cells, nor does it interfere with cellular function.

(195) Ceroid pigment is lipofuscin that has been chemically altered, probably by auto-oxidation. It is commonly found in Kupffer's cells in the liver after hepatocellular injury. Lipofuscin is liberated from dying liver cells and taken up by sinusoidal phagocytes that convert it to ceroid pigment.

(199) In liver diseases that disrupt the flow of bile, such as large bile duct obstruction, profound cholestasis ensues, and bile infarcts may occur. In this setting, Kupffer's cells mop up the spilled bile and become laden with bilirubin, the major bile pigment.

(198, 200, 201) Hematin is a hemoglobin-derived pigment whose precise chemical composition is unknown. It is most commonly found within mononuclear phagocytes after a massive hemolytic crisis such as that which may occur in malaria or a hemolytic transfusion reaction. In conditions characterized by increased destruction of red blood cells such as hereditary spherocytosis (see Chapter 7, Question 1), large deposits of hemosiderin are found in mononuclear phagocytes. Hemosiderin pigment represents aggregates of ferritin micelles that accumulate in a local or systemic excess of iron. Iron excess can result from any one of a number of conditions, including increased absorption of dietary iron, impaired utilization of iron, hemolytic anemias, or blood transfusions (an exogenous iron load).

(196, 197, 202) Carbon is the pigment encountered in sinus histiocytes of the lungs and peribronchial lymph nodes of smokers. In tattooed skin, carbon is injected into the dermal tissues and taken up by dermal macrophages. The hyperpigmentation that occurs in Addison's disease, a condition caused by adrenal insufficiency, is seen microscopically as an accumulation of melanin in epidermal keratinocytes. Increased melanocytic production of melanin in Addison's disease is probably the result of increased ACTH released from the pituitary gland. One end of this molecule is homologous to melanocyte stimulating hormone (*pp. 24–26*).

203. (A); 204. (E); 205. (B); 206. (B); 207. (A); 208. (C); 209. (D); 210. (C); 211. (C); 212. (C)

The type of inflammatory cell infiltrate found in injured tissues is primarily determined by the nature of the underlying pathologic process, namely, immunologic or inflammatory. There is much overlap in the cellular responses evoked by these two processes, however. Although lymphocytes, monocytes, and plasma cells characteristically predominate in most responses that are immunologically mediated, the same cell types predominate in inflammatory responses of a chronic nature. Neutrophilic infiltrates are usually associated with acute inflammatory reactions, but they are also present in necrotizing immunologic responses mediated by complement-fixing antibody or immune complexes.

(203 and 207) Neutrophils are the predominant inflammatory cell type seen in infarcted myocardium 48 to 72 hours after injury and represent an acute inflammatory response to the necrotic tissue. Neutrophils are also the predominant cell type present in the early phases of polyarteritis nodosa. Neutrophils are attracted by chemotactic cleavage fragments of complement activated by circulating immune complexes, the underlying cause most vasculitides (*pp. 572, 608*).

(204) Although its name implies that it is an acute inflammatory reaction, acute viral hepatitis B is an immunologically mediated disease. It is caused by a cellular immune response to virally infected hepatocytes. The effector cells in this disease are lymphocytes, and they are the predominant cell type seen in the affected liver (*pp. 928–929*).

(205) Sarcoidosis is a disease of unknown cause that produces lesions identical to those of a delayed hypersensitivity response. Noncaseating granulomas composed of epithelioid histiocyes (macrophages) occur in virtually any tissue or organ in patients with this disease (*pp. 427–429*).

(206) Primary pulmonary tuberculosis is characterized by the formation of a granulomatous focus (monocyte/macrophage aggregates) subjacent to the pleura in the upper part of the lower lobe or lower part of the upper lobe accompanied by granuloma formation in the draining hilar nodes *(p. 376)*.

(209) Although primary syphilis is an acute bacterial infection caused by the spirochete *Treponema pallidum,* the associated inflammatory response is characteristically composed principally of plasma cells. This rather unusual feature is an important clue in the histopathologic diagnosis of this infection *(p. 369)*.

(208, 210, 211, 212) Eosinophilic inflammation is characteristic of anaphylactic type hypersensitivity responses and parasitic infections. Both Löeffler's syndrome and bronchial asthma are examples of type I allergic reactions in the lung with prominent eosinophilic infiltrates. Paragonimiasis or lung fluke infection is just one of innumerable examples of parasitic infections that induce florid eosinophilic inflammatory infiltrates. For unknown reasons, eosinophils are also the characteristic inflammatory cell type associated with reflux esophagitis *(pp. 424, 776, 794, 832)*.

213. (A); **214.** (E); **215.** (B); **216.** (B); **217.** (D); **218.** (F); **219.** (F); **220.** (D)

Cytokines are soluble chemical mediators that serve to direct activities both of cells of the immune system and other cell types during induction and regulation of immune responses. Most of these factors are made by activated T cells, but some are also produced by other cell types.

(213 and 214) Interleukin-1 (IL-1), for example, is produced by virtually all cells, including activated T cells. Tumor necrosis factor (TNF) is a product of macrophages, T cells, and NK cells. Both IL-1 and TNF are mediators of inflammation, have many of the same biologic effects, and act synergistically. IL-1 and TNF activate T cells, B cells, and endothelial cells. They induce acute-phase reactions associated with infection or injury: fever, granulocytosis, ACTH and corticosteroid release, and shock. They also share with IL-2 and γ-interferon (IFN-γ) the ability to activate macrophages.

(215 and 216) Interleukin-2 (IL-2), on the other hand, is made only by activated T cells. IL-2 stimulates the growth of activated T and B cells, but unlike IL-1, TNF, or IFN-γ, IL-2 also promotes the growth of NK cells (see Questions 217, 219, and 220).

(217 and 220) Interferons were originally noted for their antiviral activity. Sensitized T cells are induced to produce IFN-α, -β, and -γ during viral infections. These interferons inhibit intracellular viral replication and therefore constitute an important host defense mechanism in viral infection. IFN-γ also has the unique ability among the cytokines to induce class II histocompatibility antigens on the surfaces of macrophages and many other cells that do not normally express class II HLA molecules.

(218 and 219) No cytokine has the ability to directly kill bacteria, and neither IL-1, IL-2, TNF, or IFN-γ

stimulates the growth of mast cells. Activated T cells do produce cytokines with mast cell growth factor activity, however: interleukin-3 and interleukin-4 *(pp. 58–59, 168–169)*.

221. (A); **222.** (D); **223.** (B); **224.** (A); **225.** (B); **226.** (C); **227.** (A)

(221) Both CD8+ cytotoxic T cells and natural killer (NK) cells are capable of destroying tumor cells and virally infected cells. CD4+ helper T cells do not attack and destroy such cells directly. Indirectly, however, helper T cells abet cytotoxic immune responses by promoting the generation and/or activation of CD8+ T cells and NK cells.

(222) None of these cell types is phagocytic.

(223, 224, 225) Both CD4+ helper T cells and CD8+ cytotoxic T cells are small lymphocytes, and small lymphocytes do not contain granules in their cytoplasm. In contrast to T cells, NK cells are larger and characteristically contain cytoplasmic granules. Although NK cells have been described as large granular lymphocytes, they are believed to be a cell type that is distinct from mature T cells, B cells, or macrophages. Unlike T cells, NK cells possess receptors for the Fc fragment of IgG. One mechanism by which NK cells effect cellular killing is through binding of their Fc receptors to antibody-coated target cells, a phenomenon known as antibody-dependent cellular cytotoxicity (ADCC). A separate mechanism requires direct interaction with the target cell but is not dependent on antibodies.

(226 and 227) Both class I and class II HLA antigens are involved in the regulation of responses of distinct subsets of T cells. Class I HLA molecules primarily regulate CD8+ cytotoxic T-cell function, whereas class II antigens regulate responses of CD4+ helper T cells. For example, cytotoxic T cells can only recognize and lyse virally infected cells that have self class I antigens on their surface. Helper T cells can only recognize antigen when presented simultaneously with self class II molecules on the surface of macrophages or dendritic cells. Although NK cells can detect and destroy virus-infected cells, they are not dependent on recognition of both viral neoantigens and HLA gene products to achieve their cytotoxic effect *(pp. 165–170)*.

228. (D); **229.** (E); **230.** (C); **231.** (B); **232.** (D); **233.** (B); **234.** (A); **235.** (A); **236.** (E); **237.** (C); **238.** (E); **239.** (B)

Disease processes and tissue injuries of specific type are usually associated with a characteristic pattern of inflammation that helps the pathologist to identify and diagnose them.

(228 and 232) Cat-scratch lymphadenitis and brucellosis characteristically produce granulomatous inflammation in involved tissues. Granulomas of cat-scratch lymphadenitis are distinctive in the later phases of the disease because of their coalescence to form large stellate structures that contain neutrophils and necrotic debris in their centers. Chronic brucellosis causes well-formed granulomas, with or without central necrosis, that may occur in organs throughout the body. Thus, it can be difficult to differentiate from tuberculosis. Granulomatous inflammation in infectious diseases is the result of cell-mediated hypersensitivity in which activated, sensitized T cells release lymphokines and other effector molecules that attract macrophages and mediate granuloma formation *(pp. 364, 367–368)*.

(229 and 234) The immune system is also the major host defense against viral infections. Inflammatory responses usually have only a minor or secondary role. Thus, the cellular infiltrates that are seen in acute viral pneumonia and acute viral hepatitis are composed predominantly of the mononuclear cells that constitute the effector cells of the immune system: lymphocytes, plasma cells, and monocytes. These same cell types also predominate in chronic inflammatory reactions. Therefore, even though they are acute in nature, viral pneumonia and viral hepatitis elicit cellular responses that are identical to those in chronic inflammatory conditions *(pp. 312, 784, 928–929)*.

(230, 237, 238) Acute appendicitis and acute ascending cholangitis are examples of suppurative (purulent) inflammation. Bacterial invasion, usually following luminal obstruction, is thought to play a major part in both of these processes. Masses of polymorphonuclear leukocytes are attracted to the site of infection, producing purulent exudate (pus). In contrast to the suppurative cholangitis produced by the bile duct obstruction and ascending infection, nonsuppurative inflammation of bile ducts is the hallmark of primary biliary cirrhosis. In this disease, bile duct inflammation and destruction are immunologically mediated (a direct immunologic attack on bile ducts), and mononuclear cell infiltrates in and around the walls of the intrahepatic bile ducts (nonsuppurative cholangitis) are characteristic *(pp. 903, 939)*.

(231, 233, 239) Fibrinous inflammation is characterized by the exudation of large amounts of plasma proteins, including fibrinogen, and the precipitation of large masses of fibrin. Cellular infiltrates may be minimal in this type of inflammation, which occurs primarily as a result of alterations in vascular integrity and increased permeability. Examples of this type of inflammation include rheumatic pericarditis, uremic pericarditis, and adult hyaline membrane disease (adult respiratory distress syndrome with diffuse alveolar damage). In diffuse alveolar damage, the amount and type of accompanying cellular inflammation may vary somewhat, but the hyaline membranes that are the characteristic histologic features of this disorder are composed predominantly of fibrin *(pp. 69, 649–650, 760)*.

(234 and 235) Serous inflammation is characterized by an outpouring of watery fluid representing either a leakage of serum from blood vessels or the secretion products of serous cells. Skin blisters resulting from mechanical friction or shallow thermal burns are common examples of serous inflammation. This type of inflammation is most often seen in mild injuries and often occurs early in the development of other types of acute inflammatory reactions before cellular infiltrates become prominent *(p. 68)*.

240. (E); **241.** (D); **242.** (E); **243.** (E); **244.** (A); **245.** (C); **246.** (D)

A large number of chemical agents are known to induce cancers in experimental animals and to induce neoplastic transformation of cells in vitro. Many human cancers are also linked by strong epidemiologic evidence to chemical carcinogens.

(240) Aflatoxin B1, a compound produced by some strains of the fungus *Aspergillus flavus*, is a contaminant of improperly stored grains and peanuts. It has been linked to the induction of hepatocellular carcinoma *(pp. 272, 959)*.

(241 and 246) Beta-naphthylamine is an azo dye that is commonly used in the aniline dye and rubber industries. This chemical has been known to increase by 50-fold the incidence of bladder cancer among exposed industrial workers. Some azo dyes have been used as food coloring agents such as those that color margarine yellow or maraschino cherries red, but these substances are now federally regulated because of the concern about their carcinogenic potential. Benzidine, an aromatic amine, is a common chemical used by biochemists, dye workers, and wood chemists. This chemical has also been shown by epidemiologic studies to be linked to bladder cancer in men *(pp. 269, 272, 1091)*.

(242) Busulfan is an alkylating agent commonly used in the chemotherapy of lymphoid neoplasms, leukemia, and other forms of cancer. Like the other chemotherapeutic alkylating agents, however, it represents a double-edged sword. Although the alkylating agents exert their therapeutic effect by damaging DNA in tumor cells, they are also capable of damaging the DNA of normal cells. Thus, alkylating agents may function as direct-acting carcinogens and most commonly induce lymphoid malignancies and leukemias *(p. 271)*.

(243) Vinyl chloride is a chemical used in the manufacture of rubber, polyvinyl resins, and organic chemicals. It is associated with a rare tumor of the liver, hepatic angiosarcoma. This highly aggressive neoplasm has also been linked to arsenic or Thorotrast exposure *(pp. 269, 959)*.

(244) Metals such as chromium and nickel that may be volatilized and inhaled in industrial environments have been linked to an increased incidence of lung cancer among exposed workers *(p. 496)*.

(245) Nitrosamines have been linked to carcinoma of the stomach and less strongly to carcinoma of the pancreas. These compounds appear to be derived from a dietary source. Nitrites used as food preservatives may combine with amines from digested proteins in the acid environment of the stomach to form nitrosamines. Thus, foods that are high in nitrites, such as processed meat and frankfurters, have been regarded as suspect *(pp. 272, 855)*.

247. (E); **248.** (E); **249.** (A); **250.** (B); **251.** (D); **252.** (E); **253.** (C)

The diagnosis, either clinical or histologic, of many types of neoplasms can be greatly aided by the detection of an associated tumor cell product. When dealing with an anaplastic tumor showing little or no evidence of differentiation, the identification of cell elements or products that are known to be restricted to certain cell types can be essential in diagnosing the histogenetic origin of the malignancy. Effective treatment often hinges on the precise identification of tumor type, and immunohistochemical methods must be used to identify such tumor markers in biopsy tissue.

(249) Hepatomas and yolk sac tumors of germ cell origin are examples of tumors that characteristically produce alpha-fetoprotein (AFP). Because metastatic tumor is by far more common than primary malignancy in the liver, the presence of AFP can help to positively identify the less common primary hepatoma. In 85% of cases, hepatomas produce substantial amounts of this substance *(p. 303)*.

(250) Like many well-differentiated adenocarcinomas, colon cancers commonly produce a glycoprotein normally found in embryonic tissues of the gut known as carcinoembryonic antigen (CEA). Blood levels of CEA are often elevated in patients with colonic carcinoma and decline below detectable levels after complete resection of the primary tumor. Monitoring of the blood levels of CEA after surgical resection has been used clinically to detect possible recurrences of the tumor *(pp. 302–303)*.

(251) The production of large amounts of human chorionic gonadotropin (HCG) is characteristic of choriocarcinoma, a malignant tumor of placental or germ cell origin. Detection of HCG is commonly used in the initial diagnosis of this malignancy or in diagnosing recurrences. Although multinucleate, syncytiotrophoblastic-type cells can occur in such diverse tumors as seminoma or gastric carcinoma, these cells usually fail to generate the high serum levels of HCG so commonly found with choriocarcinoma *(pp. 1112, 1167)*.

(253) In addition to hormones and oncofetal antigens, the identification of intermediate filaments can be helpful in determining the tissue of origin of a tumor. Desmin, for example, is a cytoskeletal intermediate filament found only in skeletal muscle cells. Thus, detection of desmin in the cytoplasm of an anaplastic sarcoma can help to identify it as a neoplasm with skeletal muscle differentiation (e.g., rhabdosarcoma), and tumors of other mesenchymal cell types can then be eliminated from the differential diagnosis *(p. 301)*.

(247, 248, 252) Lymphomas, neuroblastomas (primitive neural malignancies), and medullary carcinomas of the thyroid (malignancies of C-cell origin) do not produce any of the substances listed as choices. They can be identified by other specific markers, however. Lymphomas are often distinguished by their expression of lymphocyte-specific cell surface antigens recognized by monoclonal antibodies. Neuroblastoma commonly produces neuron-specific enolase. Medullary carcinoma of the thyroid can be identified by its production of calcitonin and/or amyloid *(pp. 539, 718, 1238–1239)*.

254. (B); 255. (E); 256. (A); 257. (A); 258. (B); 259. (E); 260. (E); 261. (E); 262. (D); 263. (E)

(256 and 257) Although oncogenic viruses are known to be capable of inducing malignant tumor formation in

a wide variety of animals including primates, the evidence linking viruses to carcinogenesis in humans is severely limited and usually indirect. Perhaps the best-known association at present is that between the Epstein-Barr virus and the African type of Burkitt's lymphoma. This virus is also associated with undifferentiated nasopharyngeal carcinoma *(pp. 276–278)*.

(254) Human papillomavirus (HPV) is now known to be an important factor in the etiology of uterine cervical carcinoma, precancerous cervical dysplasia, and cervical condylomata (warts). HPV DNA is present in these lesions in the vast majority of cases, and certain subtypes (HPV 16, 18, and 31) are more often present in malignant lesions than other subtypes. The exact role of HPV in oncogenesis is not yet clear, but it is now believed that these viruses act as promoters that act in concert with initiator cocarcinogens (possibly other viruses, bacteria, or environmental agents) to produce cervical cancer *(pp. 275–277, 1142)*.

(258) HPV is also linked to other types of squamous cell carcinoma, those which arise in the cutaneous or mucosal warts produced by this virus. As in the uterine cervix, most of the lesions produced by HPV are benign. However, anogenital mucosal warts (condylomata acuminata) occasionally give rise to squamous cell carcinoma, and in the rare clinical disease known as epidermodysplasia verruciformis, HPV-induced cutaneous warts often progress to squamous cell carcinoma *(p. 277)*.

(262) The evidence linking hepatitis B virus (HBV) to hepatocellular carcinoma is substantial, although not strong enough to ascribe a direct causal role to the virus. It is likely that HBV acts in concert with other factors (e.g., dietary or environmental) to effect malignant transformation of hepatocytes. There is also strong evidence linking the naturally occurring chemical carcinogen aflatoxin with hepatoma induction, and it may be that these two carcinogenic agents act in concert in some cases *(pp. 278, 959)*.

(261 and 263) It is of interest that none of the influences related to induction of hepatoma has any bearing on the development of cholangiocarcinoma or angiosarcoma of the liver. Both of these tumors have been linked with previous exposure to Thorotrast, formerly used in radiography of the biliary tract, but neither one is known to be causally related to viral infection *(p. 959)*.

(255, 259, 260) Although breast cancer can be virally induced in mice by a retrovirus known as the mouse mammary tumor virus (MMTV), there is no conclusive evidence that human breast cancer is virally induced. Recently, however, DNA sequences in the human genome have been discovered to be homologous to proviral sequences of MMTV, and reverse transcriptase (an enzyme unique to RNA retroviruses) has been reported in breast cancer tissue.

Although a number of viruses are capable of inducing sarcomas in animals of various species (in hamsters, sarcomas can be induced by various strains of adenovirus), human sarcomas are not known to be virally caused.

At least two forms of human lymphoma/leukemia have been shown to be virally induced, however. The causative agent of adult T-cell lymphoma/leukemia is the C retrovirus known as HTLV-1. This virus is a close relative of human immunodeficiency virus (HIV) (see Question 55), the causal agent of acquired immunodeficiency syndrome, and like HIV can be transmitted sexually or parenterally by blood transfusions or contaminated needles. Epstein-Barr virus (EBV) is strongly linked to the pathogenesis of Burkitt's lymphoma, a B-cell malignancy that is the most common childhood tumor in Central Africa and New Guinea. Unlike HTLV, which alone is capable of malignant transformation of the affected cells, EBV probably requires additional factors (cocarcinogens or promoters) to produce malignancy (*pp. 276–279, 281, 717–718*).

264. (E); 265. (A); 266. (A); 267. (A); 268. (A); 269. (C); 270. (A); 271. (E); 272. (A); 273. (E)

A paraneoplastic syndrome is a symptom complex occurring in a patient with a malignant tumor that can be ascribed neither to the effects of tumor spread nor to the production of indigenous tumor hormones. Paraneoplastic syndromes occur in about 15% of patients with advanced malignancies. They can be difficult to control clinically and, depending on the type of syndrome, can even cause the death of the patient.

(265, 266, 267, 268, 270, 272) Bronchogenic carcinoma is the most common form of underlying malignancy in many of the major types of paraneoplastic syndromes. Hypercalcemia, caused by the elaboration of parathyroid hormone by the tumor, occurs most commonly with oat cell or squamous cell carcinomas of the lung. Hyponatremia, caused by tumor cell secretion of antidiuretic hormone, is also encountered most commonly in patients with bronchogenic carcinoma. Hypertrophic osteoarthropathy with clubbing of the fingers is noted almost exclusively in patients with bronchogenic carcinoma. The less well understood cancer-associated dermatomyositis and myasthenia gravis syndromes occur most commonly in lung cancer patients. Although the nephrotic syndrome, thought to be induced by immune complexes containing tumor antigens, may occur with gastric or colon carcinomas among other malignancies, it is most often caused by lung cancer.

(269) When polycythemia occurs as a paraneoplastic syndrome, it is most often caused by the elaboration of erythropoietin by renal cell carcinoma. This syndrome

also occurs occasionally in association with cerebellar hemangioma and hepatocellular carcinoma, however.

(264, 271, 273) None of the tumor types listed as choices in the question constitutes the major form of underlying cancer associated with the paraneoplastic syndromes of acanthosis nigricans, anemia, or hypoglycemia. Gastric carcinoma is the tumor most often associated with the malignant form of acanthosis nigricans. Although the causal mechanism is unknown, carcinoma of thymic origin is the most common type of tumor associated with the paraneoplastic syndrome of anemia. Hypoglycemia, usually caused by the production of insulin or an insulin-like substance by tumor cells, occurs most commonly and curiously with sarcomas, especially fibrosarcoma (*pp. 294–296*).

274. (C); 275. (B); 276. (D); 277. (E); 278. (D); 279. (E); 280. (E); 281. (A); 282. (E)

(274, 275, 278, 281) The surface markers listed as choices in the question are all primarily T cell associated, and all are molecules related to specific cell functions. The CD3 molecule is part of the T-cell antigen receptor (TCR) complex (both the α/β and γ/δ TCRs are noncovalently bound to CD3) and functions in T-cell antigen recognition. The CD4 molecule (on helper/inducer T cells) binds to class I histocompatibility (HLA) molecules. The CD8 molecule (on suppressor/cytotoxic T cells) binds to class II HLA molecules. Both CD4 and CD8 facilitate cell-to-cell contact and interactions between T cells and other cells. The CD25 molecule is the receptor for interleukin-2, the cytokine made by activated T cells that stimulates the growth of activated T, B, and natural killer (NK) cells and directly activates monocytes and NK cells. Thus, CD25 has a key role in the amplification of an immunologic reaction (*pp. 165–167*).

(276 and 277) The receptor for complement (C3b) is CD11b; it is present on monocytes, granulocytes, and some NK cells. The CD16 molecule is a low-affinity receptor for the Fc portion of IgG and is primarily NK cell associated (*p. 165*).

(279 and 280) The CD molecules are not part of histocompatibility complexes at all. As discussed previously, CD4 and CD8 are receptors for HLA class II and HLA class I molecules, respectively (*pp. 170–171*).

(282) The B-cell antigen receptor is monomeric IgM present on the surface of the B cell; it has the same specificity as the immunoglobulin that is secreted by the plasma cell derived from that B cell (*p. 167*).

2

Pediatric and Genetic Diseases

DIRECTIONS: For Questions 1 to 12, choose the ONE BEST answer to each question.

1. The leading cause of death in infancy (under 1 year of age) is:

A. Congenital anomalies
B. Hyaline membrane disease
C. Pneumonia
D. Accident
E. Malignant neoplasms

2. Five minutes after birth, an infant appears pale and blue, has a heart rate of 90, and has slow irregular respirations. His muscles are limp, and he makes no response to passage of a nasal catheter. His Apgar score is:

A. 0
B. 1
C. 2
D. 3
E. 4

3. Which one of the following statements about the therapy of Rh incompatibility (Rh hemolytic disease) is correct?

A. Anti-gamma globulin antibody is administered to the affected infant of a sensitized mother after birth
B. Anti-gamma globulin antibody is administered in utero to the affected fetus of a sensitized mother
C. Anti-D immunoglobulin is given to a nonsensitized mother just before delivery
D. Anti-D immunoglobulin is given to a sensitized mother before birth
E. Anti-D immunoglobulin is given to a sensitized mother throughout the last trimester of pregnancy

4. The lesion pictured in Figure 2–1 arose on the face of a young child and grew rapidly to a large red-blue mass. This lesion:

A. Is known as a choristoma
B. Will most likely regress spontaneously
C. Is best treated by surgical excision
D. Is best treated by radiation therapy
E. Tends to metastasize to local lymph nodes

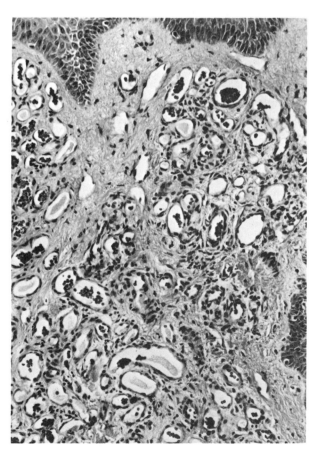

Figure 2–1

5. Conditions associated with impaired intrauterine fetal growth and low birth weight include all of the following EXCEPT:

A. First pregnancy
B. Chromosomal disorders of the fetus
C. Small placentas
D. Toxemia of pregnancy
E. Maternal alcohol abuse

6. Congenital malformations are associated with all of the following conditions EXCEPT:

A. Fetal chromosomal abnormalities
B. Maternal thalidomide use
C. Rubella infection in the first 8 weeks of pregnancy
D. Cytomegalovirus infection in the second trimester of pregnancy
E. Heavy cigarette smoking throughout pregnancy

7. In severe cases of erythroblastosis fetalis, all of the following findings are characteristic EXCEPT:

A. Anasarca
B. Yellow pigmentation of the brain
C. Extramedullary hematopoiesis
D. Enlarged placenta
E. Dark urine

8. All of the conditions listed below are commonly associated with the disease process illustrated by the micrograph of the pancreas in Figure 2–2 EXCEPT:

A. Diabetes mellitus
B. Meconium ileus
C. Male infertility
D. *Pseudomonas* pneumonia
E. Vitamin K deficiency

9. Malignancies that commonly occur in children younger than 5 years of age include all of the following EXCEPT:

A. Leukemia
B. Wilms' tumor
C. Retinoblastoma
D. Rhabdomyosarcoma
E. Osteosarcoma

10. Principal characteristics of the group of genetic disorders known as the mucopolysaccharidoses include all of the following EXCEPT:

A. Hepatomegaly
B. Muscle weakness
C. Skeletal deformities
D. Coronary artery disease
E. Cardiac valvular lesions

11. All of the following statements about congenital heart disease are true EXCEPT:

A. Most of the cases are associated with chromosomal abnormalities
B. Males are more commonly affected
C. The most common clinical presentation is cyanosis
D. Impaired growth and development are common
E. Affected individuals are at increased risk of developing any disease of childhood

12. All of the following are features of Down's syndrome EXCEPT:

A. Trisomy of chromosome 21
B. Normal parental karyotypes
C. Mental retardation
D. Higher frequency with increased maternal age
E. Average life expectancy of about 5 years

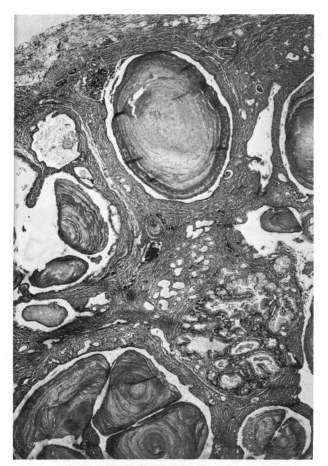

Figure 2–2

DIRECTIONS: For Questions 13 to 19, ONE or MORE of the completions given correctly finishes the incomplete statement. Choose:

A—if only *1, 2, and 3* are correct
B—if only *1 and 3* are correct
C—if only *2 and 4* are correct
D—if only *4* is correct
E—if all are correct

13. A 2000-gm infant delivered at 39 weeks' gestational age:
   1. Is considered preterm
   2. Has weight appropriate for gestational age
   3. Is at high risk for hyaline membrane disease
   4. Has a greater than 95% chance of survival
      A. 1,2,3   B. 1,3   C. 2,4   D. 4 Only   E. All

Questions 14, 15, and 16 refer to Figure 2–3.

14. The condition shown in Figure 2–3 is associated with:
   1. Diabetes in the mother
   2. Infants of male sex
   3. Delivery by cesarean section
   4. Preterm delivery
      A. 1,2,3   B. 1,3   C. 2,4   D. 4 Only   E. All

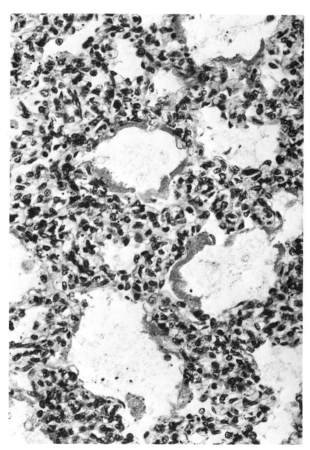

Figure 2–3

15. The major complication(s) in infants recovering from this condition is/are:
   1. Patent ductus arteriosus
   2. Intraventricular cerebral hemorrhage
   3. Necrotizing enterocolitis
   4. Respiratory infection
      A. 1,2,3   B. 1,3   C. 2,4   D. 4 Only   E. All

16. The major complication(s) of the *therapy* for this disorder is/are:
   1. Retrolental fibroplasia
   2. Toxic alveolar damage
   3. Bronchopulmonary dysplasia
   4. Viral pneumonia
      A. 1,2,3   B. 1,3   C. 2,4   D. 4 Only   E. All

17. Enzymatic deficiencies that produce progressive mental deterioration and lead to death in infancy include:
   1. Galactosemia
   2. Niemann-Pick disease
   3. Tay-Sachs disease
   4. McArdle's syndrome
      A. 1,2,3   B. 1,3   C. 2,4   D. 4 Only   E. All

18. The sudden infant death syndrome:
   1. Usually occurs in infants with congenital malformations
   2. Is associated with maternal narcotic abuse
   3. Tends to occur in infants who are postmature at birth
   4. Usually occurs between the ages of 2 and 4 months
      A. 1,2,3   B. 1,3   C. 2,4   D. 4 Only   E. All

19. Neurofibromatosis (von Recklinghausen's disease) is associated with:
   1. Mental retardation
   2. Scoliosis
   3. Hemangioblastomas of the central nervous system
   4. Pigmented macular skin lesions
      A. 1,2,3   B. 1,3   C. 2,4   D. 4 Only   E. All

DIRECTIONS: For Questions 20 to 39, you are to decide whether EACH choice is TRUE or FALSE.

For each of the following statements about erythroblastosis fetalis (hemolytic disease of the newborn), choose whether it is TRUE or FALSE.

20. ABO hemolytic disease requires no prior sensitization of the mother

21. Most antibodies generated in Rh hemolytic disease are of the IgM type

22. ABO hemolytic disease occurs almost exclusively in infants of type O mothers

23. Maternal Rh sensitization occurs more readily when the fetus is also ABO incompatible

24. The magnitude of the antibody response in Rh hemolytic disease is independent of the dose of the immunizing antigen

For each of the following statements about the ductus arteriosus, choose whether it is TRUE or FALSE.

25. Functional closure normally occurs within the first 24 hours of postnatal life

26. Closure is delayed in premature infants

27. Prostaglandins are essential to normal closure

28. Patent ductus arteriosus presents with cyanosis during infancy

29. Patent ductus arteriosus creates an early systolic blowing murmur

For each of the following statements about coarctation of the aorta, choose whether it is TRUE or FALSE.

30. It occurs commonly in Turner's syndrome

31. It occurs as a solitary congenital defect in an otherwise normal child most of the time

32. Preductal coarctation causes right ventricular hypertrophy in utero

33. Notching of the inner surfaces of the ribs on x-ray is associated with preductal coarctation

34. The lesion often recurs after surgical resection

For each of the following statements about tetralogy of Fallot, choose whether it is TRUE or FALSE.

35. The severity of clinical symptoms is most directly related to the degree of right ventricular outflow obstruction

36. A patent ductus arteriosus is requisite to survival in most cases

37. The intensity of the heart murmur is directly proportional to the severity of the right ventricular outflow obstruction

38. Polycythemia is a common complication

39. Early corrective surgery is the treatment of choice

DIRECTIONS: For Questions 40 to 61, the set of lettered headings is followed by a list of numbered words or phrases. For each numbered word or phrase choose:

    A—if the item is associated with (A) only
    B—if the item is associated with (B) only
    C—if the item is associated with *both* (A) and (B)
    D—if the item is associated with *neither* (A) nor (B)

For each of the characteristics listed below, choose whether it describes phenylketonuria, alkaptonuria, both, or neither.
    A. Phenylketonuria
    B. Alkaptonuria
    C. Both
    D. Neither

40. A defect in tyrosine metabolism causes the disease

41. Affected infants appear normal at birth

42. Urine turns black on standing

43. Untreated patients often develop mental retardation

44. Vertebral arthritis characteristically develops

For each of the characteristics listed below, choose whether it describes Marfan's syndrome, the Ehlers-Danlos syndromes, both, or neither.

    A. Marfan's syndrome
    B. Ehlers-Danlos syndromes
    C. Both
    D. Neither

45. Occur(s) as congenital but not hereditary disorder(s)

46. Characterized by a primary defect in collagen structure

47. Associated with a high frequency of aortic aneurysms

48. Characterized by long, slender extremities

49. Typically produce(s) joint inflexibility

For each of the following statements, choose whether it describes atrial septal defect, ventricular septal defect, both, or neither.

    A. Atrial septal defect
    B. Ventricular septal defect
    C. Both
    D. Neither

50. The lesion is the most common congenital cardiac defect

51. The defect is commonly first recognized in adult life

52. A small defect predisposes to bacterial endocarditis

53. Pulmonary hypertension commonly develops

54. The defect develops between the second and eighth weeks of embryogenesis

55. The defect is a feature of tetralogy of Fallot

56. Early surgical closure reduces morbidity

For each of the following characteristics, choose whether it describes tricuspid atresia, pulmonary valve atresia, both, or neither.

    A. Tricuspid valve atresia
    B. Pulmonary valve atresia
    C. Both
    D. Neither

57. Commonly associated with a hypoplastic right ventricle

58. Commonly associated with an atrial septal defect

59. Frequently associated with a ventricular septal defect

60. Accounts for as much as 15% of congenital cyanotic heart disease

61. Depends on a patent ductus arteriosus to provide blood flow to the lungs

DIRECTIONS: Questions 62 to 70 are matching questions. For each numbered item, choose the most likely associated lettered item from those provided. Each numbered item has ONLY ONE answer. Within each group, each lettered item may be the answer to one, more than one, or none of the numbered items.

For each of the sexual disorders listed below, choose whether the most common associated karyotype is 45,XO, 46,XY, 47,XXY, or none of these.

    A. 45,XO
    B. 46,XY
    C. 47,XXY
    D. None of these

62. Klinefelter's syndrome

63. Turner's syndrome

64. True hermaphroditism

65. Testicular feminization syndrome

For each of the features listed below, choose whether it is characteristic of Fabry's disease, Lesch-Nyhan syndrome, von Hippel-Lindau disease, Wilson's disease, or none of these.

    A. Fabry's disease
    B. Lesch-Nyhan syndrome
    C. Von Hippel-Lindau disease
    D. Wilson's disease
    E. None of these

66. Gout and self-mutilative behavior

67. Progressive renal failure and angiokeratomas

68. Xanthomas and accelerated atherosclerosis

69. Cirrhosis and cavitation of the brain

70. Retinal angiomas and renal cell carcinoma

Pediatric and Genetic Diseases

1. (A) In the United States, far more deaths occur in infancy (before 1 year of age) than in any other period of childhood. Among neonates (less than 4 weeks of age), survival correlates with birth weight, and the leading causes of death are asphyxia, immaturity, and hyaline membrane disease. After 4 weeks of age, however, congenital anomalies cause increasing numbers of deaths and ultimately are the leading cause of death in infancy. Pneumonia, although an important cause of mortality in infancy, causes less than half as many infant deaths as congenital anomalies. Accidents and malignant neoplasms cause only a small fraction of the total number of deaths in infancy, but in the older pediatric age-group they assume major importance. In fact, accidents are the leading cause of death among children between 1 and 14 years of age (pp. 515–516).

2. (C) The Apgar score is a useful clinical method for evaluating the physiologic condition of a newborn infant on a simple, rapid basis. Five parameters are evaluated: heart rate, respiratory effort, muscle tone, response to nasal catheter, and color. The infant is evaluated at 1 and 5 minutes of life, and each item is given a score of 0, 1, or 2. A score of 2 is normal, a score of 0 indicates absence of that function, and a score of 1 is an intermediate response. Thus, an infant with a heart rate of less than 100 (score 1), slow irregular respirations (score 1), and absence of muscle tone, pink color, or response to a nasal catheter (scores of 0) would have an overall Apgar score of 2. The Apgar score correlates well with the chances of survival during the first 28 days of life. Infants with Apgar scores of 0 or 1 at 5 minutes have a 50% risk of mortality during the first months of life. Prognosis improves with increasing Apgar scores, and mortality is almost 0 when the score is 7 or greater (pp. 518–519).

3. (C) The principle of the therapeutic approach to Rh incompatibility is to prevent maternal sensitization to the D antigen. Thus, before delivery, anti-D immunoglobulin is administered to the nonsensitized, Rh-negative mother. The administered antibody coats the fetal red blood cells that leak into the maternal circulation. Thus, the antigenic determinants become masked and fail to stimulate the maternal immune system. This treatment must be given for the first and every subsequent pregnancy of the unsensitized mother. There is no theoretical or practical use for this treatment in the sensitized mother (pp. 527–528).

4. (B) The lesion pictured in the micrograph (see Fig. 2–1) is a benign tumor of blood vessels known as a capillary hemangioma. Hemangiomas are the most common tumors of infancy. Because this lesion is benign and tends to regress spontaneously, it does not require surgical excision or radiation therapy and, of course, does not metastasize. A choristoma is the name applied to microscopically normal cells or tissues that are present in an abnormal location (e.g., a pancreatic rest in the duodenal submucosa). Although benign, a hemangioma is a true tumor and would therefore not be classifiable as a choristoma (p. 538).

5. (A) Low birth weight in small-for-gestational-age infants is frequently the result of impaired intrauterine growth. Impaired growth in utero may be caused by various fetal, placental, or maternal factors. Fetal conditions that commonly reduce growth potential despite an adequate supply of nutrients from the mother include chromosomal disorders, congenital anomalies, and congenital infections. Small placentas and other placental conditions (infections, tumors, or vascular lesions) may produce placental insufficiency and retard intrauterine growth. In the vast majority of cases, however, impaired intrauterine growth is caused by maternal conditions that limit or interfere with fetal nourishment or oxygenation. In this category, maternal vascular diseases such as toxemia of pregnancy or chronic systemic hypertension are common underlying causes. Additional important maternal causes of impaired intrauterine growth include alcohol abuse, cigarette smoking, and narcotic abuse. First pregnancy, however, is not in itself associated with impaired intrauterine fetal growth. On the contrary, it is more likely that the small uterus of a first pregnancy may constrain a normally growing fetus and cause fetal deformation (*pp. 516–517*).

6. (E) Congenital malformations are structural defects that are present at birth. Major malformations result from a defect in embryogenesis and are present in as many as 2% of newborn infants. The cause of most (65 to 70%) congenital malformations in humans is unclear, but the remainder are known to be related to either genetic or environmental factors. Fetal chromosomal abnormalities are among the most common genetic causes of congenital malformation. Environmental causes include infection, drugs, chemicals, and irradiation. Maternal thalidomide use is an infamous cause of malformation. Rubella and cytomegalovirus infections are two of the most common infections known to cause congenital malformations. Although heavy cigarette smoking throughout pregnancy is associated with impaired intrauterine growth (infants are small for gestational age), there is no definitive evidence that it leads to congenital malformations (*pp. 519–523*).

7. (E) In cases of severe erythroblastosis fetalis (see Questions 20 to 24), hemolysis is extensive, and the oxygen-carrying capacity of the blood is severely impaired. Thus, the heart may suffer hypoxic damage, leading to circulatory failure. Circulatory failure, in turn, exacerbates the anemia-induced hypoxic damage to other organs. The liver, with its high metabolic rate, is especially prone to injury, and hepatic failure with resultant edema (anasarca) often ensues. Unconjugated hyperbilirubinemia, the hallmark of any hemolytic disease with jaundice, has severe consequences in neonates that would not occur in older children or adults. In neonates, unconjugated bilirubin, which is markedly lipophilic, passes readily through the immature blood-brain barrier, causing toxic damage to the brain and spinal cord. The brain becomes edematous and has a characteristic bright yellow pigmentation (kernicterus). Kernicterus is the most serious complication of erythroblastosis fetalis. The marked increase in erythropoietic activity in this hemolytic state characteristically induces extramedullary hematopoiesis in the spleen and liver and possibly other tissues as well. Enlarged, heavy, edematous placentas are also highly characteristic of severe erythroblastosis fetalis with liver damage, hypoalbuminemia, and fetal edema.

Dark urine is a consequence of spillover into the urine of water-soluble conjugated bilirubin. This occurs in disorders in which bilirubin is conjugated but not excreted (e.g., cholestatic jaundice). In erythroblastosis fetalis, however, jaundice is caused by excess production of unconjugated bilirubin and is not productive of dark urine (*pp. 527–530*).

8. (A) Although the pathologic changes in the pancreas pictured in the micrograph (see Fig. 2–2) are characteristic of cystic fibrosis, they make it difficult to identify the tissue. Markedly dilated pancreatic ducts plugged with inspissated secretions dominate the pathologic picture. The obstruction leads to atrophy of the exocrine pancreas and its replacement by fibrous tissue. As is typical of any form of pancreatic ductal obstruction with secondary pancreatic atrophy, the endocrine pancreas is largely spared. Diabetes mellitus, therefore, is not commonly associated with cystic fibrosis or any other form of pancreatic ductal obstruction. The major defect in cystic fibrosis is the production in glandular structures of a highly cystic mucus that is difficult to mobilize and that tends to form plugs. Tissues that are organized around mucin-secreting tubal structures such as the bronchial tree, the gastrointestinal mucosa, and the excretory ducts of the male genital system are primarily involved in this disease process. In newborns with this disease, small bowel obstruction known as meconium ileus may occur as a consequence of abnormal gastrointestinal mucus secretion and the absence of pancreatic amylases. Obstruction of wolffian duct derivatives (the epididymis and vas deferens) produces azoospermia and infertility in 95% of males with this disease. Pulmonary abnormalities are present in almost every case of cystic fibrosis. The bronchial tree becomes plugged with tenacious mucous secretions. Superimposed infections give rise to severe chronic bronchitis and marked bronchiectasis. *Pseudomonas aeruginosa* and *Staphylococcus aureus* are the two most common pathogens responsible for lung infections in this setting. Deficiency of vitamin K, a fat-soluble vitamin, often occurs as part of the malabsorption syndrome that results from the loss of pancreatic exocrine secretions (*pp. 533–536*).

9. (E) Although benign tumors are far more common in infancy and childhood than malignant tumors, several malignancies exhibit sharp peaks in incidence in children younger than 5 years of age. Primary among these are leukemia (particularly acute lymphocytic leukemia), Wilms' tumor (nephroblastoma), retinoblastoma, and rhabdomyosarcoma as well as neuroblastoma, hepatoblastoma, teratoma, and ependymoma. Osteosarcoma is virtually nonexistent in this age-group and characteristically occurs in children 10 to 15 years of age. Knowledge of the characteristic age distribution in childhood neoplasms can be helpful in diagnosing malignant processes in early childhood (*pp. 539–540*).

10. (B) The mucopolysaccharidoses are a group of genetic disorders resulting from deficiencies of specific lysosomal enzymes involved in the degradation of mucopolysaccharides. Mucopolysaccharides typically accumulate in the mononuclear phagocyte system, causing hepatosplenomegaly. Accumulation in endothelial cells, intimal smooth muscle cells, and fibroblasts throughout the body is also common. The cardiovascular system is usually involved, especially the coronary arteries and valves. Skeletal and facial deformities also occur: Typically, the head is large and long and the nose is broad and flat. Muscle weakness is not a characteristic symptom of the mucopolysaccharidoses, but it is one of the cardinal symptoms of glycogen storage diseases *(pp. 149–152)*.

11. (A) Only about 5% of cases of congenital heart disease are associated with chromosomal abnormality. Yet some genetic factors appear to play a part in the etiology of congenital heart disease, because about one-third of affected individuals have one or more relatives with congenital heart disease. In addition, congenital heart disease appears more frequently in males, suggesting a sex-linked genetic influence. Although congenital heart disease covers a spectrum of disorders, most of the anomalies produce some degree of cyanosis and commonly lead to impaired growth and development of the affected child. In addition to the direct consequences of the cardiac defect, afflicted children are at higher risk of developing any of the acquired diseases of childhood *(pp. 618–619)*.

12. (E) Down's syndrome is the most common chromosomal disorder, affecting about 1 in 700 newborns in the United States. Approximately 95% of affected individuals have three complete copies of chromosome 21 and a chromosome count of 47. About 4% have 46 chromosomes with an extra copy of genetic material from the long arm of chromosome 21 translocated to another acrocentric chromosome, such as 14 or 22 (translocation variant). Parents of affected individuals have normal karyotypes, however. Full expression of Down's syndrome requires triplication of only a single region (band 21q22) of the long arm of chromosome 21, a band large enough to include several hundred genes. Mapping of the genes in this "obligate Down's region" will hopefully provide new insight into the pathogenesis of this syndrome.

Major features of the Down's syndrome include severe mental retardation, distinctive facies (flat facial profile, oblique eyelids, and epicanthal folds), occurrence of congenital heart disease in about 40%, and a 20-fold increased risk of developing acute leukemia in childhood. The incidence of the disease increases dramatically with maternal age (1 in 1150 live births for mothers younger than 20 years; 1 in 25 births for mothers older than 45). With medical care, individuals with Down's syndrome have an average life expectancy of 30 years, and 25% live to age 50 *(pp. 129–132)*.

13. (D) Only infants delivered before the 37th or 38th week of gestation are considered preterm. Infants born between the 38th and 42nd weeks of gestation are considered term infants. Their birth weight is considered appropriate for gestational age if it falls between the 10th and 90th percentiles of weights within that gestational age-group. For a term infant at 39 weeks, an appropriate birth weight would range from approximately 2300 to 3600 gm, and a 2000-gm infant would be considered small for that gestational age.

Classifying infants on the basis of both their birth weight and their gestational age in this way is more accurately predictive of infant morbidity and mortality than classification by either parameter alone. For example, 2000-gm infants born at 34 weeks of gestation have an 8% mortality rate, and yet an infant of the same birth weight born at 39 weeks of gestation has only a 2% risk of mortality. Certain causes of infant morbidity are associated only with preterm delivery (irrespective of birth weight) and result from functional and structural immaturity of various organ systems. Hyaline membrane disease of the newborn, caused by functional immaturity of type II pneumocytes, is a prime example. A full-term infant would not be at increased risk for hyaline membrane disease *(pp. 515–518)*.

14. (E) The micrograph of the lung (see Fig. 2–3) illustrates the classic microscopic features of respiratory distress syndrome (RDS) of the newborn. This disorder is the result of structural and functional immaturity of the lungs, almost always occurring in infants delivered before term. The fundamental defect in RDS is deficient surfactant production by immature type II pneumocytes. As a consequence, the work of expanding the air spaces increases dramatically, and widespread atelectasis ensues. The resultant hypoxemia and acidosis not only further impair surfactant production but lead to pulmonary vasoconstriction and hypoperfusion. Capillary endothelial cells then suffer anoxic damage, and plasma proteins (particularly fibrinogen) leak into the alveolar spaces to form thick hyaline membranes, the characteristic pathologic feature of this disorder.

Respiratory distress syndrome of the newborn occurs six times more frequently in infants of diabetic mothers than in those of normal mothers. In these infants, the reactive hyperinsulinemia of the fetus counteracts the normal inductive effects of corticosteroids on surfactant synthesis. The respiratory distress syndrome occurs twice as often in male infants as female, owing to the relatively early maturation of the lungs of females. Delivery by cesarean section when performed before the 38th week of gestation is also associated with a higher risk of RDS in infants. However, it is unclear whether the procedure itself is the cause of the problem or whether it is merely a case of "guilt by association" with antepartum problems (e.g., hemorrhage, toxemia) that are indications for cesarean section. By far the most common association with RDS of newborns, however, is preterm delivery *(pp. 523–527)*.

15. (A) In general, infants with RDS have an excellent chance of recovery if ventilatory therapy is successful in maintaining their life for the first 3 to 4 days. Unfortunately, however, recovery from RDS is associated with several complications. Most significantly, the infant is at increased risk of patent ductus arteriosus (PDA), intraventricular cerebral hemorrhage, and necrotizing enterocolitis. PDA results from delayed closure of the ductus because of immaturity, hypoxia, and acidosis. Intraventricular hemorrhage is a consequence of anoxia and immaturity of the brain as well as the disproportionately large amount of cerebral blood flow through the periventricular circulation where the vessel walls are fragile. The pathogenesis of necrotizing enterocolitis is less well understood but is thought to be related to intestinal ischemia resulting from hypoxia and secondary bacterial invasion. Interestingly, it is the extrapulmonary consequences of hypoxia that pose the greatest risk to life in the recovery phase of neonatal RDS. Although respiratory infection may occur in this setting, it is not a major complicating factor. Pneumonia in neonates is usually a consequence of complications of pregnancy or labor with resultant aspiration of infected amniotic fluid by the fetus (*p. 526*).

16. (A) Therapy for RDS consists primarily of delivery of high concentrations of oxygen and mechanically assisted ventilation. Although these measures are potentially lifesaving, there is a precarious balance between their therapeutic effects and their toxic complications. Ironically, oxygen in high concentration is itself a cause of the respiratory distress syndrome (hyaline membrane disease/diffuse alveolar damage). Toxic alveolar damage results from destruction of cell lipids and proteins mediated by oxygen free radicals (superoxides) (see Chapter 6, Question 3). In infants, a second form of lung disease known as bronchopulmonary dysplasia may result from oxygen toxicity and mechanical ventilation. This disorder is characterized by fibrotic thickening of the peribronchial and alveolar walls with epithelial hyperplasia and squamous metaplasia of the large airways, prolonging respiratory distress for as long as 3 to 6 months.

Retrolental fibroplasia is a consequence of oxygen toxicity in which arterial hyperoxia causes spasm of the retinal vessels and ischemic necrosis and fibrosis of the retina. The tragic result is blindness.

Viral pneumonia is not usually a consequence of therapy of RDS of the newborn. However, viral pneumonia is itself a cause of diffuse alveolar damage and RDS in any age-group, and neonates treated with oxygen and ventilatory support can develop any of the complications described earlier (*p. 526*).

17. (A) Galactosemia, Niemann-Pick disease, and Tay-Sachs disease all produce progressive mental deterioration in affected infants. Although benign variants of galactosemia exist, the most common form involves a lack of galactose-1-phosphate uridyl transferase with resultant galactosemia and progressive mental retardation. The pathophysiologic basis of the mental retardation in galactosemia is poorly understood. In Niemann-Pick disease and Tay-Sachs disease, however, it is the accumulation of sphingomyelin and GM_2 gangliosides, respectively, in the central nervous system of affected infants that leads to the progressive mental retardation characteristic of these diseases. McArdle's syndrome does not involve the central nervous system at all. It is a condition produced by a deficiency of phosphorylase in striated muscle, and in general its only symptoms are

muscle weakness after periods of physical activity (*pp. 145–148, 532–533*).

18. (C) The sudden infant death syndrome (SIDS) is an enigmatic disorder. Its very definition reflects the almost complete lack of understanding of this process: "the sudden and unexpected death of an infant who was either well or almost well prior to death, and whose death remains unexplained after the performance of an adequate autopsy." There is no evidence that these deaths occur more frequently in infants with congenital malformations than in normal infants. Epidemiologic studies have shown that the risk of SIDS is increased if the mother has abused narcotics or smoked cigarettes. SIDS also occurs more frequently in infants who are premature and are the offspring of young mothers. Most infants stricken by SIDS are between the ages of 2 and 4 months and usually die at home during the night after a period of sleep. It is currently thought that SIDS results from an instantaneous interruption of some basic physiologic function, either cardiac or respiratory, but the cause of the dysfunction is still far from clear (*pp. 536–537*).

19. (C) Neurofibromatosis (von Recklinghausen's disease) is a syndrome with two major features: multiple neural tumors (neurofibromas) throughout the body and pigmented skin lesions. Skeletal abnormalities such as scoliosis also commonly occur in this syndrome. Notably, patients with this syndrome are usually of normal mentality. Hemangioblastomas of the central nervous system do not occur in von Recklinghausen's disease but are characteristic of another rare autosomal disorder known as von Hippel-Lindau disease (*pp. 139–140*).

20. (True); 21. (False); 22. (True); 23. (False); 24. (False)

When the red blood cells of a fetus display antigenic determinants inherited from the father that differ from those of the mother, a maternal immune reaction against the fetal erythrocyte antigens may occur. The maternal antibodies cross the placenta and cause hemolysis in her infant (erythroblastosis fetalis). Although in theory many erythrocyte antigens could produce this phenomenon, in practice only ABO and Rh antigens cause significant amounts of hemolytic disease of the newborn.

(20 and 21) One of the major differences between the immunologic diseases produced by ABO antigens and by Rh antigens is the role of prior maternal sensitization. In Rh hemolytic disease, an Rh-negative mother is exposed to the red blood cells of the Rh-positive infant during delivery when the infant erythrocytes leak into the maternal circulation. The IgG antibodies formed in response to this exposure cross the placenta and cause disease in Rh-positive fetuses of subsequent pregnancies. Antibodies to A and B antigens, in contrast, occur naturally in all individuals lacking one or both (type O blood) of these antigens. No previous sensitization is required.

(22) Naturally occurring antibodies to A and B antigens are mostly of the IgM type and do not cross the placenta. Individuals with type O blood, however, often make IgG antibodies to these antigens as well. Thus, hemolytic disease occurs almost exclusively in infants of mothers with type O blood. Luckily, disease produced by ABO incompatibility is rarely severe.

(23) The incidence of maternal immunization against Rh antigens is greatly reduced if concurrent ABO incompatibility exists. This is thought to occur because leaked fetal red blood cells are promptly coated with agglutinating IgM antibodies against A and/or B antigens and rapidly removed from the maternal circulation by the mononuclear phagocyte system before sensitization to Rh antigen can occur. (24) Besides ABO incompatibility, another important factor modulating the maternal immune response is the dose of the immunizing antigen. The magnitude of the subsequent response is directly proportional to the magnitude of exposure to the immunogen. Thus, obstetric complications that increase the risk of placental hemorrhage (e.g., placenta previa, cesarean section, or toxemia of pregnancy) increase the risk of immunization *(pp. 527–530)*.

25. (True); **26.** (True); **27.** (False); **28.** (False); **29.** (False)

(25) The ductus arteriosus is a vascular channel that connects the pulmonary artery with the aorta and serves to divert blood flow from the pulmonary vascular system during intrauterine life. Normally, during the first day of postnatal life, muscular contraction of the ductus arteriosus occurs and produces functional closure of the conduit.

(26) In premature infants, this muscular contraction and functional closure are delayed. (27) Physiologic stimuli that cause the ductus to remain open include low arterial oxygen tensions and vasodilators, including prostaglandins. Vasodilatory prostaglandins, then, would delay normal closure.

(28) Most commonly, patent ductus arteriosus (PDA) produces no functional defect at birth. During infancy, when the shunt is left to right, there is no cyanosis. It is only with the ultimate production of pulmonary hypertension and reversal of the shunt from right to left that cyanosis develops.

(29) The murmur of PDA is a harsh, continuous sound that is described as machinery-like *(pp. 623–624)*.

30. (True); **31.** (False); **32.** (True); **33.** (False); **34.** (False)

(30) Coarctation (constriction) of the aorta is the third most common congenital cardiovascular anomaly and accounts for about 10 to 15% of all congenital cardiovascular defects. Females with Turner's syndrome often have coarctation of the aorta. However, the defect, overall, is two to three times more common in males.

(31) Although coarctation of the aorta may sometimes occur as a solitary defect, in 75% of the cases it occurs in association with other congenital cardiovascular defects.

(32) The position of the defect has a profound effect

on the prognosis. Coarctations located proximal to the ductus arteriosus carry an ominous prognosis. In such cases, the right side of the heart must supply the entire systemic circulation through the ductus arteriosus. Consequently, right ventricular hypertrophy occurs early, often in utero. Postpartum survival depends on the patency of the ductus arteriosus, but heart failure commonly supervenes, and many infants die in the neonatal period.

(33) When the coarctation is located distal to the ductus arteriosus (postductal coarctation), blood flow to the head and upper extremities is unimpaired, but blood flow to the lower half of the body depends on the development of collateral flow that bypasses the aortic obstruction. Blood is frequently diverted through the intercostal arteries, a common collateral bypass route. As they undergo enlargement, the intercostal arteries tend to produce erosion of the inner surface of the ribs that commonly appears radiographically as notching. (34) Surgical correction is the definitive treatment and is curative in most cases. The defect does not tend to recur once it has been surgically resected *(pp. 624–625)*.

35. (True); **36.** (False); **37.** (False); **38.** (True); **39.** (True)

(35) Of the four features that compose the tetralogy of Fallot—(1) ventricular septal defect, (2) an overriding aorta, (3) right ventricular outflow obstruction, and (4) right ventricular hypertrophy—it is the degree of obstruction to the outflow from the right ventricle that determines the severity of the clinical symptoms.

(36) The right ventricular outflow obstruction, which usually consists of a narrowing of the infundibulum of the right ventricle (with or without pulmonary valvular stenosis), limits flow through the pulmonary arterial system. Patency of the ductus arteriosus does not alleviate this physiologic deficit and therefore does not affect survival.

(37) The heart murmur of tetralogy of Fallot is produced by the right ventricular outflow obstruction and is inversely proportional to its severity.

(38) Reduction of flow through the pulmonary system and shunting of blood through the ventricular septal defect lead to profound cyanosis. The low oxygen tension is a stimulus to erythropoietin production, and thus polycythemia is a common part of the clinical picture.

(39) Corrective surgery should be performed as soon as possible in patients with tetralogy of Fallot, because the right ventricular outflow obstruction (infundibular narrowing) tends to increase with time. Untreated, most patients die before age 10 from cyanosis and congestive heart failure *(p. 620)*.

40. (C); **41.** (C); **42.** (B); **43.** (A); **44.** (B)

(40) Phenylketonuria (PKU) and alkaptonuria both are diseases that are caused by inborn errors of tyrosine metabolism. (41) The defect in PKU is a total lack of hepatic phenylalanine hydroxylase, preventing the conversion of phenylalanine to tyrosine. The defect in

alkaptonuria is the lack of homogentisic oxidase, blocking the metabolism of phenylalanine-tyrosine at the level of homogentisic acid. In both diseases, affected infants appear normal at birth.

(**42**) In alkaptonuria, homogentisic acid accumulates in the body and spills over into the urine. If the urine is allowed to stand, the homogentisic acid oxidizes, and the urine turns black. (**44**) The retained homogentisic acid in the body characteristically binds to connective tissues, tendons, and cartilage, producing a characteristic blue-black pigmentation (ochronosis) and arthritis.

(**43**) The buildup of dietary phenylalanine in infants with phenylketonuria has more profound consequences. Unless treated with dietary restriction, hyperphenylalaninemia leads to mental deterioration and retardation in most patients *(pp. 143–144, 530–531).*

45. (D); 46. (C); 47. (C); 48. (A); 49. (D)

(**45**) Marfan's syndrome and Ehlers-Danlos syndromes are hereditary disorders of connective tissue. Marfan's syndrome is an uncommon autosomal dominant syndrome. The Ehlers-Danlos syndromes encompass seven variants with distinctive modes of inheritance. Of these seven variants, only one type is X-linked; three are autosomal dominant, and three are autosomal recessive.

(**46**) Both Marfan's syndrome and the Ehlers-Danlos syndromes are characterized by a primary defect in collagen structure. Reduced tensile strength of connective tissue is the result. The precise biochemical defects in these disease processes have not been elucidated.

(**47**) In both syndromes, aortic aneurysms occur with a high frequency and constitute the major life-threatening complication. (**48**) The skeletal abnormalities of Marfan's syndrome are, however, distinctive. Individuals with Marfan's syndrome characteristically have long, slender extremities with particular elongation of the fingers and tall stature. (**49**) Although joint disorders are characteristic of both Marfan's and Ehlers-Danlos syndromes, they are typified by joint ligament laxity and hypermobility of the joints rather than the inflexibility that occurs in most other joint diseases *(pp. 138–139, 155–157).*

50. (B); 51. (A); 52. (B); 53. (C); 54. (C); 55. (B); 56. (B)

(**50 and 51**) Atrial septal defect (ASD) is the most frequent congenital cardiac anomaly to remain asymptomatic through childhood. ASD is usually first recognized in the adult. Overall, however, ventricular septal defect (VSD) is the most common congenital cardiac anomaly. VSD is commonly symptomatic in childhood, even from birth, depending on the size of the defect.

(**52**) Infective endocarditis is rare with ASD of any size. Small or moderate-sized VSD, however, poses a well-defined risk of superimposed bacterial endocarditis. (**53**) The end result of septal defects in the heart, whether atrial or ventricular, is a left-to-right shunt that increases flow through the pulmonary system and ultimately induces pulmonary hypertension and respiratory difficulty.

(**54**) By the eighth week of gestational life, both the atrial and septal walls of the heart have normally completed their development. Defects in the development of either the atrial septum or the ventricular septum are thus produced between the second and eighth weeks of embryogenesis. (**55**) VSD is frequently associated with other structural cardiac anomalies. VSD constitutes one of the four cardiac defects in the syndrome known as tetralogy of Fallot, in which it is accompanied by an overriding aorta, right ventricular outflow obstruction, and right ventricular hypertrophy (see Question 35).

(**56**) Surgical closure of an ASD is not generally indicated during infancy. Most ASDs are well tolerated during the first decade of life before pulmonary hypertension develops. Thus, the threat to life during infancy is less than that of the operative mortality associated with surgical closure. Ventricular septal defects that are functionally significant, however, may lead to right ventricular enlargement and pulmonary hypertension with cyanosis. They may, furthermore, predispose to infective endocarditis. The benefits of surgical closure in this case would offset the risk of operative mortality *(pp. 621–623).*

57. (C); 58. (C); 59. (A); 60. (B); 61. (C)

(**57 and 58**) Tricuspid valve atresia and pulmonary valve atresia are both commonly associated with a hypoplastic right ventricle and an atrial septal defect. (**59**) In addition, tricuspid valve atresia is frequently associated with a ventricular septal defect. (**60**) Although neither is a common congenital cardiac defect, pulmonary valve stenosis or atresia accounts for 5 to 15% of congenital cardiac defects, whereas tricuspid atresia accounts for only about 2%. (**61**) Because both tricuspid atresia and pulmonary atresia severely reduce flow through the pulmonary arterial system, a septal defect and patent ductus arteriosus are necessary to provide blood flow to the lungs *(pp. 621, 625).*

62. (C); 63. (A); 64. (D); 65. (B)

(**62**) Cytogenetic disorders involving sex chromosomes occur more frequently than those involving autosomal aberrations. One of the most common is Klinefelter's syndrome, with an approximate incidence of 1 in every 600 male births. The characteristic karyotype of Klinefelter's syndrome is 47,XXY, although numerous multiple X chromosome variants and mosaics may also occur. Because the major manifestation of Klinefelter's syndrome is hypogonadism, the disorder is rarely diagnosed before puberty.

(**63**) Turner's syndrome, occurring approximately once in every 3000 female births, is generally associated with a 45,XO karyotype. The major manifestation of Turner's syndrome is gonadal (ovarian) dysgenesis, but the disorder is commonly recognized at birth by the accompanying characteristic manifestations, webbing of the neck and peripheral lymphedema.

(**64**) True hermaphroditism is a rare disorder that is most often associated with a 46,XX karyotype, although some mosaics have been described. The disorder is characterized by the presence of both ovarian and testicular tissue; external genitalia are usually ambiguous.

(65) The syndrome of testicular feminization is characteristically associated with a 46,XY karyotype. This disorder is a form of male pseudohermaphroditism and is characterized by a female phenotype with good breast development but absence of uterus and tubes. Bilateral inguinal testes are usually present (*pp. 133–136*).

66. (B); 67. (A); 68. (E); 69. (D); 70. (C)

(66) The Lesch-Nyhan syndrome is an X-linked disorder that is characterized by a deficiency of hypoxanthine-guanine phosphoribosyl transferase, an enzyme involved in purine metabolism. Without this enzyme, there is deficient production of the nucleotides that inhibit the enzyme governing the rate-limiting step of de novo uric acid synthesis. Thus, uric acid is synthesized in excess, and gout is produced. A variety of neurologic problems whose pathogenesis is less well understood also occur. Principal among them are self-mutilation, aggressive behavior, mental retardation, spastic cerebral palsy, and choreoathetosis.

(67) Fabry's disease is an X-linked disorder of ceramide trihexoside (a glycosphingolipid) metabolism, resulting in the systemic accumulation of this compound. Although the cardiovascular system, the central nervous system, and the reticuloendothelial systems all are affected, the kidney is the most severely involved organ, and most patients die of progressive renal failure in middle life. However, another aspect of Fabry's disease may dominate the clinical picture—namely, red-blue elevated skin nodules known as angiokeratomas. Histologically, an angiokeratoma consists of a dermal cavernous hemangioma with hyperkeratotic thickening of the overlying epidermis. Although they are a characteristic

finding in Fabry's disease, their relationship to the underlying storage disorder is obscure.

(68) Xanthomas and accelerated atherosclerosis are the features of familial hypercholesterolemia, an autosomal dominant disorder that is possibly the most common disease with mendelian inheritance. Familial hypercholesterolemia results from loss of feedback control mechanisms that regulate cholesterol synthesis. Deposition of cholesterol in skin (xanthomas), coronary arteries, peripheral vessels, and other organs typically results. Death at an early age due to coronary artery disease and myocardial infarction is a common consequence.

(69) Wilson's disease is a rare inborn error of copper metabolism. Excess deposits of copper accumulate in the brain, liver, and cornea to produce the three characteristic pathologic consequences of this disorder: degenerative changes in the brain with focal cavitation, liver damage with cirrhosis, and the pathognomonic green-brown ring at the limbus of the cornea (Kayser-Fleischer ring). Characteristically, hepatic disease occurs long before the ocular or neurologic disease becomes clinically evident. The disease is important to recognize because it can be treated effectively with a low-copper diet and chelating agents.

(70) Von Hippel-Lindau disease is a rare autosomal dominant disorder characterized by the occurrence of multiple benign and malignant neoplasms throughout the body. The most commonly occurring tumors in this disorder are retinal and cerebellar hemangioblastomas. Renal cell carcinomas, adrenal pheochromocytomas, angiomas of the liver and kidney, and adenomas of the kidney and epididymis are also common. Renal cell carcinomas occur in about 25% of cases, and in this subgroup are the major cause of death (*pp. 140–143, 154, 956–957, 1356–1357*).

Nutritional Diseases

DIRECTIONS: For Questions 1 to 14, choose the ONE BEST answer to each question.

1. All of the following conditions are frequently associated with secondary malnutrition EXCEPT:

A. Diabetes mellitus
B. Membranous nephritis
C. Cystic fibrosis
D. Anticonvulsant drug therapy
E. Hypothyroidism

2. All of the following statements about vitamin A are true EXCEPT:

A. Deficiency causes blindness
B. Liver disease causes deficiency
C. Toxicity causes liver disease
D. Deficiency causes squamous metaplasia in glandular epithelia
E. Toxicity is associated with increased infections

3. Hypovitaminosis A occurs in association with all of the following conditions EXCEPT:

A. Pseudomembranous colitis
B. Chronic pancreatitis
C. Whipple's disease
D. Abetalipoproteinemia
E. Celiac sprue

4. Deficiency of vitamin D is associated with all of the following conditions EXCEPT:

A. Strict vegetarianism
B. Celiac disease (nontropical sprue)
C. Cirrhosis
D. Hypoparathyroidism
E. Chronic renal failure

5. All of the following statements about vitamin E are true EXCEPT:

A. It is abundant in both animal and vegetable dietary sources
B. Deficiency occurs with abetalipoproteinemia

C. Deficiency causes neurologic damage
D. Toxicity reactions are unknown in humans
E. It reduces complications of oxygen/ventilatory therapy in infants with the respiratory distress syndrome

6. All of the following statements about thiamine deficiency (beriberi) are true EXCEPT:

A. It is associated with diets of polished rice
B. It is associated with diuretic therapy
C. It is associated with diets of raw fish
D. It is common among alcoholics
E. It is common among patients with pancreatic insufficiency

7. Absorption of vitamin B_{12} is dependent on all of the following factors EXCEPT:

A. Intrinsic factor
B. R-binder proteins
C. Pancreatic proteases
D. Bile salts
E. Calcium

8. At the cellular level, deficiency of vitamin B_{12} causes all of the following EXCEPT:

A. Increased intrinsic factor production
B. Folate deficiency
C. Synthesis of abnormal fatty acids
D. Reduced adenine synthesis
E. Reduced thymidine synthesis

9. Patients with scurvy frequently develop defects of all of the following functions EXCEPT:

A. Phagocytotic activity of macrophages
B. Iron absorption
C. Collagen cross-linking
D. Formation of hydroxyproline
E. Platelet adhesion

10. Neurologic dysfunctions are known to result from deficiencies of all of the following nutrients EXCEPT:

    A. Pyridoxine (vitamin B_6)
    B. Niacin
    C. Copper
    D. Vitamin B_{12}
    E. Folate

11. All of the following statements about iron as a nutrient are true EXCEPT:

    A. Daily requirements are greater for young women than for young men
    B. Normally, most dietary iron is not absorbed
    C. In the Western world, deficiency in adult males is often due to gastrointestinal blood loss
    D. Deficiency causes a drop in the transferrin iron-binding capacity (TIBC)
    E. Deficiency causes abnormal mitochondrial and cytochrome function

12. All of the following conditions increase in incidence with obesity ("overnutrition") EXCEPT:

    A. Hypertension
    B. Diabetes mellitus
    C. Hyperlipidemia
    D. Gallstones
    E. Rheumatoid arthritis

13. All of the following actions are associated with synthetic retinoids EXCEPT:

    A. Effectively treat severe acne
    B. Induce regression of premalignant squamous metaplasia
    C. Effectively treat basal cell carcinoma
    D. Increase the incidence of urinary tract cancers
    E. Increase the incidence of fetal malformations when taken during pregnancy

14. Which of the following statements about vitamin K deficiency is TRUE?

    A. Deficiency causes defects in both the intrinsic and extrinsic coagulation pathways
    B. Deficiency produces defects in platelet functioning
    C. Deficiency is associated with strict vegetarian diets
    D. Intestinal bacteria produce enough vitamin K to prevent deficiency under normal conditions
    E. Deficiency develops less frequently in breast-fed infants than in bottle-fed infants

DIRECTIONS: For Questions 15 to 17, ONE or MORE of the completions given correctly finishes the incomplete statement. Choose:
    A—if only *1, 2, and 3* are correct
    B—if only *1 and 3* are correct
    C—if only *2 and 4* are correct
    D—if only *4* is correct
    E—if all are correct

15. Vitamins that are ingested in an inactive form and require metabolic conversion to an active form include:

    1. Vitamin K
    2. Vitamin E
    3. Vitamin C
    4. Vitamin D

    A. 1,2,3 B. 1,3 C. 2,4 D. 4 Only E. All

16. Pellagra is associated with which of the following conditions?

    1. Diets consisting primarily of maize
    2. Cirrhosis
    3. Functioning carcinoid tumors
    4. Hartnup disease

    A. 1,2,3 B. 1,3 C. 2,4 D. 4 Only E. All

17. Which of the following conditions is/are associated with a vitamin B_{12} deficiency?

    1. Strict vegetarianism
    2. Achlorhydria
    3. Crohn's disease
    4. Jejunal resection

    A. 1,2,3 B. 1,3 C. 2,4 D. 4 Only E. All

18. Which of the following nutritional deficiencies cause(s) impaired immunologic function?

    1. Zinc deficiency
    2. Vitamin B_6 (pyridoxine) deficiency
    3. Iron deficiency
    4. Vitamin C deficiency

    A. 1,2,3 B. 1,3 C. 2,4 D. 4 Only E. All

19. Which of the following nutrients is/are involved in free radical scavenging (antioxidant) reactions?

    1. Vitamin E
    2. Selenium
    3. Beta carotene
    4. Vitamin D

    A. 1,2,3 B. 1,3 C. 2,4 D. 4 Only E. All

20. Which of the following biochemical reactions involve(s) copper-containing enzymes?

    1. Synthesis of neurotransmitters

    2. Formation of cross-linkages in collagen
    3. Synthesis of myelin
    4. Synthesis of melanin

      A. 1,2,3 B. 1,3 C. 2,4 D. 4 Only E. All

DIRECTIONS: For Questions 21 to 58, the set of lettered headings is followed by a list of numbered words or phrases. For each numbered word or phrase choose:

    A—if the item is associated with (A) only
    B—if the item is associated with (B) only
    C—if the item is associated with *both* (A) and (B)
    D—if the item is associated with *neither* (A) nor (B)

For each of the characteristics listed below, choose whether it describes kwashiorkor, marasmus, both, or neither.

    A. Kwashiorkor
    B. Marasmus
    C. Both
    D. Neither

21. Total caloric intake is adequate

22. Affected infants appear cachectic and ravenously hungry

23. Edema is usually present

24. Desquamative skin lesions are pathognomonic

25. Fatty change is usually seen in the liver

26. Intercurrent parasitic infection is common

27. T-lymphocyte function is depressed

For each of the characteristics listed below, choose whether it describes rickets, osteomalacia, both, or neither.

    A. Rickets
    B. Osteomalacia
    C. Both
    D. Neither

28. Osteoid mineralization is retarded

29. Endochondral ossification is retarded

30. Osteitis fibrosa frequently occurs concomitantly

31. The disease has a hereditary autosomal recessive form

32. The disease has a hereditary X-linked form

33. Tetracycline administration is useful for treatment

For each of the characteristics listed below, choose whether it relates to calcium, phosphate, both, or neither.

    A. Calcium
    B. Phosphate
    C. Both
    D. Neither

34. Decreased serum levels induce synthesis of 1,25-$(OH)_2D_3$

35. Intestinal absorption is increased by vitamin D

36. Renal reabsorption is increased by vitamin D

37. Increased renal excretion occurs in Fanconi's syndrome

38. Lamellar osteoid seams appear in bone in deficiency states

39. Anticonvulsant drugs cause decreased intestinal absorption

40. Serum levels affect calcitonin secretion

For each of the characteristics listed below, choose whether it describes disease caused by alcohol, thiamine deficiency, both, or neither.

    A. Alcoholic disease
    B. Thiamine deficiency
    C. Both
    D. Neither

41. Produces a dilated cardiomyopathy

42. Causes cirrhosis

43. Associated with transketolase deficiency

44. Produces skeletal muscle weakness

45. Associated with the Wernicke-Korsakoff syndrome

For each of the following conditions, choose whether it is associated with vitamin B_{12} deficiency, folate deficiency, both, or neither.

    A. Vitamin B_{12} deficiency
    B. Folate deficiency
    C. Both
    D. Neither

46. Occurs in pernicious anemia

47. Occurs commonly in alcoholism

48. Typically produces glossitis

49. Typically produces sideroblasts in the bone marrow

50. Results in hypersegmentation of neutrophils

51. Reduces fertility

For each of the physiologic processes listed below, choose whether it requires vitamin C, vitamin D, both, or neither.

    A. Vitamin C
    B. Vitamin D
    C. Both
    D. Neither

52. Osteoid production

53. Osteoid mineralization

54. Bone resorption

55. Bone remodeling

56. Cartilage resorption in endochondral bone growth

57. Tooth formation

58. Wound healing

DIRECTIONS: Questions 59 to 85 are matching questions. For each numbered item, choose the most likely associated lettered item from those provided. Each numbered item has ONLY ONE answer. Within each group, each lettered item may be the answer to one, more than one, or none of the numbered items.

For each of the vitamins listed below, choose whether its principal storage site is within striated muscle, adrenal cortex, liver, all body tissues in even distribution, or none of these.

    A. Striated muscle
    B. Adrenal cortex
    C. Liver
    D. Evenly distributed in all tissues
    E. None of the above

59. Vitamin A

60. Vitamin B_1 (thiamine)

61. Vitamin D

62. Folate

63. Vitamin B_6 (pyridoxine)

64. Vitamin C

65. Riboflavin

For each of the following characteristics, choose whether it is associated with riboflavin, niacin, pyridoxine, all of these, or none of these.

    A. Riboflavin
    B. Niacin
    C. Pyridoxine (vitamin B_6)
    D. All of the above
    E. None of the above

66. The molecule is a coenzyme in cellular oxidative metabolism

67. The human body is capable of endogenous synthesis of the vitamin

68. Dietary intake of tryptophan determines the dietary requirement for the vitamin

69. It is particularly important in tryptophan metabolism

70. A deficiency state causes a macrocytic anemia

71. A deficiency state causes a dermatitis

72. A deficiency state is associated with dementia

73. Parenteral administration commonly produces toxic effects

For each of the hematologic abnormalities listed below, choose whether it is associated with iron deficiency, vitamin B_{12} deficiency, starvation, none of these, or all of these.

    A. Iron deficiency
    B. Vitamin B_{12} deficiency
    C. Starvation
    D. All of the above
    E. None of the above

74. Increased hemolysis

75. Increased osmotic fragility of erythrocytes

76. Hypochromic, microcytic anemia

77. Normochromic, macrocytic anemia

78. Hypochromic, normocytic anemia

For each of the characteristics listed below, choose whether it is associated with zinc, copper, selenium, all of these, or none of these.

    A. Zinc
    B. Copper
    C. Selenium
    D. All of the above
    E. None of the above

79. It functions as a component of a metalloenzyme

80. Deficiencies are common in patients receiving long-term total parenteral nutrition

81. In children, deficiency causes growth retardation

82. Deficiency causes anemia

83. Deficiency causes cardiomyopathy

84. It is required for the formation of cross-linkages in collagen

85. It is required for the formation of cross-linkages in elastin

Nutritional Diseases

1. (E) Diabetes mellitus causes derangements in the metabolism of all foodstuffs including fats, carbohydrates, and proteins; these derangements may produce secondary deficiencies of these basic nutrients. In addition, loss of minerals and electrolytes may occur in the urine as glycosuria induces an osmotic diuresis.

Membranous nephropathy, as a cause of the nephrotic syndrome, is associated with excessive protein losses and secondary protein malnutrition.

Almost all individuals with cystic fibrosis have pancreatic exocrine insufficiency from ductal plugging and secondary acinar atrophy. The decrease in pancreatic enzyme secretion results in deficient enzymatic hydrolysis of ingested nutrients, especially fats. Fat malabsorption, in turn, results in deficiencies of essential fatty acids and fat-soluble vitamins A, D, E, and K.

Anticonvulsant medications (e.g., phenytoin and phenobarbital) are associated with various secondary vitamin deficiency states, although the mechanisms by which these are produced remain largely unknown. Folate, vitamin D, and vitamin K are the nutrients most often depleted by long-term anticonvulsant therapy.

Although hypothyroidism may rarely produce a malabsorptive syndrome, it is not usually associated with secondary malnutrition. Hyperfunction of the thyroid, in contrast, frequently produces a clinical picture of malnutrition. This is the result of numerous factors, including anorexia, increased metabolic demands, and diarrhea with nutrient losses (*pp. 449, 535, 1001–1002, 1034–1035*).

2. (B) Vitamin A is known to be requisite to (1) the processes of maturation and differentiation of epithelial cells, both glandular and squamous, and (2) the production of photosensitive pigments in the retina. Deficiencies of the vitamin lead to decreased production of rhodopsin in rods (impairing vision in dim light) and iodopsin in cones. Protracted deficiency leads to conjunctival and corneal desiccation and erosion, impeding transmission of light and predisposing to infection. Subsequent scarring or extrusion of the lens produces blindness. Indeed, it is the leading cause of blindness in many Asian countries.

Although most hypovitaminosis A is caused by dietary deficiency, it can also occur with diseases that lead to decreased absorption or transport of the vitamin. Transportation of mobilized vitamin A stores in the blood and uptake by peripheral tissues is dependent on retinol-binding protein (RBP), a protein that is synthesized by the liver. Thus, decreased RBP production in chronic liver disease and cirrhosis leads to inadequate circulating levels of vitamin A and produces hypovitaminosis A. Loss of RBP via the urine (e.g., in the nephrotic syndrome) has the same effect. Cirrhosis may also compromise hepatic retinyl ester stores (the principal reservoir of vitamin A in the body). Decreased uptake of vitamin A occurs in any disease interfering with fat absorption (pancreatic, biliary tract, or small intestinal disease) (see Question 3).

Vitamin A toxicity may be either acute or chronic. Acute toxicity produces symptoms suggestive of a brain tumor: headache, stupor, vomiting, and papilledema. Chronic toxicity begins with anorexia, nausea, vomiting, cutaneous desquamation, and pruritus. Liver injury with hepatomegaly and fibrosis (sometimes severe enough to produce portal hypertension) occurs with more protracted disease.

In deficiency states, glandular epithelia (e.g., gastrointestinal, respiratory, and genitourinary mucosae) undergo squamous metaplasia. Squamous metaplasia in the bronchial tree destroys the natural host defense provided by ciliated epithelial surfaces and increases susceptibility to respiratory tract infection. Furthermore, the mortality rate from infection is increased in

Asian children with vitamin A deficiency. Vitamin A toxicity, on the other hand, is not associated with increased infections *(pp. 439–441).*

3. (A) Vitamin A is a fat-soluble vitamin. Therefore, a primary deficiency of the vitamin may occur in any disease causing impaired absorption of fat. In chronic pancreatitis, the resultant pancreatic insufficiency leads to defective intraluminal hydrolysis, solubility, and subsequent absorption of fat.

Whipple's disease, an acquired small bowel disease of suspected infectious etiology, causes fat malabsorption. In this disease, the small bowel mucosa is distended by infiltrates of macrophages with periodic acid-Schiff (PAS)-positive granules that contain bacillary bodies (the suspected infectious agent) on electron microscopic examination.

The mucosal absorptive cell is the site of the primary defect in abetalipoproteinemia. This form of malabsorption is hereditary rather than acquired. It is characterized by an inability to synthesize beta lipoproteins required for the export of triglycerides from intestinal absorptive cells. Thus, fats accumulate within the mucosal cells, and severe hypolipidemia and consequent hypovitaminosis A result.

Celiac sprue is a hypersensitivity enteropathy caused by a reaction to gluten (wheat protein). Severe small bowel mucosal injury is produced, and malabsorption of many nutrients, including fats and fat-soluble vitamins, results.

Pseudomembranous colitis (most commonly caused by *Clostridia difficile*) is not usually associated with defects in nutrient absorption. The disease process is entirely limited to the mucosa of the colon, and nutrient absorption in the small bowel takes place normally. Therefore, absorption, transport, or storage of vitamin A is unaffected *(pp. 439, 876, 889–890).*

4. (D) Vitamin D is a biochemical relative of cholesterol, and its principal dietary sources are animal products. Strict vegetarian diets can therefore lead to vitamin D deficiency. This is especially true if endogenous sources of vitamin D are inadequate, as they are for most people living in the northern hemisphere, where exposure to sunlight is limited. Because dietary vitamin D is absorbed in the small intestine like other fats, diseases such as celiac sprue (nontropical sprue) that severely reduce the bowel's absorptive surface compromise uptake of vitamin D. The liver has three key roles in vitamin D metabolism: (1) synthesis of serum transport proteins for vitamin D, (2) storage of the vitamin, and (3) 25-hydroxylation of vitamin D_3, the first step in the metabolic conversion of vitamin D_3 (endogenous or exogenous) to its metabolically active form. Thus hepatic parenchymal disease, such as cirrhosis, is often associated with a vitamin D deficiency state. The second step in conversion of D_3 to its active form, 1-hydroxylation, takes place in the kidney. Severe renal parenchymal disease with chronic renal failure therefore can lead to a functional vitamin D deficiency.

The parathyroid glands have no direct effect on vitamin D metabolism. Indirectly, however, hypoparathyroidism would be expected only to stimulate vitamin D metabolism in response to the consequent fall in serum calcium concentration *(pp. 441–446, 1247–1248).*

5. (D) Vitamin E (actually, like vitamin A, vitamin E encompasses several different chemically related compounds) is a fat-soluble vitamin widely distributed in both plant and animal dietary sources. Deficiencies can result, however, from diseases causing severe fat malabsorption, such as abetalipoproteinemia (see Question 3). Clinically, the deficiency state is characterized by neurologic damage, but hypovitaminosis E is typically present for years before becoming clinically evident. Pathologically, axonal degeneration in the posterior columns and neuron loss from the dorsal root ganglia are the most common changes.

The primary biologic role of vitamin E is that of an antioxidant. It is especially important in the neutralization of free radicals that are continuously generated (and highly destructive) at the cellular level. The therapeutic value of vitamin E has been demonstrated for several diseases known to be caused or complicated by oxidative injury. In particular, vitamin E has proved effective in the treatment of bronchopulmonary dysplasia and retrolental fibroplasia in infants with the respiratory distress syndrome treated with high oxygen concentrations and ventilatory support.

Vitamin E toxicity occurs with massive overdoses (e.g., megadose vitamin consumption) and is characterized by a variety of gastrointestinal disturbances, platelet dysfunction, and coagulation defects. In infants, vitamin E therapy has been associated with necrotizing enterocolitis *(pp. 447–448).*

6. (E) Thiamine (vitamin B_1) deficiency is the cause of a disease known as beriberi. Primary dietary deficiency of thiamine occurs in populations whose diet consists largely of polished rice or milled grains, because the discarded husks contain most of the grains' thiamine. Increased losses of this water-soluble vitamin with diuretic therapy also cause deficiencies. Thiamine losses also occur as a consequence of direct enzymatic degradation of the vitamin by thiaminases contained in raw foods such as fish, shellfish, or meat. A diet consisting mainly of these foods therefore may cause beriberi. Alcoholism is the most universal cause of beriberi. Poor general nutrition with decreased thiamine intake, coupled with increased losses from vomiting and ethanol-induced diuresis, forms the basis for thiamine deficiency in alcoholic patients. Because thiamine is readily absorbed in the upper intestinal tract without the aid of pancreatic enzymes, pancreatic insufficiency is not associated with thiamine deficiency *(pp. 450–452).*

7. (D) Absorption of vitamin B_{12} is a complex process requiring the interaction of a number of factors. When ingested, the vitamin is attached to animal protein from which it is released in the acid-peptic milieu of the stomach. It then complexes with a secreted gastric protein known as R-binder protein, which has a high affinity for cobalamin at a low pH. Pancreatic proteases in the duodenum, in turn, release cobalamin from the R-binder protein. The vitamin then combines with the glycoprotein synthesized by gastric parietal cells known as intrinsic factor. Specific mucosal cell receptors in the ileum bind the intrinsic factor-vitamin B_{12} complex, but the process requires calcium and a pH greater than 5.6. Once bound, the complex is then taken up and transported across the ileal mucosal cell to the blood, completing vitamin B_{12} absorption. None of the steps in this absorptive process, however, is known to require the presence of bile salts (*pp. 455–456*).

8. **(A)** Metabolic derivatives of vitamin B_{12} are required for two important biochemical reactions: (1) the conversion of methylmalonyl coenzyme A to succinyl coenzyme A and (2) conversion of homocysteine to methionine. The first is essential to fatty acid synthesis and the second to both adenine and pyrimidine synthesis. Thus, in vitamin B_{12} deficiency, abnormal fatty acids are synthesized, and purine and thymidine synthesis is reduced. In the reaction generating methionine, tetrahydrofolate is also produced from its methylated form. With the decrease in this vitamin B_{12}-dependent reaction, folate is "trapped" in the form of methyltetrahydrofolate, and a functional folate deficiency is created. Although the availability of vitamin B_{12} is dependent on the production of intrinsic factor, vitamin B_{12} is not known to exert any feedback control on the elaboration of intrinsic factor by gastric parietal cells. Therefore, vitamin B_{12} deficiency would not be expected to increase intrinsic factor production (*pp. 455–456, 681*).

9. **(E)** Scurvy, the disease produced by vitamin C deficiency, is an uncommon disorder, because vitamin C is abundant in most foods, easily absorbed throughout the small bowel, and stored in substantial quantity in most tissues. The deficiency state reflects the loss of the primary functions of vitamin C in the body—namely, its participation in several steps of collagen metabolism. Vitamin C is required for collagen cross-linking and the hydroxylation of proline as well as other biochemical events in collagen synthesis. Deficiency of vitamin C has also been found to depress both motility and phagocytotic activity in macrophages and neutrophils, creating an immunologic defect. Iron absorption is also adversely affected by deficiency of vitamin C, because the vitamin is known to facilitate uptake of inorganic (non-heme) iron. Although scurvy is associated with hemorrhagic diatheses, these are the result of vascular fragility caused by defective collagen in blood vessel walls. Platelet functions, however, are not known to be affected by vitamin C deficiency (*pp. 456–458*).

10. **(E)** Many nutritional deficiencies have profound effects on the nervous system; these effects may occasionally dominate the clinical presentation. Pyridoxine (vitamin B_6) is known to participate (as a coenzyme) in numerous metabolic functions in the brain, including the synthesis of neurotransmitters. Consequently, pyridoxine deficiency states produce peripheral neuropathies and occasionally convulsions. Furthermore, pyridoxine-deficient mothers may produce mentally retarded infants. Niacin deficiency is typically associated with degeneration of the ganglion cells of the brain and spinal cord tracts. Ganglion cell degeneration produces dementia that, along with diarrhea and dermatitis, forms the classic symptom triad (the three D's) of pellagra. Copper is an essential component of metalloenzymes involved in the synthesis and maintenance of myelin and the metabolism of neurotransmitters. Copper deficiencies therefore produce various central nervous system abnormalities.

Both vitamin B_{12} and folate deficiencies produce megaloblastic anemia, but only vitamin B_{12} deficiency is associated with neurologic abnormalities. Vitamin B_{12} deficiency produces peripheral neuropathy and degeneration of the posterior and lateral spinal columns. The pathogenesis of these lesions is not completely understood but may be related to the derangement of cobalamin-dependent fatty acid biosynthesis and incorporation of abnormal fatty acids into the lipids of myelin. The neurologic manifestations of vitamin B_{12} deficiency help to distinguish it from folate deficiency, which it resembles hematologically (*pp. 455, 681–685*).

11. **(B)** The total iron content of the body is normally a closely regulated constant. In general, iron is efficiently recycled by the body, and daily losses of iron from sloughing of various epithelial cells (skin, gastrointestinal, and genitourinary) are constant and quite small. Additional losses in young adult females occur with menses and pregnancy. Therefore, women of reproductive age require approximately twice as much iron daily as their male counterparts. Because normal losses are small, iron balance is maintained by restricting intestinal absorption of dietary iron (most of which takes place in the duodenum). Enterocytes constitute a "mucosal barrier" to iron absorption by regulating uptake of iron from the gut lumen and transfer to the plasma. Only about 5 to 10% of the iron of the average Western diet is normally absorbed.

In the Western world, deficiencies in adult males often reflect occult bleeding from an infectious, inflammatory, or neoplastic process in the gastrointestinal tract. In nonindustrialized countries, however, deficiencies are usually caused by dietary lack. Early manifestations of deficiency are (1) the depletion of iron stores indicated by a decrease in serum ferritin and (2) decreased iron transport with low serum iron levels and *increased* transferrin-binding capacity. Iron deficiency causes qualitative and/or quantitative abnormalities of all normal iron-containing compounds, including mitochondrial enzymes involved in ATP synthesis, cytochromes, flavoproteins, and hemoglobin. Thus, the overall metabolic abnormalities of iron deficiency are as much a consequence of abnormalities in enzyme and mitochondrial function as of anemia (*pp. 459–461, 685–688*).

12. (E) In the United States, obesity is the single most common nutritional disorder. Obesity is known to predispose to a number of diseases that carry significant risks of morbidity and even mortality. Among the conditions that occur with increased frequency in obesity are hypertension, adult-onset diabetes mellitus, hyperlipidemia, and cholelithiasis (gallstones). Although degenerative osteoarthritis from increased stress on weight-bearing joints may be associated with obesity, there is no correlation between obesity and rheumatoid arthritis, a disease caused by immunologic injury (*pp. 462–463*).

13. (D) Synthetic retinoids (vitamin A analogs) have antiproliferative and differentiation-promoting effects on both squamous and glandular epithelia. They are highly effective, if not curative, in the treatment of many bothersome and disfiguring nonneoplastic skin diseases, such as severe acne, rosacea, and psoriasis. Several premalignant and malignant skin diseases such as actinic keratosis, keratoacanthoma, and basal cell carcinoma can also be treated effectively with synthetic retinoids. These compounds have the further ability to induce regression of a wide variety of premalignant metaplastic, hyperplastic, and/or dysplastic lesions in other epithelia, such as bronchial, oropharyngeal, cervical, and bladder mucosa. There is also evidence to suggest that retinoids (natural or synthetic) may also be effective in preventing the development or inducing the regression of many epithelial malignancies (carcinomas). Tumors of the urinary bladder, for example, have been reported to be susceptible to the anticancer effects of retinoids in both laboratory animals and humans. In sharp contrast to other forms of chemotherapy, retinoids themselves are not thought to be carcinogenic. They are not without their downside, however. Their use is contraindicated in pregnancy, because they are known to cause an increase in fetal malformations. They can also cause acute toxic reactions and other complications (*pp. 440–441*).

14. (A) Vitamin K is a cofactor for a hepatic carboxylase that converts the inactive proenzyme forms of clotting factors II (prothrombin), VII, XI, and X to their functionally active state. Vitamin K-dependent carboxylation of these factors is required for calcium-binding activity. Factor VII is activated in the extrinsic pathway, factor XI in the intrinsic pathway, and factors X and II in both (in the final common pathway). Thus, inactivity of these vitamin K-dependent clotting factors would cause defects in both pathways. However, vitamin K deficiency would not be expected to affect platelet function, because the vitamin plays no known role in platelet biology.

The dietary form of vitamin K is phylloquinone, or vitamin K_1, which is especially plentiful in leafy green vegetables. Therefore, strict vegetarianism, although associated with deficiencies of most other fat-soluble vitamins, is not expected to cause a vitamin K deficiency. Intestinal bacteria also contribute to the daily supply by synthesizing menaquinone (vitamin K_2) but do not provide enough of this compound to meet the full vitamin K requirements without dietary supplementation. In infancy, when intestinal bacterial colonization is incomplete and hepatic reserves of vitamin K are small, the risk of developing vitamin K deficiency is increased by breast-feeding, because human breast milk contains less vitamin K than cow's milk (*pp. 448–449*).

15. (D) Vitamin K and vitamin E (fat-soluble vitamins) and vitamin C (a water-soluble vitamin) all are obtained from dietary sources in their active form and require no metabolic conversion for biologic activity in humans. Vitamin K_1 (phylloquinone) is obtained primarily from leafy green vegetables in the diet, whereas vitamin K_2 (menaquinone) is synthesized by microorganisms in the gastrointestinal tract. Vitamin E is also obtained from leafy green vegetables as well as cooking oils and whole grains. Although alpha-tocopherol is the major dietary form of vitamin E, there are actually eight compounds (four tocopherols and four tocotrienols) that have vitamin E activity. All of these are absorbed directly from the diet and are usable in their absorbed form. Vitamin C (ascorbate) is an acid available in many foodstuffs including fruits, vegetables, liver, fish, and milk. It too is absorbed directly in its biologically active form. Vitamin D, however, is absorbed from dietary sources (a variety of animal products) in the form of cholecalciferol, also called vitamin D_3. Vitamin D_3 requires two metabolic conversions in order to acquire full biologic activity. Cholecalciferol is first hydroxylated at the 25-carbon position in the liver and again at the 1-carbon position in the kidney, producing $1,25\text{-}(OH)_2D_3$, the active vitamin D hormone (see Question 4) (*pp. 441–443, 447–448, 456*).

16 (E) Pellagra is the disease state resulting from a deficiency of niacin, a vitamin that is widely distributed in most foods. Deficiencies are primarily encountered among populations whose diets consist primarily of maize. Although maize contains adequate amounts of niacin, it also has a high leucine content. It is now known that leucine acts as an antagonist in the synthesis of nicotinamide adenine dinucleotide (NAD) and its phosphorylated analog NADP, the two major metabolic coenzymes of which niacin is a component. Thus a disorder identical to niacin deficiency develops as a consequence of increased leucine content in the diet. Pellagra is also encountered in patients with chronic debilitating diseases such as cirrhosis. Because niacin is also synthesized endogenously from tryptophan, diseases that produce tryptophan depletion may cause pellagra. Active carcinoid tumors, for example, greatly increase the utilization of tryptophan, from which they synthesize serotonin; thus, patients with the carcinoid syndrome may also develop pellagra. Hartnup disease may also be complicated by pellagra, because this disease causes decreased intestinal absorption of tryptophan (*pp. 453–454*).

17. (A) Vitamin B$_{12}$ (cobalamin) is a metallo-organic compound for which the only dietary sources are meats and dairy products. Because fruits and vegetables are devoid of vitamin B$_{12}$, strict vegetarian diets often produce deficiency states. Achlorhydria results from any process that is destructive to gastric parietal cells such as chronic gastritis or pernicious anemia. Because parietal cells produce intrinsic factor as well as hydrochloric acid, decreased vitamin B$_{12}$ absorption as well as achlorhydria results from their destruction. Crohn's disease causes small intestinal mucosal injury, resulting in an inadequate absorptive surface. Deficiencies of many nutrients may occur secondarily. However, vitamin B$_{12}$ deficiency is especially common, since the ileum (the primary site of vitamin B$_{12}$ absorption) is the region of the small bowel most frequently affected in Crohn's disease.

Because the ileum is the major site of vitamin B$_{12}$ absorption, jejunal resection alone in an otherwise normal individual (e.g., for a jejunal tumor, volvulus, reduplication) is not expected to produce vitamin B$_{12}$ deficiency *(pp. 455–456)*.

18. (A) Nutritional deficiencies that have been found to alter immune function include those of zinc, vitamin B$_6$, and iron. For example, impaired T-cell function and antibody synthesis have been noted with pyridoxine deficiency, and impaired cell-mediated immunity has been found to result from iron deficiency. Although debate persists about the immune-stimulating function (e.g., interferon production, blastogenesis, cell-mediated immunity) of increased vitamin C intake, evidence is lacking that deficiency of this vitamin (scurvy) actually causes immune dysfunction *(pp. 456–459, 461)*.

19. (A) Free radicals are highly reactive chemical species with an unpaired electron in an outer orbit. Most are derived from oxygen and are generated in many different biologic and pathologic processes. Free radicals are highly injurious to cells. Normally, they are controlled by enzymes that break them down and antioxidant molecules that either block their initiation or inactivate ("scavenge") them. Several essential nutrients are either constituents of antioxidant compounds or are themselves antioxidants.

The major role of vitamin E is that of an antioxidant. It is the only lipid-soluble antioxidant, and it has an important role in terminating peroxide-generated autocatalytic chain reactions that result in loss of unsaturated fatty acids from phospholipids and extensive membrane damage.

Beta carotene, a provitamin A derived from plants, also has antioxidant, free radical-scavenging activity.

Selenium is a component of glutathione peroxidase, an enzyme that catalyzes the conversion of hydroxyl radicals or peroxide to water by releasing hydrogen from reduced glutathione. Thus, glutathione peroxidase protects against injury from these toxic, partially reduced oxygen species.

Vitamin D is an essential nutrient that plays a major role in the maintenance of normal plasma levels of calcium and phosphorus, but it is not an antioxidant *(pp. 12, 441, 447, 462)*.

20. (E) Copper is an essential trace mineral that is a component of various metalloenzymes. Copper-containing enzymes include (1) dopamine-beta-hydroxylase, involved in the synthesis of neurotransmitters; (2) lysyl oxidase, involved in the cross-linking of collagen fibrils; and (3) tyrosinase, involved in melanin production. Copper-containing enzymes are involved with the synthesis and/or maintenance of myelin. Other copper-containing proteins in the body include ceruloplasmin, erythrocuprein, hepatocuprein, cerebrocuprein, cytochrome *c* oxidase, and monoamine oxidase *(p. 461)*.

21. (A); 22. (B); 23. (A); 24. (A); 25. (C); 26. (C); 27. (C)

(21) Marasmus and kwashiorkor are opposite ends of the spectrum of protein-energy malnutrition (PEM). Marasmus is characterized by a marked deficiency in total caloric intake. Kwashiorkor, in contrast, is the consequence of a critical deficiency of protein despite sufficient caloric intake.

(22) Both diseases are most frequently encountered in children and in their classic forms are readily distinguishable. On one hand, marasmic children appear obviously wasted but have a voracious appetite. **(23)** On the other hand, children with kwashiorkor appear bloated (edematous) and are often anorectic. **(24)** Also characteristic of kwashiorkor but not uniformly present are skin lesions characterized by pigment changes and desquamation.

(25) Fatty change in the liver is a common finding in both kwashiorkor and marasmus. **(26)** Also common to both conditions is intercurrent parasitic infection with such organisms as ascarids, *Trichuris, Strongyloides,* and amebae. Infectious processes exacerbate PEM by further increasing metabolic demand for calories and proteins already in inadequate supply. **(27)** PEM predisposes to infections largely through its effects on the immune system. It primarily causes premature thymic atrophy and depressed T-cell function, but mild defects in B-cell humoral immune responses may also be produced *(pp. 436–438)*.

28. (C); 29. (A); 30. (C); 31. (C); 32. (C); 33. (D)

(28) Deficiency of vitamin D can cause skeletal disease in children (rickets) or in adults (osteomalacia). Both disorders are characterized by retarded or inadequate mineralization of newly formed osteoid in bone.

(29) The major distinguishing feature between the two conditions is the defective endochondral ossification of epiphyseal cartilage that occurs in rickets. This distinction is somewhat artificial, however, because it is merely a reflection of ongoing bone growth in children, whose epiphyses have not yet closed.

(30) In both disorders, the lack of vitamin D has profound effects on the regulation of serum calcium concentration. Resultant hypocalcemia stimulates the parathyroid glands to increase production of parathormone, and parathormone in turn induces osteoclastic resorption of mineralized bones. Scalloping and thinning of cancellous and cortical bone are produced along with fibrosis of the marrow (osteitis fibrosa).

(**31 and 32**) Two hereditary diseases characterized by defects in vitamin D metabolism produce rickets and osteomalacia: an autosomal recessive form (vitamin D-dependent rickets) and an X-linked dominant hereditary form (vitamin D-resistant rickets). With the decreasing incidence of dietary vitamin D deficiency in developed nations, these diseases, especially the latter, have emerged as relatively important causes of rickets and osteomalacia.

(**33**) Because of its chelating property, tetracycline can be used to distinguish mineralized from unmineralized osteoid and to quantitate the rate of bone mineralization. In mineralized osteoid, the incorporated antibiotic can be visualized by its fluorescence under ultraviolet light and the amount of mineralized osteoid measured at a known time after administration of the drug. Thus tetracycline is an aid to the diagnosis and evaluation of rickets and osteomalacia but has no known therapeutic effect on these disease processes (*pp. 441–447*).

34. (C); 35. (C); 36. (A); 37. (B); 38. (A); 39. (C); 40. (A)
(**34**) Although the role of phosphate in vitamin D metabolism is poorly understood, it is known to parallel calcium in some of its effects. Hypophosphatemia as well as hypocalcemia stimulates synthesis of 1,25-$(OH)_2D_3$. Conversely, elevated serum levels of either phosphate or calcium increase production of the less metabolically active form of the vitamin, 24,25-$(OH)_2D_3$. (**35**) Vitamin D in turn has at least one parallel function in both calcium and phosphate homeostasis: control of uptake from dietary sources. Vitamin D increases intestinal absorption of both elements, although it apparently does so through independent mechanisms for each.

(**36**) In the role of conservation of renal losses, however, vitamin D affects only calcium handling. The active form, 1,25-$(OH)_2D_3$, increases the reabsorption of calcium in the distal renal tubules but has no known effect on the renal handling of phosphate.

(**37**) Increased phosphate loss occurs in several forms of renal tubular disorders including Fanconi's syndrome and renal tubular acidosis. The resultant hypophosphatemia stimulates synthesis of 1,25-$(OH)_2D_3$, and intestinal absorption of phosphate increases (see Questions 34 and 35). If losses exceed uptake, however, defects in bony mineralization characterized by widened osteoid seams ensue.

(**38**) In hypophosphatemic states, osteoid seams composed only of woven osteoid are seen in the bone, but in hypocalcemic states lamellar as well as woven osteoid is characteristically present. Excessive woven osteoid results from defective mineralization of newly laid down osteoid matrix. Lamellar osteoid, however, is produced by mobilization of the mineral phase of lamellar bone

in response to the parathormone generated in a hypocalcemic state.

(**39**) The intricate mechanisms that control calcium and phosphate homeostasis can be compromised in various ways by drugs. Virtually all anticonvulsant medications, for example, increase hepatic degradation of vitamin D. Thus, intestinal absorption of both calcium and phosphate is affected. In addition, anticonvulsants act directly on intestinal absorptive cells to inhibit calcium transport.

(**40**) Parathormone and calcitonin affect calcium homeostasis only. These hormones raise or lower serum calcium levels in response to hypo- or hypercalcemia, respectively but, unlike vitamin D, are not directly involved in regulation of phosphorus (*pp. 441–447*).

41. (C); 42. (A); 43. (C); 44. (C); 45. (C)
(**41**) Both alcoholism and beriberi can cause a dilated cardiomyopathy. Alcoholic cardiomyopathy is thought to result from the direct toxic effects of alcohol and its metabolites on cardiac muscle. Beriberi heart disease is probably the result of metabolic derangements in the myofibers induced by thiamine deficiency. The two disorders have many similar manifestations and can be difficult to differentiate from each other. (**42**) Cirrhosis is a manifestation of alcoholic disease alone; it is not caused by beriberi.

(**43**) In the Western world, chronic alcoholic patients are frequently affected by beriberi. Beriberi in alcoholic patients appears to be the result of a combination of factors: poor general nutrition and an apparent increased incidence of hereditary transketolase abnormality in chronic alcoholic patients compared with the general population. Thiamine is a cofactor for transketolase, an enzyme involved in the pentose phosphate pathway of carbohydrate metabolism. Thus, a transketolase abnormality predisposes to clinical manifestations of beriberi.

(**44**) Both disorders may also be associated with skeletal muscle weakness, although the pathogenesis may differ in the two conditions. In alcoholism, muscle weakness may result either from the direct toxic effect of ethanol on skeletal muscle fibers (rhabdomyolysis) or from an alcohol-induced polyneuropathy. In beriberi, however, weakness is primarily the result of the peripheral neuropathy caused by myelin degeneration, a characteristic feature of many thiamine deficiency states.

(**45**) Wernicke-Korsakoff encephalopathy is thought to be caused primarily by thiamine deficiency but, in the Western world, is most often encountered in alcoholic patients with beriberi. Clinically, it is characterized by mental confusion, nystagmus, extraocular palsies, and ataxia. Pathologically, degeneration of the mammillary bodies is the most common finding. Although thiamine administration is frequently therapeutic, only about 20% of affected individuals recover completely with thiamine treatment, raising the possibility that some disease is alcoholic in origin (*pp. 450–452*).

46. (A); 47. (C); 48. (C); 49. (D); 50. (C); 51. (A)
(**46**) Pernicious anemia refers specifically to the meg-

aloblastic anemia resulting from gastric atrophy, decreased intrinsic factor production, and impaired vitamin B$_{12}$ absorption.

(47) Alcoholism may cause deficiencies of both vitamin B$_{12}$ and folate for several reasons. The general nutritional intake, including that of vitamin B$_{12}$ and folate, is inadequate in many alcoholic patients. Alcohol-associated gastritis and pancreatitis may also lead to defective vitamin B$_{12}$ absorption, which requires gastric intrinsic factors and pancreatic proteases.

(48) Glossitis is a feature of both vitamin B$_{12}$ and folate deficiencies. Because both these elements are necessary for the metabolic events of cell division, rapidly dividing cells in the bone marrow and gastrointestinal tract (including oral mucosal cells) are characteristically affected.

(49) The primary manifestation of both vitamin B$_{12}$ and folate deficiencies is megaloblastic anemia with prominent megaloblasts (not sideroblasts) in the bone marrow. Sideroblastic anemias constitute a separate group of disorders characterized by hypochromic, microcytic erythrocytes and red blood cell precursors (sideroblasts) containing granules of non-heme iron in their cytoplasm. Sideroblastic anemias have a number of causes, but the common defect is impaired iron utilization. The defect in megaloblastic anemias is defective DNA synthesis (see Question 8).

(50) In megaloblastic anemia due to either folate or vitamin B$_{12}$ deficiency, the defect in DNA metabolism is reflected in the myeloid and megakaryocytic series as well as in the erythroid series. Thus, neutrophils are also larger than normal and have hypersegmented nuclei (see Chapter 7, Question 2).

(51) Two defects occur in vitamin B$_{12}$ deficiency that do not occur in folate deficiency: greatly reduced fertility in either sex and peripheral neuropathy (*pp. 455–456*).

52. (A); 53. (B); 54. (B); 55. (C); 56. (C); 57. (C); 58. (A)

(52) Vitamin C is essential to the synthesis of all collagen (see Question 9) and is, therefore, requisite to the production of osteoid, a specialized type of collagen.

(53) The process of mineralization of osteoid, however, is regulated by vitamin D through its effects on calcium and phosphorus metabolism.

(54) Bone resorption is also dependent on vitamin D, because only previously mineralized bone can be resorbed by osteoclasts.

(55) Bone remodeling is the combined result of both bone formation and resorption; thus, both vitamin C and vitamin D are required.

(56) In endochondral bone formation, cartilage at the expanding edge of the epiphysis is replaced by osteoid, which is then mineralized. In this process, the cartilage must first undergo provisional mineralization before it can be resorbed and replaced by osteoid. Like mineralization of osteoid, mineralization of cartilage is a vitamin D-dependent process.

(57) Tooth enamel formation is also a complex process requiring both collagen matrix synthesis and subsequent

mineralization. Therefore, tooth enamel formation, like normal bone formation, is dependent on both vitamins.

(58) Only vitamin C is essential for wound healing, because this is a process based almost completely on collagen and new vessel (hence vascular wall and basement membrane collagen) formation (*pp. 80, 443–445, 456*).

59. (C); 60. (A); 61. (C); 62. (C); 63. (A); 64. (B); 65. (D)

Recognition of the primary tissue storage sites for vitamins is important because disease involving those tissues can lead to depletion of vitamin stores and subsequent deficiency states.

(59, 61, 62) The liver is the primary storage site for folate and for the fat-soluble vitamins including vitamins A and D.

(60 and 63) Two of the water-soluble B vitamins, B$_1$ (thiamine) and B$_6$ (pyridoxine), are stored primarily in striated muscle.

(64) Vitamin C is unique among the adrenal cortex as its primary site of storage (*pp. 439, 450, 456*).

(65) Riboflavin, another of the B vitamins, appears to have no primary tissue storage site and is distributed evenly among the body tissues. (64) Vitamin C is unique among the vitamins in having the adrenal cortex as its primary site of storage (*pp. 439, 450, 456*).

66. (D); 67. (B); 68. (B); 69. (C); 70. (E); 71. (D); 72. (B); 73. (B)

(66) Riboflavin, niacin, and pyridoxine all are B vitamins that function as coenzymes in various important reactions in cellular oxidative metabolism. (67) Niacin is unique among the B vitamins because it can be synthesized endogenously from tryptophan. (68) Thus, the dietary requirements for niacin vary inversely with the tryptophan content of the diet, and a niacin deficiency state (pellagra) usually reflects a deficiency of both niacin and tryptophan. (69) Many of the biochemical reactions in tryptophan metabolism, in turn, require pyridoxine as a cofactor. (70) Experimental deficiency states of any one of these three vitamins—riboflavin, niacin, or pyridoxine—may produce anemia. Clinically, however, anemia rarely occurs in association with deficiencies of these nutrients. Moreover, when anemias do occur, they are usually normocytic. (Macrocytic anemias are associated with deficiencies of two other B vitamins: cyanocobalamin [vitamin B$_{12}$] and folate.) (71) Dermatitis is a characteristic clinical feature of the deficiency states of all three vitamins. (72) Dementia, however, is associated only with niacin deficiency. It is usually accompanied by a desquamative dermatitis and diarrhea (the "three D's" of pellagra) and may be followed by death. (73) Because they are water soluble and can be rapidly eliminated in the urine, B vitamins do not produce persistent toxic disorders. However, parenteral administration of niacin commonly produces transient toxic effects such as abdominal pain and peripheral vasodilatation. Toxic reactions are not associated with either riboflavin or pyridoxine (*pp. 452–455*).

74. (E); 75. (E); 76. (A); 77. (B); 78. (C)

(**74**) Iron deficiency, vitamin B_{12} deficiency, and starvation all produce anemia. The anemia in all three cases is based primarily on red blood cell production and maturation defects rather than increased erythrocyte destruction. Increased hemolysis is not a feature of any of these conditions; (**75**) nor is osmotic fragility associated with these anemias. Osmotic fragility reflects a defect (usually hereditary) in the red blood cell membrane. No membrane defects are known to be produced in the anemias of nutritional deficiency.

(**76**) Iron deficiency is manifested by insufficient production of hemoglobin. Red blood cells are pale and decreased in size, constituting a hypochromic, microcytic anemia.

(**77**) Vitamin B_{12} deficiency produces a defect in DNA synthesis. Red blood cell precursors grow in size as their cytoplasm develops, but they cannot divide. Hemoglobin production is not affected, however. Megaloblasts produce abnormally large erythrocytes, and the resultant anemia is characterized as normochromic, macrocytic.

(**78**) For reasons less well understood, the characteristic anemia of starvation is hypochromic and normocytic. Normal red blood cell morphology is not typical of any of these deficiency states, although normochromic, normocytic anemia may appear in starvation (*pp. 438, 455, 459*).

79. (D); 80. (D); 81. (A); 82. (B); 83. (C); 84. (B); 85. (B)

(**79**) Deficiencies of zinc, copper, or selenium can have profound effects on cellular metabolism, because these elements are critical components of numerous essential metalloenzymes. (**80**) Because deficiencies of these elements are common among patients receiving long-term unsupplemented total parenteral nutrition, they are of ever-increasing clinical importance. (**81**) Zinc deficiency causes retardation of growth and defective sexual maturation in children and adults. (**82**) Of these elements, only copper deficiency is known to cause anemia, however. The copper-requiring protein ceruloplasmin is critical to the oxidation of iron required for heme synthesis. (**83**) Deficiency of selenium has been associated with a congestive myopathy known as Keshan disease, which is endemic in selenium-deficient areas of China. The disorder has also been described in patients receiving parenteral nutritional support. (**84, 85**) Copper is the metallic element in the metalloenzyme lysyl oxidase, which is essential to formation of cross-linkages in both elastin and collagen (*pp. 461–462*).

Infectious Diseases

DIRECTIONS: For Questions 1 to 5, choose the ONE BEST answer to each question.

1. Which of the following is the most common cause of childhood diarrhea?

A. *Yersinia enterocolitica*
B. Rotavirus
C. *Giardia lamblia*
D. *Escherichia coli*
E. *Campylobacter jejuni*

2. Sexually transmitted chlamydiae produce all of the following problems EXCEPT:

A. Pelvic inflammatory disease
B. Acute epididymitis
C. Genital elephantiasis
D. Condylomata lata
E. Rectal strictures

3. Ulcerated lesions on the penis occur in the acute form of all of the following sexually transmitted infectious diseases EXCEPT:

A. Herpes genitalis infection
B. Syphilis
C. Chancroid
D. Granuloma inguinale
E. Gonorrhea

4. Which of the following diseases is a veterinarian at LEAST risk of contracting?

A. Listeriosis
B. Brucellosis
C. Leptospirosis
D. Toxoplasmosis
E. Glanders

5. Trichomoniasis causes lesions referred to as:

A. Raspberry tongue
B. Strawberry mucosa
C. Strawberry gallbladder
D. Anchovy paste abscesses
E. None of these

DIRECTIONS: For Questions 6 to 15, ONE or MORE of the completions given correctly finishes the incomplete statement. Choose:
   A—if only *1, 2, and 3* are correct
   B—if only *1 and 3* are correct
   C—if only *2 and 4* are correct
   D—if only *4* is correct
   E—if all are correct

6. Mumps in adults:

1. Is caused by a DNA virus
2. Produces pancreatitis
3. Produces diagnostic cell inclusions
4. Usually produces orchitis

   A. 1,2,3   B. 1,3   C. 2,4   D. 4 Only   E. All

7. Infectious causes of atypical pneumonia (diffuse alveolar damage/adult respiratory distress syndrome) include:

1. *Legionella pneumophila*
2. *Pneumocystis carinii*
3. *Mycoplasma pneumoniae*
4. Influenza virus

   A. 1,2,3   B. 1,3   C. 2,4   D. 4 Only   E. All

8. Body lice are the principal vectors of transmission of the organisms causing:

    1. Bubonic plague
    2. Relapsing fever
    3. Q fever
    4. Epidemic typhus

      A. 1,2,3 B. 1,3 C. 2,4 D. 4 Only E. All

9. Ticks are the principal vectors of transmission of the organisms causing:

    1. Lyme disease
    2. Rocky Mountain spotted fever
    3. Babesiosis
    4. Chagas' disease

      A. 1,2,3 B. 1,3 C. 2,4 D. 4 Only E. All

10. Organisms that typically invade blood vessel walls include:

    1. *Pseudomonas* species
    2. *Aspergillus*
    3. *Rickettsia*
    4. *Plasmodium*

      A. 1,2,3 B. 1,3 C. 2,4 D. 4 Only E. All

11. Gonococcal infection is correctly described as:

    1. Having an asymptomatic carrier state
    2. A cause of Fitz-Hugh–Curtis syndrome
    3. A cause of septic arthritis
    4. The most common cause of pelvic inflammatory disease

      A. 1,2,3 B. 1,3 C. 2,4 D. 4 Only E. All

12. Wound infections are one of the most important sources of:

    1. Tetanus
    2. Diphtheria
    3. Gas gangrene
    4. Botulism

      A. 1,2,3 B. 1,3 C. 2,4 D. 4 Only E. All

13. Bacteria that typically induce granuloma formation include:

    1. *Brucella suis* (brucellosis)
    2. *Pseudomonas mallei* (glanders)
    3. *Francisella tularensis* (tularemia)
    4. *Yersinia pestis* (plague)

      A. 1,2,3 B. 1,3 C. 2,4 D. 4 Only E. All

14. Amebiasis is a protozoal infection that:

    1. Is most often asymptomatic
    2. Most often affects the left colon
    3. Produces flask-shaped ulcers
    4. Produces mucosal pseudopolyps

      A. 1,2,3 B. 1,3 C. 2,4 D. 4 Only E. All

15. Which of the following diseases is/are acquired by ingestion of raw or undercooked animal flesh (meat or fish)?

    1. Schistosomiasis
    2. Liver fluke infection
    3. Filariasis
    4. Tapeworm infection

      A. 1,2,3 B. 1,3 C. 2,4 D. 4 Only E. All

DIRECTIONS: For Questions 16 to 20, you are to decide whether EACH choice is TRUE or FALSE.

For each of the following statements about infectious mononucleosis, choose whether it is TRUE or FALSE.

16. It is caused by the Epstein-Barr virus

17. The abnormal circulating mononuclear cells are infected T lymphocytes

18. Microscopic changes produced in the liver resemble those seen in viral hepatitis

19. Microscopic changes produced in the lymph nodes resemble those seen in Hodgkin's disease

20. Heterophil antibodies are virtually diagnostic

DIRECTIONS: For Questions 21 to 38, the set of lettered headings is followed by a list of numbered words or phrases. For each numbered word or phrase choose:

A—if the item is associated with (A) only
B—if the item is associated with (B) only
C—if the item is associated with *both* (A) and (B)
D—if the item is associated with *neither* (A) nor (B)

For each of the diseases listed below, choose whether it is caused by streptococci, staphylococci, both, or neither.

A. Streptococci
B. Staphylococci
C. Both
D. Neither

21. Impetigo

22. Erysipelas

23. Erythema nodosum

24. Carbuncles

25. Toxin-induced food poisoning

26. Toxic shock syndrome

27. Glomerulonephritis

28. Scarlet fever

For each of the statements listed below, choose whether it describes lepromatous leprosy, tuberculoid leprosy, both, or neither.

A. Lepromatous leprosy
B. Tuberculoid leprosy
C. Both
D. Neither

29. The causative organism has never been cultivated in vitro

30. Lesions typically contain large numbers of organisms

31. Hypergammaglobulinemia often occurs

32. Nerve involvement is typical

33. Affected individuals are not infectious

For each of the features listed below, choose whether it is characteristic of nocardiosis, actinomycosis, both, or neither.

A. Nocardiosis
B. Actinomycosis
C. Both
D. Neither

34. Infection rarely occurs in normal (immunocompetent) individuals

35. Person-to-person spread is the major mode of transmission

36. Abscesses are characteristically produced

37. "Sulfur granules" are typically seen in lesions

38. The causative agent is strictly anaerobic

DIRECTIONS: Questions 39 to 113 are matching questions. For each numbered item, choose the most likely associated lettered item from those provided. Each numbered item has ONLY ONE answer. Within each group, each lettered item may be the answer to one, more than one, or none of the numbered items.

For each of the following features of respiratory viruses, choose whether it describes adenovirus, influenza virus, coxsackievirus, rhinovirus, or none of these.

A. Adenovirus
B. Influenza virus
C. Coxsackievirus
D. Rhinovirus
E. None of these

39. Major cause of the common cold

40. Associated with the Guillain-Barré syndrome

41. Associated with Reye's syndrome in aspirin-treated children

42. Causes herpangina

43. Most common cause of croup (lethal bronchiolitis) in infants

44. Causes epidemic hemorrhagic keratoconjunctivitis

45. Produces characteristic inclusion bodies in infected cells

For each of the features of childhood infectious disease listed below, choose whether it is characteristic of measles (rubeola), German measles (rubella), chicken-pox (varicella zoster), all of these, or none of these.

    A. Measles (rubeola)
    B. German measles (rubella)
    C. Chickenpox (varicella zoster)
    D. All of these
    E. None of these

46. The causative organism is an RNA virus

47. The disease is highly contagious by droplet aspiration

48. Koplik's spots are clinically diagnostic

49. Warthin-Finkeldey multinucleate cells are pathognomonic

50. Maternal disease is associated with congenital malformations

51. Skin lesions are characteristically pustular

52. Giant cell pneumonia is sometimes produced

53. A latent phase of infection is a common consequence

54. Recovery confers lifelong immunity

For each of the infectious disorders listed below, choose whether it is caused by viral, chlamydial, bacterial, or protozoal infection or none of these.

    A. Viral infection
    B. Chlamydial infection
    C. Bacterial infection
    D. Protozoal infection
    E. None of the above

55. Yellow fever

56. Cold sores

57. Psittacosis

58. Legionnaires' disease

59. Bubonic plague

60. Smallpox

61. Oral thrush

62. Whooping cough

63. Diphtheria

64. Cat-scratch disease

65. Athlete's foot

66. Hydatid disease

67. Sleeping sickness

68. Poliomyelitis

For each of the bacterial organisms listed below, decide whether it causes pathogenicity in humans by one of the mechanisms listed below or whether it acts by none of these mechanisms.

    A. Formation of a phagocyte-resistant capsule
    B. Production of leukocyte-killing substances
    C. Avoidance of immune mechanisms by programmed antigenic variation
    D. Interference with normal phagosome function
    E. None of these

69. Pneumococcus *(Streptococcus pneumoniae)*

70. *Borrelia recurrentis*

71. *Mycobacterium tuberculosis*

72. *Clostridium perfringens*

73. *Vibrio cholerae*

74. *Brucella suis*

75. *Clostridium botulinum*

For each of the characteristics listed below, choose whether it describes *Escherichia coli*, *Proteus mirabilis*, *Pseudomonas aeruginosa*, all of these, or none of these.

    A. *Escherichia coli*
    B. *Proteus mirabilis*
    C. *Pseudomonas aeruginosa*
    D. All of the above
    E. None of the above

76. A source of endotoxin

77. Grows best in anaerobic conditions

78. Not a cause of infectious enterocolitis

79. Cause of urinary tract infection

80. Cause of gram-negative pneumonia

81. Associated with epidemics in burn units

82. Not associated with suppurative infections of the abdominal cavity

For each of the features listed below, choose whether it is characteristic of primary syphilis, secondary syphilis, tertiary syphilis, all of these stages, or none of these.

    A. Primary syphilis
    B. Secondary syphilis
    C. Tertiary syphilis
    D. All of these
    E. None of these

83. A generalized skin eruption typically occurs

84. The syphilitic gumma is the histologic hallmark

85. Obliterative endarteritis is the histologic hallmark

86. Treponemes are extremely difficult to demonstrate in lesions

87. Tabes dorsalis develops

88. Charcot's joints develop

89. Hutchinson's teeth develop

For each of the characteristics listed below, choose whether it describes *Candida albicans*, *Mucor*, *Aspergillus fumigatus*, *Cryptococcus neoformans*, or none of these.

    A. *Candida albicans*
    B. *Mucor*
    C. *Aspergillus fumigatus*
    D. *Cryptococcus neoformans*
    E. None of these

90. Most common cause of human fungal infection

91. Typically forms pseudohyphae

92. Rarely, if ever, infects immunologically normal individuals

93. India ink preparations aid in identification

94. Most frequent clinical manifestation is meningitis

95. Causes hypersensitivity pneumonitis without lung infection

96. Causes oral infection in infants who are bottle-fed

For each of the features listed below, choose whether it is characteristic of blastomycosis, coccidioidomycosis, histoplasmosis, all of these, or none of these.

    A. Blastomycosis
    B. Coccidioidomycosis
    C. Histoplasmosis
    D. All of these
    E. None of these

97. Most prevalent in the southwest of the United States

98. Acquired from inhalation of contaminated soil

99. Causative fungus grows in tissue as a yeast form

100. Commonly produces asymptomatic primary disease

101. Commonly produces skin involvement in disseminated disease

102. Causes granulomatous lung disease

103. Occasionally causes sclerosing mediastinitis

For each of the features listed below, choose whether it is characteristic of malaria, babesiosis, Chagas' disease, all of these, or none of these.

    A. Malaria
    B. Babesiosis
    C. Chagas' disease
    D. All of these
    E. None of these

104. Mosquitoes transmit the disease

105. Pigment is typically found in phagocytes

106. Sickle cell hemoglobin limits parasitemia

107. Myocarditis is common in adult infection

108. Progressive brain dysfunction occurs in the late stage of disease

For each of the characteristics listed below, choose whether it describes infection by *Ascaris lumbricoides*, hookworm, *Strongyloides*, pinworm, or none of these.

    A. *Ascaris lumbricoides*
    B. Hookworm
    C. *Strongyloides*
    D. Pinworm
    E. None of these

109. Causes childhood night itch

110. Typically invades striated muscle

111. Diagnosed by duodenal aspiration

112. Causes mechanical obstruction of the gastrointestinal tract

113. Causes disease by sucking blood

4

Infectious Diseases

1. **(B)** Rotaviruses are the most common cause of childhood diarrhea in the United States, where they account for more than half of all cases. Fortunately, the disease is mild and self-limited. Bacterial or parasitic forms of childhood enteritis are not nearly as common in the United States as in other parts of the world. Although less common, they are often more debilitating than viral enteritides. For example, *Yersinia enterocolitica*, now recognized as a major cause of bacterial enteritis in the pediatric age-group, is a highly invasive and virulent enteric pathogen that causes severe and potentially lethal disease. *Campylobacter jejuni* is a major gastrointestinal pathogen that affects both adults and children and is responsible for about 10% of diarrhea and dysentery in the United States. *Giardia lamblia* and enteropathic *Escherichia coli* are common causes of traveler's diarrhea but rare causes of childhood diarrhea *(pp. 317, 356–357, 400)*.

2. **(D)** Chlamydial urethritis and cervicitis caused by *Chlamydia trachomatis* are now two of the most common forms of chlamydial disease in the United States. In females, chlamydial infection is an increasingly more common cause of pelvic inflammatory disease. In males, it causes nongonorrheal urethritis and may extend to produce acute epididymitis. Genital elephantiasis and rectal strictures are two of the more unusual sequelae of lymphogranuloma venereum, a venereally transmitted disease caused by three of the eight known serotypes of *C. trachomatis*. Lymphogranuloma venereum should not be confused with granuloma inguinale, a venereal disease caused by the bacterium *Calymmatobacterium donovani*. Condylomata lata are not produced by chlamydia; they are the characteristic papular lesions found on the penis or vulva in secondary syphilis, a disease caused by *Treponema pallidum (pp. 326–328, 372)*.

3. **(E)** Ulcerated lesions characteristically occur on the penis in a number of venereal infections, including herpes genitalis infection, syphilis, chancroid, and granuloma inguinale. Obviously then, among patients with an ulcerated penile lesion, bacteriologic, serologic, or immunohistochemical testing may be required to make a diagnosis. However, gonorrhea, the most common venereal disease in the United States, does not produce a penile ulcer. In males, gonococcal infection produces a mucopurulent exudate from the anterior urethra and meatus. The meatus becomes hyperemic, edematous, and obviously inflamed, but does not ulcerate *(pp. 319–320, 369–370, 372–373)*.

4. **(A)** For obvious reasons, veterinarians are among those at greatest risk of developing infections from organisms that are harbored by domestic animals. Brucelli are gram-negative intracellular coccobacilli that originate in livestock and dogs. Most infections arise from animal contact; thus, veterinarians and meat packers are at greatest risk. Leptospirae are zoonotic bacteria that infect both wild and domestic animals (principally dogs). Infection usually occurs from contact with animals or contaminated soil, and veterinarians, farmers, and trappers are among those at highest risk. Toxoplasmosis, caused by the protozoan *Toxoplasma gondii*, is most often contracted from domestic cats, which are the definitive host of this parasite. Glanders may occur as either an acute febrile illness or a chronic granulomatous disease. It is caused by *Pseudomonas mallei*, a gram-negative bacillus that is harbored by horses, mules, and donkeys. Although *Listeria monocytogenes*, the gram-positive bacillus that causes listeriosis, is harbored by many mammals and fowl, it is principally an opportunistic agent in human disease. Its chief victims are pregnant women and their fetuses, the elderly, the sick,

or the immunosuppressed. Thus, in contrast to the other zoonotic agents just discussed, *Listeria* does not normally pose an increased threat of infection to veterinarians (*pp. 362, 364–366, 410–411*).

5. (B) Trichomoniasis is a common venereal parasitic infection caused by the flagellate *Trichomonas vaginalis.* Infection occurs most commonly in the vagina of postpubertal females and in the urethra of males. The affected mucosa is typically erythematous, edematous, and spotted with small blisters or granules, and its appearance is referred to as strawberry mucosa. Raspberry tongue is associated with scarlet fever and refers to the bright red tongue and its edematous papillae in the early stage of the disease dominated by pharyngitis and tonsillitis. Strawberry gallbladder refers to the gross appearance of the gallbladder mucosa in cholesterolosis. In this condition, the gallbladder mucosa is diffusely erythematous and studded with small yellow "seeds," which are actually collections of cholesterol-laden macrophages in the lamina propria. The anchovy paste abscess occurs in amebiasis with liver involvement. In the liver, the contents of amebic abscesses, made up of hemorrhage and digested liver cell debris, appear grossly as a chocolate-colored pasty material resembling anchovy paste (*pp. 341, 398, 401, 973*).

6. (C) Mumps is an acute contagious disease caused by a single-stranded RNA paramyxovirus. It most commonly occurs in children but may occur in adults. Reoviruses are a family of double-stranded RNA viruses whose major pathogenic species is the rotavirus, the agent responsible for most childhood diarrhea. The mumps virus principally involves the parotid gland, producing the characteristic inflammation and swelling. Other glandular organs, principally the pancreas and the testes, are often affected as well. Mumps pancreatitis tends to be mild and self-limited. In contrast to mumps parotitis, which is most often bilateral, mumps orchitis in adults is most frequently unilateral and therefore rarely leads to male sterility. Like other RNA viruses, mumps virus does not produce characteristic cell inclusions by which it can be identified microscopically (*pp. 316–317*).

7. (E) If bronchopneumonia (usually caused by bacteria and characterized by purulent exudative inflammation in the lung) is considered "typical," then infections characterized by a pattern of diffuse alveolar damage with hyaline membranes are considered "atypical." Organisms commonly associated with atypical pneumonia are respiratory viruses (e.g., influenza virus, respiratory syncytial virus, adenovirus), *Legionella* species (*Legionella pneumophila*, etc.), *Mycoplasma pneumoniae*, and *Pneumocystis carinii*. Although bronchopneumonia is always infectious in origin, diffuse alveolar damage can be produced by toxic injury, shock, and other noninfectious causes (*pp. 313, 315, 760, 784*).

8. (C) Body lice are the principal vectors of transmission of the organisms causing relapsing fever and typhus

fever. Relapsing fever is caused by a zoonotic bacterium known as *Borrelia recurrentis;* it is transmitted from person to person by body lice and has no known animal reservoir. Epidemic typhus is caused by *Rickettsia prowazekii*, which, like all rickettsiae, is a small, bacteria-like obligate intracellular parasite. It is transmitted from person to person by human head and body lice. Bubonic plague, caused by *Yersinia pestis*, is transmitted to humans by fleas from infected rodents. Q fever, a rickettsial infection, is transmitted to humans by the respiratory route from infected animals and requires no arthropod vector (*pp. 330, 333, 362–363, 366*).

9. (A) Ticks transmit numerous infectious diseases, including Lyme disease, Rocky Mountain spotted fever, and babesiosis. Lyme disease, an inflammatory disease characterized by skin rash and migratory polyarthritis, is believed to be caused by a treponema-like spirochete. Rocky Mountain spotted fever is a rickettsial disease, whereas babesiosis is caused by a protozoan that is a close relative of plasmodia. Although these diseases are caused by disparate classes of organisms, they all are transmitted to humans by ticks. Chagas' disease, in contrast, is caused by an intracellular protozoan (a trypanosome) and is transmitted from person to person or from animals to humans by "kissing bugs" (triatomidae or reduviid bugs) (*pp. 332, 366–367, 406, 407–408*).

10. (A) Infectious diseases caused by organisms that typically invade vessel walls are usually characterized by hemorrhage and thrombosis and are thus particularly destructive. *Pseudomonas aeruginosa, Aspergillus* species, and rickettsial organisms are prototypic examples of organisms that readily invade vessels. Plasmodia, the protozoal organisms that cause malaria, typically induce thromboses of small vessels, but they do not do so by direct vascular invasion. Rather, they produce changes in the infected erythrocyte membranes that increase red blood cell stickiness and induce clumping. Plugging of small vessels results, and tissue hypoxia or ischemic necrosis is produced (*pp. 330, 346–347, 389–390, 403–404*).

11. (E) Gonorrhea (venereal infection by *Neisseria gonorrhoeae*, also known as "clap") is the most common reportable communicable disease in the United States. Although it usually produces acute exudative and purulent inflammation, infection can be asymptomatic. In females it is the most common cause of pelvic inflammatory disease. Spread into the peritoneum can result in perihepatitis, producing stabbing right upper quadrant pain known as the Fitz-Hugh–Curtis syndrome. Gonococcal bacteremia may result in gonococcal arthritis produced either by seeding of joints by organisms or as a result of immunologically mediated processes in the absence of culturable organisms. The frequency of gonococcemia and gonococcal arthritis in women is increasing (*p. 344*).

12. (A) Wound infections are the primary source of disease produced by *Clostridium tetani, Corynebacte-*

rium diphtheriae, and *Clostridium perfringens. Clostridium tetani* is an anaerobic organism that thrives in the devitalized tissue of penetrating wounds and produces a powerful neurotoxin that causes the convulsive contractions of voluntary muscles that characterize tetanus. Diphtheria used to occur primarily as a communicable childhood upper respiratory tract infection with systemic manifestations resulting from exotoxin production by the causative agent, *C. diphtheriae* (see Question 63). Vaccination has made diphtheria a rare childhood disease, and most infection now occurs from neglected skin wounds in adults. Gas gangrene is a severe form of necrotizing anaerobic infection caused by gas-producing *C. perfringens*. The infection is most frequently the result of invasion of traumatic surgical wounds. Botulism is a severe paralyzing illness caused by the powerful neurotoxin produced by *Clostridium botulinum*. Although botulism can be caused by wound infection, this occurs only rarely. By far the most common cause of botulism is ingestion of contaminated foods containing the preformed botulinum neurotoxin *(pp. 351, 358–360)*.

13. (E) Although a granulomatous response is commonly associated with mycobacteria, spirochetes, fungi, and parasites, several bacterial organisms also elicit granulomatous responses in the host. Principal among these are *Brucella suis, Pseudomonas mallei, Francisella tularensis*, and *Yersinia pestis*. Thus, the respective infectious diseases caused by these organisms—brucellosis, glanders, tularemia, and plague—are typically associated with granulomas in affected organs *(pp. 362–365)*.

14. (B) Amebiasis is a protozoal disease caused by *Entamoeba histolytica*. Infection is primarily limited to the lumen of the colon, but systemic spread of the organism may occur. Although amebiasis is a well-known cause of dysentery, infection far more commonly produces an asymptomatic carrier state, which is principally responsible for transmission of the disease. The colitis produced most often affects the cecum and ascending colon but occasionally involves the sigmoid, rectum, or appendix. The organisms produce mucosal ulcerations with a classic flask-shaped contour (a narrow neck and a broad base) when viewed in tissue sections. In contrast to idiopathic ulcerative colitis, in amebiasis the colonic mucosa between ulcerations is characteristically normal and does not show pseudopolyp formation *(pp. 397–399)*.

15. (D) Tapeworm infection is usually contracted by ingestion of undercooked meat or fish containing encysted larvae. Schistosomiasis, a trematode infection, is transmitted by water contact with the free-swimming, four-tailed cercarial forms of the organism released by infected snails. They burrow quickly through the skin, maturing into young worms. Liver fluke infection is acquired by eating contaminated watercress containing the metacercarial form of the parasite. Filariasis, a group of roundworm infections, is transmitted to humans by insect bites *(pp. 417, 420, 422–423, 424–427)*.

16. (True); 17. (False); 18. (True); 19. (True); 20. (True)

(16) Infectious mononucleosis is a benign lymphoproliferative disease caused by the Epstein-Barr virus, a member of the herpes family and the same virus implicated in the cause of the malignant lymphoproliferative disease known as African Burkitt's lymphoma.

(17) After an initial replicative phase within the salivary epithelial glands, the Epstein-Barr virus infects the B lymphocytes in lymphoid tissues. Because B cells possess surface receptors for the virus, they are the primary target of infection. On their surface, infected B cells display virus-directed antigens that are recognized by T cells. The activated T lymphocytes appear in the peripheral blood as atypical mononuclear cells (mononucleosis cells) but represent response to the infection rather than virally transformed cells.

(18) The diagnosis of infectious mononucleosis can be difficult, because the disease may mimic other disorders both clinically and pathologically. The microscopic changes produced in the liver resemble those of viral hepatitis, with mononuclear inflammation of the portal tracts and focal hepatocellular necrosis. **(19)** Affected lymph nodes have markedly expanded paracortical (T cell) zones that occasionally contain large binucleate cells resembling Reed-Sternberg cells. Thus, a histologic appearance resembling that in Hodgkin's disease is produced. **(20)** A helpful diagnostic feature is the presence of heterophil antibodies (sheep erythrocyte agglutinins). These are present in about 90% of cases and can be easily detected with a commercially available spot kit (Monospot test). The test is both sensitive and specific; only rare false-positive results occur in patients with lymphoma or hepatitis *(pp. 323–325)*.

21. (C); 22. (A); 23. (A); 24. (B); 25. (B); 26. (B); 27. (A)

(21) Streptococci and staphylococci are two of the most common and versatile human bacterial pathogens. Impetigo, a common superficial infection of the skin characterized by erosive lesions covered by honey-colored crust, can be caused by either streptococci or staphylococci *(p. 341)*.

(22) Erysipelas is a disorder characterized by a rapidly spreading edematous and erythematous cutaneous infection, usually on the face. It is caused by group A beta-hemolytic streptococcal infection *(p. 341)*.

(23) Erythema nodosum, the most common type of panniculitis, is commonly associated with beta-hemolytic streptococcal infection. Erythema nodosum may occur in association with other infectious diseases, such as tuberculosis, leprosy, coccidioidomycosis, or histoplasmosis, but is not associated with staphylococcal infection *(p. 1299)*.

(24) Carbuncles are deep-seated suppurative lesions of the skin and subcutaneous tissues. They spread laterally beneath the deep subcutaneous fascia and then erupt onto the skin surface, forming multiple adjacent skin sinuses. Carbuncles typically appear on the upper back and posterior neck and are caused by staphylococcal infection *(p. 338)*.

(**25 and 26**) Food poisoning and toxic shock syndrome are two examples of diseases caused by staphylococcal toxin production. Staphylococcal food poisoning results from the ingestion of a preformed enterotoxin without invasive staphylococcal enterocolitis. Toxic shock syndrome is caused by unique toxins produced by staphylococci that propagate in blood-soaked vaginal tampons during menstruation. In contrast to staphylococci, streptococci are not known to produce exotoxins; they commonly produce disease by suppurative spreading infection or via the complications of a host hypersensitivity response *(p. 339)*.

(**27**) Poststreptococcal glomerulonephritis is a fairly common renal glomerular disease that is produced by streptococcal-antistreptococcal immune complexes *(pp. 339, 1030)*.

(**28**) Scarlet fever is an acute febrile disease caused by *Streptococcus*. It is characterized by pharyngitis or tonsillitis and an erythematous rash caused by an erythrogenic toxin. The disease is rare before age 3 or after age 15. Although the disease is self-limited, it requires prompt treatment to prevent poststreptococcal complications such as glomerulonephritis *(p. 341)*.

29. (C); 30. (A); 31. (A); 32. (C); 33. (B)

(**29**) Leprosy is an indolent, chronic debilitating disease caused by *Mycobacterium leprae*. Infection typically takes one of two forms, lepromatous leprosy or tuberculoid leprosy, depending on the response of the host. The causative agent has never been successfully cultured in vitro from patients with either form of the disease.

(**30 and 33**) Large numbers of organisms are typically demonstrable in the lesions of lepromatous leprosy, the form of the disease characterized by a poor cellular immune response to the invading organism. In contrast, tuberculoid leprosy is characterized by a brisk cellular immune response with granuloma formation and a paucity of demonstrable organisms. Thus, only the lepromatous form of the disease is contagious.

(**31**) Although patients with lepromatous leprosy fail to produce an adequate cellular immune response, they often have polyclonal hypergammaglobulinemia thought to be due to the dearth of suppressor T cells together with massive lepra antigen exposure. With the production of large amounts of antilepra antibody in lepromatous leprosy, antigen-antibody complexes often form, producing immune complex-mediated disorders such as erythema nodosum or vasculitis.

(**32**) Regardless of the type of host response and subsequent form of disease, leprosy typically involves the peripheral nerves and the skin *(pp. 380–383)*.

34. (A); 35. (D); 36. (C); 37. (B); 38. (B)

(**34**) The Actinomycetales are fungus-like bacteria closely related to mycobacteria. *Nocardia* and *Actinomyces* are the most important human pathogens in this group of organisms. Unlike actinomycetes, which are not opportunistic and infect healthy individuals, *Nocardia* primarily infects patients who are immunosuppressed or chronically ill.

(**35**) There is no evidence of person-to-person spread in either nocardiosis or actinomycosis; all infections appear to be derived endogenously.

(**36**) Both organisms characteristically produce abscesses in the tissues they affect. Nocardiosis most often involves the lung and typically causes single or chronic necrotizing walled-off abscesses. Actinomycosis most frequently involves the cervicofacial soft tissues, forming abscesses that lead to sinus formation. Abdominal actinomycosis resulting from invasion of the intestinal mucosa and bowel wall penetration typically forms a localized peritoneal abscess. Similarly, thoracic actinomycosis causes lung abscesses or empyemas.

(**37**) A distinguishing feature of the actinomycotic abscess is its content of grossly visible yellowish colonies called "sulfur granules." These are composed of intertwined radiating filaments of bacteria.

(**38**) A further distinguishing feature between nocardiosis and actinomycosis is the culture requirements of the causative organism. Unlike *Nocardia*, which is an aerobe similar to *Mycobacterium tuberculosis*, actinomycetes are strict anaerobes that are difficult to culture *(pp. 383–384)*.

39. (D); 40. (C); 41. (B); 42. (C); 43. (E); 44. (A); 45. (A)

(**39**) Viral diseases of the respiratory tract are the most common and least preventable of all human infectious diseases. Among the myriad species and serotypes responsible, adenovirus, influenza virus, coxsackievirus, and rhinovirus are among the most important. Rhinovirus is the major cause of the common cold. Although it is the cause of the single most frequent infectious disease, it seldom produces serious sequelae.

(**40 and 42**) Coxsackieviruses produce many patterns of disease besides upper respiratory tract infections. Coxsackievirus B can cause the Guillain-Barré syndrome and myocarditis. Coxsackievirus A can cause herpangina, a blistering inflammation of the pharynx.

(**41**) Influenza viruses are the leading causes of lower respiratory tract infection ("flu"). In addition, they can cause serious extrapulmonary complications such as Reye's syndrome in aspirin-treated children (see Chapter 9, Question 2).

(**43**) Also of particular importance among viral respiratory pathogens affecting infants and children are the parainfluenza and respiratory syncytial viruses, which produce croup (lethal bronchiolitis) or pneumonia. Adenoviruses can also cause croup but do so infrequently.

(**44**) Adenoviruses produce a number of febrile respiratory syndromes of varying severity but are also commonly associated with eye infections, particularly acute conjunctivitis. The more severe adenovirus-induced keratoconjunctivitis may occur in sharp outbreaks related to inadequately chlorinated swimming pools.

(**45**) Among the major respiratory viruses, only adenovirus produces characteristic inclusion bodies that are diagnostic by light microscopy. Other viral agents that produce characteristic inclusion bodies and may involve the respiratory tract include herpesvirus and measles (rubeola) *(pp. 313, 315–316)*.

46. (A); **47.** (D); **48.** (A); **49.** (A); **50.** (B); **51.** (E); **52.** (A); **53.** (C); **54.** (D)

(46) Measles, German measles, and chickenpox are three common viral infections of childhood with various acute and chronic consequences. Measles (like mumps) is caused by a single-stranded RNA paramyxovirus. German measles is caused by a single-stranded DNA virus of the togavirus family; chickenpox is caused by the virus varicella zoster, a double-stranded DNA herpesvirus.

(47) All of these diseases are highly contagious by droplet aspiration and hence spread rapidly among unimmunized children and nonimmune adults.

(48) Measles infection produces several unique clinical and pathologic features. The earliest diagnostic sign is the appearance of small blistering, ulcerating lesions, known as Koplik's spots, on the cheek mucosa near the opening of Stensen's ducts. Their appearance may precede the skin rash. (49) A pathognomonic histologic feature of measles is the Warthin-Finkeldey cells found in involved lymphoid organs. These multinucleated giant cells characteristically contain eosinophilic nuclear and intracytoplasmic inclusion bodies. (52) Another unique and sometimes life-threatening complication of measles infection is an interstitial pneumonia characterized by the abundance of giant cells for which it is named (giant cell pneumonia).

(50) In contrast to measles or chickenpox, German measles is a relatively mild childhood infection with few if any serious sequelae. Its major importance is its ability to produce congenital malformations in the offspring of affected mothers, a feature not associated with either measles or chickenpox.

(51) Although skin lesions occur in all three of these systemic viral diseases, none are pustular in character. Measles and German measles produce a maculopapular rash, and chickenpox characteristically causes macular lesions that rapidly progress to a vesicular stage without forming pustules.

(53 and 54) Although recovery from all three of these childhood infections confers lifelong immunity to reinfection, only varicella zoster causes latent disease. After the production of chickenpox, the virus may remain latent for years in the sensory dorsal root ganglia. With advancing age or immunosuppression, the virus may become reactivated and cause a localized vesicular eruption (shingles) in the distribution of the corresponding dermatomes (pp. 317–318, 320–321).

55. (A); **56.** (E); **57.** (B); **58.** (C); **59.** (C); **60.** (A); **61.** (E); **62.** (C); **64.** (C); **65.** (E); **66.** (E); **67.** (D); **68.** (A)

(55) Yellow fever is an arthropod-borne hemorrhagic fever caused by a single-stranded RNA togavirus. The yellow fever virus characteristically produces severe hepatocellular damage with resultant jaundice, a feature that has given the disease its name (pp. 313, 325).

(56) Cold sores are skin or mucosal vesicles (usually on the face, lips, and/or nostrils) caused by herpes simplex type I virus (HSV I), a double-stranded DNA virus. Herpes simplex type II (genital herpes) virus also causes these lesions, but much less commonly than HSV I. On primary infection transmitted by local contact (e.g., kissing), the virus replicates within epithelial cells. Infected cells develop intranuclear (Cowdry type A) inclusion bodies and undergo lysis, producing an inflamed vesicle. The virus may then enter a latent phase, inhabiting sensory ganglia reached via travel along sensory nerve pathways. Reactivation (by mechanisms still largely unknown) of latent disease causes recurrence of skin lesions (pp. 320–321).

(57) Psittacosis is a disease caused by a chlamydial organism found in contaminated excreta from infected birds. Chlamydiae are obligate intracellular organisms and produce intracytoplasmic inclusions (elementary bodies) in infected cells. Thus, elementary bodies can be identified in the alveolar cells of patients with this acute flu-like illness (pp. 326–327).

(58) Legionnaires' disease is an acute, potentially fatal atypical pneumonia produced by a gram-negative bacterial pathogen (*Legionella*) that was recognized anew by microbiologists after the epidemic in Philadelphia in 1976 (pp. 347–348).

(59) Bubonic plague is a periodically epidemic, systemic febrile disease caused by *Yersinia pestis*, a gram-negative bacillus. The disease is fortunately rare in the United States, but the organism is harbored by many wild animals, principally rodents, and occurs occasionally in the western United States, where squirrels are the principal reservoir (pp. 362–363).

(60) Smallpox is a highly contagious febrile illness characterized by vesicular/pustular skin eruptions (pockmarks). It is caused by variola virus, a double-stranded DNA virus that infects only humans. Variola virus is a close relative of vaccinia virus, the cause of cowpox, and immunization with vaccinia confers immunity to smallpox. In 1798, Edward Jenner first published his historic discovery that inoculation of pustular material from cowpox lesions protected against smallpox. Since then, the worldwide practice of inoculation of vaccinia (*vaccination*) has eradicated this once epidemic disease (p. 318).

(61) Oral thrush is candidiasis of the oral cavity. It is one of the most common forms of candidal infection and occurs most commonly in bottle-fed newborns and immunosuppressed or antibiotic-treated adults (p. 388).

(62) Whooping cough is an acute, highly contagious respiratory disease of childhood caused by *Bordetella pertussis*, a gram-negative coccobacillus. The organisms attach to the brush border of the bronchial epithelium, where they replicate without invading. They release an exotoxin that causes systemic symptoms (lymphocytosis, malaise, weight loss) and paroxysms of violent coughing (followed by loud inspiratory "whoops"). Recovery and immunity depend on secretory IgA antibodies that prevent bacterial adhesion to the respiratory mucosa (p. 350).

(63) Diphtheria is an acute communicable childhood disease caused by *Corynebacterium diphtheriae*, a gram-positive bacillus. The organisms cause ulcerating

pseudomembranous lesions of the respiratory tree via direct invasion and systemic complications (primarily cardiac and neural injury) via phage-mediated exotoxin. Systemic complications can be prevented with early diagnosis and administration of diphtheria antitoxin. Active immunization with toxoid (modified toxin) prevents the disease *(pp. 351–352)*.

(64) Cat-scratch disease is a self-limited localized lymphadenopathy caused by streptobacilli of the genus *Rothia* that colonize the teeth of cats. Coalescent granulomas with central abcess formation (stellate granulomas) in affected lymph nodes similar to those seen in lymphogranuloma venereum are characteristic *(pp. 367–368)*.

(65) Athlete's foot is a fungal infection of the plantar skin caused by a dermatophyte known as *Tinea pedis*. Dermatophytic fungi (there are several types) infect only the nonviable keratinaceous structures of skin (stratum corneum, hair, and nails) and are troublesome but not dangerous *(pp. 396, 1309)*.

(66) Hydatid disease is caused by the canine tapeworm *Echinococcus*, for which humans are an intermediary host. Ingested eggs hatch in the duodenum, and embryos penetrate the mucosa, enter the portal veins, travel to the liver and, from there, to other parts of the body (e.g., brain, heart, lungs). After long periods of growth, large parasitic cysts (hydatids) containing the pathognomonic hooklet-bearing scolices are formed, most commonly in the liver. The cysts expand in a tumorous manner, compress vital structures, provoke hypersensitivity immune responses, spawn daughter cysts, and/or become secondarily bacterially infected. Cysts may require surgical removal (the preferred form of therapy), but aspiration or biopsy is contraindicated because of the danger of rupture or spillage of cyst contents *(p. 421)*.

(67) "Sleeping sickness" is the common name for African trypanosomiasis caused by the protozoans *Trypanosoma rhodesiense* and *Trypanosoma gambiense*. The disease begins with parasitemia after a bite by an infected tsetse fly and an acute febrile illness with pupura and disseminated intravascular coagulation. Chronic bouts of fever with lymphadenopathy and splenomegaly follow. The final stage of the disease is characterized by a demyelinating panencephalitis that produces increasing lethargy and leads to death in coma *(p. 406)*.

(68) Poliomyelitis is a systemic disease of varying severity that predominantly affects the central nervous system and can produce permanent paralysis. It is caused by poliovirus, a single-stranded RNA virus (one of the enteroviruses) belonging to the family Picornaviridae. Once a devastating scourge, poliomyelitis has been virtually eradicated in industrialized countries by immunization programs using either inactivated or oral vaccines *(p. 313)*.

69. (A); 70. (C); 71. (D); 72. (B); 73. (E); 74. (D); 75. (E)

(69) Bacterial agents have evolved numerous clever ways of combating human biologic defense mechanisms. Some organisms, like the pneumococcus, are particularly resistant to engulfment by neutrophils by virtue of their slippery hydrophilic polysaccharide capsules.

(70) Others, like *Borrelia recurrentis*, the agent of relapsing fever, elude immunologic defense mechanisms by continuously changing their antigenic surface determinants. This genetically programmed variation in surface antigens allows each successive generation of organisms to survive while the preceding generations are immunologically exterminated.

(71 and 74) Granuloma-forming facultative intracellular bacteria such as *Mycobacterium tuberculosis* and *Brucella suis* have evolved mechanisms to escape destruction after ingestion by phagocytes. By unknown mechanisms, they interfere with the fusion of phagocytic vacuoles and lysosomes, thus forestalling the enzymatic reactions that would lead to their digestion.

(72) *Clostridium perfringens* is a prime example of an organism that digests the cells of its host before it can be digested. It produces a plethora of bacterial enzymes, including a lecithinase (alphatoxin) that disrupts the plasma membranes of both white blood cells and erythrocytes.

(73 and 75) In contrast, *Vibrio cholerae* and *Clostridium botulinum* are two examples of organisms that do not need to invade the tissues of their host to produce disease. These organisms produce powerful, selective exotoxins that drastically alter the physiologic functions of their target tissues (the intestinal epithelium and the cholinergic nerves, respectively) without any tissue invasion or damage *(pp. 334–336)*.

76. (D); 77. (E); 78. (B); 79. (D); 80. (D); 81. (C); 82. (B)

(76) All gram-negative organisms have cell walls that contain lipopolysaccharide-protein complexes known as endotoxins. The release of endotoxins from disintegrating bacteria is responsible for the dramatic systemic effects of gram-negative sepsis such as high fever, increased capillary permeability with shock, and disseminated intravascular coagulation.

(77) All of the gram-negative bacilli grow best in the presence of oxygen and, except for *Enterobacter* species, are only facultatively anaerobic.

(78, 79, 80) *Escherichia coli*, *Proteus* species, and *Pseudomonas* species all are well-known causes of both urinary tract infection and gram-negative bronchopneumonia. *E. coli* is the most common cause of primary uncomplicated urinary tract infection. In addition, *E. coli* and *Pseudomonas* are intestinal pathogens as well, and both have been implicated as primary causes of necrotizing enterocolitis in infants. *E. coli* is an especially versatile enteric pathogen; different strains cause disease by either direct mucosal invasion or elaboration of toxins that cause enterocyte secretory dysfunction. No *Proteus* species is known to be enterotoxic.

(82) *E. coli* and *Proteus* are members of the family Enterobacteriaceae and are part of the indigenous intestinal flora. Enteric organisms, such as *E. coli*, *Proteus* species, and *Enterobacter,* are commonly associated with various suppurative infections within the abdominal cavity such as acute cholecystitis, diverticulitis, and cholangitis. *Pseudomonas,* in contrast, does not usually colonize the intestine and is not commonly associated with suppurative intra-abdominal processes.

(**81**) In contrast to *E. coli, Pseudomonas aeruginosa* is of low virulence for normal individuals and usually causes nosocomial and opportunistic infections. It is virtually ubiquitous in hospitals and is commonly associated with epidemic infections in burn units, nurseries, and critical care units. It is, in fact, the most common cause of skin infections and generalized sepsis in burn patients (*pp. 344–347*).

83. (B); 84. (C); 85. (D); 86. (C); 87. (C); 88. (C); 89. (E)

(**83**) Syphilis is a venereal disease caused by *Treponema pallidum.* The untreated disease has three stages, each with its own unique features. Primary syphilis is manifested only by the painless chancre that occurs on the external genitalia at the site of treponemal invasion. Secondary syphilis appears after a latent period of 2 weeks to 6 months after the primary stage. It is characterized by a generalized skin eruption that disappears spontaneously in about 4 to 12 weeks.

(**84**) It is the tertiary stage of syphilis that appears years or decades later that has the most devastating consequences. During this final stage of disease, localized destructive lesions known as syphilitic gummas appear in virtually any tissue.

(**85**) Whatever the stage of disease, the histologic hallmark of the syphilitic lesions is an obliterative endarteritis with plasma cell infiltrates. Swelling and proliferation of endothelial cells in affected arterioles and small arteries produce a characteristic concentric onion-skin appearance and luminal narrowing.

(**86**) Treponemes are characteristically extremely difficult to demonstrate in the gummas of tertiary syphilis in contrast to the ease with which they are demonstrated in the lesions of primary and secondary syphilis.

(**87**) Central nervous system involvement is also characteristic of tertiary syphilis. Two classic complications of central nervous system involvement are tabes dorsalis, a locomotor ataxia resulting from degeneration of the posterior columns of the spinal cord, and (**88**) Charcot's joint, a rapidly destructive arthritis of the knee joint resulting from spinal cord sensory loss.

(**89**) In contrast to the characteristics of adult sexually transmitted *Treponema pallidum,* Hutchinson's teeth are associated only with congenital syphilis, infection contracted in utero from the mother (*pp. 368–371*).

90. (A); 91. (A); 92. (B); 93. (D); 94. (D); 95. (C); 96. (A)

(**90**) Among the few fungal species that infect humans, *Candida albicans* (an endogenous yeast), *Mucor* (a "bread mold"), *Aspergillus fumigatus* (a ubiquitous filamentous fungus), and *Cryptococcus neoformans* (a soil-dwelling yeast) are the most important. *C. albicans* is the single most common form of human fungal disease. (**91**) The organism can be recognized by its formation of pseudohyphae, which represent concatenations of individual yeast forms.

(**92**) Although most fungal infection tends to occur in immunosuppressed or chronically debilitated patients, many fungal species are capable of causing disease in otherwise healthy individuals. Only mucormycosis seldom, if ever, occurs in healthy individuals and is most often encountered in patients with diabetes, acidosis, advanced malignancy, or some form of immunodeficiency. Examples of fungal infections occurring in healthy individuals are (1) vaginal candidiasis in women taking oral contraceptives, (2) colonizing aspergillosis (aspergilloma) occurring at the site of a previous lung abscess or infarct, and (3) cryptococcosis arising in a healthy individual exposed to contaminated bird excreta.

(**93**) *C. neoformans* is a round budding yeast about the size of an erythrocyte. It has a heavy gelatinous capsule and can be identified by a simple laboratory test known as an India ink preparation. The carbon particles of the ink serve as a contrast medium that offsets the gelatinous capsule and permits ready identification of the organism. (**94**) In contrast to the other fungi, *C. neoformans* has a special affinity for the central nervous system. This organism frequently produces meningitis as a result of seeding from a primary focus in the lung, where the infection may be mild or asymptomatic. Thus, the most common form of cryptococcal infection to come to clinical attention is meningitis.

(**95**) *Aspergillus* is distinctive among the fungi in its ability to produce disease in the absence of true infection. In some sensitized individuals, inhalation of aspergillus spores leads to a florid hypersensitivity pneumonitis. This immunologically mediated lung disease, known as bronchopulmonary aspergillosis, can produce marked pulmonary pathology in the absence of actual colonization or infiltration of the lung by organisms.

(**96**) "Oral thrush" is the name by which candidiasis of the oral cavity is commonly known (see Question 61). Although it may occur in adults undergoing broad-spectrum antibiotic therapy, it is most commonly encountered in neonates, especially those who are bottle-fed. In infants, the disease is usually self-limited and disappears when the normal microflora of the mouth develop (*pp. 386–391*).

97. (B); 98. (D); 99. (D); 100. (D); 101. (A); 102. (D); 103. (C)

(**97**) In the United States there are three major mycotic infections that occur in the normal host and establish systemic infection. They are caused by *Blastomyces dermatitidis, Coccidioides immitis,* and *Histoplasma capsulatum.* In contrast to blastomycosis and histoplasmosis, which occur most frequently in the midwestern United States, particularly in the Mississippi-Ohio River basins, coccidioidomycosis is most prevalent in the southwestern United States, especially in the San Joaquin Valley of California.

(**98**) The fungal agent in each of these diseases is

dimorphic. These fungi grow in nature as mycelium (mold)-bearing infectious spores, which are aerosolized from contaminated soil and inhaled. (99) In the host, the fungi evolve to a yeast-like phase, the pathogenic form of the organism.

(100) The diseases have many clinical as well as microbiologic features in common. Each of these infections may produce acute disease, chronic progressive disease, or no symptoms at all. In fact, asymptomatic disease is the most common outcome in all three of these disorders.

(101) In the systemic form of blastomycosis, the skin is commonly involved and may be the only site of active infection. Skin lesions typically consist of fleshy fungating ulcers that may be confused with cutaneous malignancies. Although coccidioidomycosis and histoplasmosis may cause cutaneous infection with dissemination, it is not common.

(102) The histologic hallmark of all of these fungal infections is granulomatous inflammation, and all may be counted among the causes of granulomatous lung disease. (103) Only histoplasmosis, however, is known to produce the condition known as sclerosing mediastinitis. This results from extension of the histoplasma infection from the mediastinal lymph nodes into the surrounding tissues, causing progressive scarring and contraction of mediastinal structures. This condition may appear as a mediastinal mass and can be confused with a malignancy such as lymphoma (*pp. 391–396*).

104. (A); 105. (A); 106. (A); 107. (C); 108. (E)

(104) Malaria, babesiosis, and Chagas' disease are protozoal diseases caused by *Plasmodium* species, *Babesia* species, and *Trypanosoma cruzi*, respectively. Although all of these diseases are transmitted to humans by insects, only malaria is transmitted by mosquitoes. Babesiosis is transmitted by ticks, and Chagas' disease is transmitted by "kissing bugs," or reduviid bugs.

(105) The protozoal agents of both malaria and babesiosis characteristically invade red blood cells and may be difficult to differentiate from each other. A distinguishing feature of malaria, however, is the characteristic pigment found in the cells of the monocyte-phagocyte system. The pigment represents products of heme digestion that have been released into the bloodstream on destruction of the infected erythrocytes. In babesiosis, pigment is not found in the cells of the monocyte-phagocyte system.

(106) Sickle cell hemoglobin has a protective effect in infection by plasmodia, because it forces the parasites to leave the cell when sickling begins and because erythrocytes have a shortened life span in sickle cell disease.

(107) In contrast to malaria and babesiosis, Chagas' disease is produced by an organism that does not multiply within the bloodstream. The trypanosomes invade tissues to proliferate, and the subsequent tissue injury induces inflammation. The heart is the organ most frequently involved by parasitic invasion. Thus, acute myocarditis or chronic heart disease with progressive cardiac failure is characteristic of Chagas' disease.

(108) Progressive brain dysfunction is not a feature of any of these three diseases. It is characteristic of African trypanosomiasis, so-called sleeping sickness (see Question 67) (*pp. 102 108*).

109. (D); 110. (E); 111. (C); 112. (A); 113. (B)

Worms are the largest human parasites and produce a number of distinctive diseases. Among the most common are ascariasis, hookworm disease, strongyloidiasis, and pinworm infection (enterobiasis).

(109) The pinworm, *Enterobius vermicularis*, causes "night itch" syndrome in children when the female worms migrate to the anal skin for egg laying during the night.

(110) The worm that typically invades striated muscle is *Trichinella spiralis*. Trichinosis is acquired by ingesting viable cysts present in meat that has been inadequately cooked.

(111) *Strongyloides stercoralis* is a roundworm that causes human disease principally by inhabiting the gut lumen, damaging the mucosa, and giving rise to the malabsorption syndrome. Because its eggs mature high in the intestine, duodenal aspiration or biopsy may be particularly helpful in diagnosing this form of helminth infection.

(112) *Ascaris lumbricoides* is another intestinal roundworm that tends to be a luminal dweller. In contrast to the malabsorption syndrome of strongyloidiasis, intestinal obstruction by worms tends to be more characteristic of ascariasis.

(113) Like strongyloidiasis, hookworm infection is acquired by larval penetration, migration to the lungs via the blood, and finally intestinal luminal habitation after being coughed up and swallowed by the host. Once in the small intestine, hookworms attach themselves to the mucosal villi and continuously suck blood from the underlying capillaries, causing chronic blood loss (*pp. 412–415*).

The Cardiovascular System

DIRECTIONS: For Questions 1 to 17, choose the ONE BEST answer to each question.

1. Myocardial hypertrophy is most accurately assessed by:

A. Left ventricular wall thickness
B. Histologic appearance of left ventricular myocardium
C. Weight of the heart
D. Measurement of the heart size by chest x-ray
E. None of these

2. Which of the following situations is the most common outcome of an acute myocardial infarction?

A. Sudden cardiac death
B. Recovery without complications
C. Left ventricular congestive failure
D. Cardiogenic shock
E. Cardiac arrhythmias

3. The LEAST common cause of death due to systemic hypertension is:

A. Stroke
B. Aortic aneurysm rupture
C. Heart failure
D. Renal failure
E. Berry aneurysm rupture

4. Which of the following is the LEAST important independent risk factor for myocardial infarction?

A. Cigarette smoking
B. Hyperlipidemia
C. Systemic hypertension
D. Obesity
E. Diabetes mellitus

5. Immediate consequences of a first ischemic cardiac event include all of the following EXCEPT:

A. Angina pectoris
B. Sudden death without infarction

C. Transmural infarction
D. Cardiac rupture
E. No symptoms

6. The most common cause of sudden cardiac death is:

A. Marked aortic stenosis
B. Myocarditis
C. Ischemic heart disease
D. Hypertensive heart disease
E. Conduction system abnormalities

7. After recovery from a myocardial infarction, all of the following therapeutic approaches are beneficial EXCEPT:

A. Treatment with tissue plasminogen activator (TPA)
B. Treatment with beta-adrenergic blocking agents
C. Treatment with calcium channel blocking agents
D. Aspirin administration
E. Coronary artery bypass surgery

8. Chronic ischemic heart disease is characterized by all of the following EXCEPT:

A. Diffuse subendocardial fibrosis
B. Diffuse myocardial atrophy
C. Severe stenosing coronary atherosclerosis
D. Diffuse, small myocardial scars
E. Evolution to congestive heart failure

9. Compensated hypertensive heart disease is associated with all of the following features EXCEPT:

A. Concentric thickening of the left ventricular wall
B. Increased myocardial oxygen demand
C. Normal cardiac silhouette by chest x-ray
D. Absence of clinical symptoms
E. Normal electrocardiogram

10. Microscopic features of hypertensive heart disease include all of the following EXCEPT:

A. Increased diameter of myofibers
B. Increased size of myofiber nuclei
C. Hyperchromatism of myofiber nuclei
D. Increased number of capillaries between myofibers
E. Thickening of intramyocardial arterioles

11. Cardiac changes related to aging (senile changes of unknown cause) include all of the following EXCEPT:

A. Calcific aortic stenosis
B. Mitral stenosis
C. Mitral annulus calcification
D. Cardiac amyloidosis
E. Brown atrophy of the heart

12. Common complications of prosthetic heart valves include all of the following EXCEPT:

A. Hemolytic anemia
B. Infective endocarditis
C. Mechanical malfunction of the prosthesis
D. Arrhythmias
E. Thromboembolism

13. Sterile cardiac valvular vegetations are associated with all of the following disorders EXCEPT:

A. Mitral valve prolapse
B. Systemic lupus erythematosus
C. Underlying adenocarcinoma
D. Indwelling pulmonary artery (Swan-Ganz) catheter
E. Rheumatic fever

14. All of the following statements about isolated aortic stenosis are true EXCEPT:

A. Most is rheumatic in origin
B. Congenital bicuspid valves are a risk factor
C. Concentric left ventricular hypertrophy develops
D. It is typically asymptomatic for many years
E. Heart failure is the most common cause of death

15. The sinoatrial node (the cardiac pacemaker) sends an impulse directly to:

A. The atrioventricular node
B. The bundle of His
C. The atrioventricular bundle
D. The right bundle branch
E. The left bundle branch

16. Infectious myocarditis is commonly caused by all of the following EXCEPT:

A. Coxsackie virus A
B. *Trypanosoma* (Chagas' disease)
C. Diphtheria bacillus
D. *Staphylococcus*
E. *Meningococcus*

17. All of the following features are commonly associated with hypertrophic cardiomyopathy EXCEPT:

A. A disproportionately enlarged ventricular septum
B. Aortic valve thickening
C. Myofiber disarray in the affected myocardium
D. Small left ventricular volume
E. Large left atrial volume

DIRECTIONS: For Questions 18 to 27, ONE or MORE of the completions given correctly finishes the incomplete statement. Choose:
A—if only *1, 2, and 3* are correct
B—if only *1 and 3* are correct
C—if only *2 and 4* are correct
D—if only *4* is correct
E—if all are correct

18. Cardiac toxicity is known to be produced by which of the following chemotherapeutic agents?

1. Prednisone
2. Cyclophosphamide
3. Bleomycin
4. Adriamycin

A. 1,2,3   B. 1,3   C. 2,4   D. 4 Only   E. All

19. Causes of cor pulmonale include:

1. Pulmonary embolus
2. Pickwickian syndrome

3. Emphysema
4. Patent ductus arteriosus

A. 1,2,3   B. 1,3   C. 2,4   D. 4 Only   E. All

20. Which of the following histologic features are characteristic of normal cardiac muscle?

1. Intercalated disks
2. Peripherally located nuclei
3. Branching myofibers
4. Longitudinal striations

A. 1,2,3   B. 1,3   C. 2,4   D. 4 Only   E. All

21. Which of the following statements about cardiac myxomas is/are true?

    1. They are the most common primary tumor of the heart
    2. They occur most frequently in the left ventricle
    3. They are often associated with syncopal attacks
    4. They tend to be malignant in the pediatric age-group

      A. 1,2,3 B. 1,3 C. 2,4 D. 4 Only E. All

22. Which of the following factors is/are known to exacerbate ischemic heart disease?

    1. Pregnancy
    2. Myocardial hypertrophy
    3. Anemia
    4. Tachycardia

      A. 1,2,3 B. 1,3 C. 2,4 D. 4 Only E. All

23. In a patient with myocardial hypertrophy, the diagnosis of hypertensive heart disease cannot be made if the individual has:

    1. No prior history of hypertension
    2. Coarctation of the aorta
    3. Takayasu's arteritis
    4. Aortic stenosis

      A. 1,2,3 B. 1,3 C. 2,4 D. 4 Only E. All

24. Compared with the rest of the myocardium, the subendocardial region is at higher risk of ischemic injury because:

    1. The subendocardial muscle has a higher metabolic demand than the rest of the myocardium

    2. The intermuscular vascular bed is compressed with the greatest force in this area
    3. This region is less likely to have a collateral vascular supply
    4. The intermuscular arteries in this region are more often affected by stenosing atherosclerosis

      A. 1,2,3 B. 1,3 C. 2,4 D. 4 Only E. All

25. Complications of acute infective endocarditis include:

    1. Myocardial abscesses
    2. Glomerulonephritis
    3. Acute valvular insufficiency
    4. Meningitis

      A. 1,2,3 B. 1,3 C. 2,4 D. 4 Only E. All

26. Myocardial infarction in the *absence* of coronary atherosclerosis is associated with:

    1. Cocaine abuse
    2. Coronary arteritis
    3. Vegetative endocarditis
    4. Coronary artery trauma

      A. 1,2,3 B. 1,3 C. 2,4 D. 4 Only E. All

27. Consequences of rupture of necrotic cardiac muscle after a transmural infarction include:

    1. Cardiac tamponade
    2. Acute mitral valvular insufficiency
    3. Left-to-right shunt
    4. Acute aortic valvular insufficiency

      A. 1,2,3 B. 1,3 C. 2,4 D. 4 Only E. All

    DIRECTIONS: For Questions 28 to 48, you are to decide whether EACH choice is TRUE or FALSE.

For each of the statements about ischemic heart disease (IHD) listed below, choose whether it is TRUE or FALSE.

28. In the United States, more people die of IHD every year than of all forms of cancer collectively

29. Only a minority of cases are associated with widespread, severe coronary atherosclerosis

30. Improved therapy has contributed to a declining mortality from IHD

31. Women are protected from IHD during reproductive life

32. Physical conditioning (exercise) is associated with a reduction in the rate of fatal myocardial infarction

For each of the following statements about rheumatic fever (RF), choose whether it is TRUE or FALSE.

33. The disease is caused by systemic infection and tissue invasion by group A beta-hemolytic streptococcus

34. Rheumatoid arthritis is a late complication of previously involved joint tissues

35. Rheumatic heart disease is a late complication of previously involved heart tissues

36. Rheumatic fever is more common in children than in adults

37. Culture-positive streptococcal pharyngitis is usually present at the onset of a rheumatic attack

38. Prompt antibiotic therapy of streptococcal pharyngitis is the major factor in the declining incidence of acute RF

39. Group A streptococcal infections of the skin are more likely to cause acute glomerulonephritis than acute RF

40. There is no correlation between the severity of the initial streptococcal infection and the likelihood of developing RF

41. An individual who has once had acute RF is more vulnerable to developing the disease again

42. In the absence of cardiac involvement, complete recovery without residual pathologic changes is the rule

43. Prophylactic long-term antistreptococcal therapy is required for patients who have had RF

44. Genetic predisposition is suggested by the high incidence of HLA-B27 antigens in affected individuals

For each of the following statements about carcinoid heart disease, choose whether it is TRUE or FALSE.

45. The disease is unlikely to develop in association with intestinal carcinoid tumors unless liver metastases are present

46. The disease predominantly affects the left side of the heart

47. The characteristic lesion is an endocardial plaque rich in elastic fibers

48. The disease usually produces insufficiency of affected valves

DIRECTIONS: For Questions 49 to 92, the set of lettered headings is followed by a list of numbered words or phrases. For each numbered word or phrase choose:

    A—if the item is associated with (A) only
    B—if the item is associated with (B) only
    C—if the item is associated with *both* (A) and (B)
    D—if the item is associated with *neither* (A) nor (B)

For each of the features listed below, decide whether it describes atherosclerotic aneurysm, syphilitic aneurysm, both, or neither.

    A. Atherosclerotic aneurysm
    B. Syphilitic aneurysm
    C. Both
    D. Neither

49. Marked dilatation of the aorta is NOT a common feature

50. The thoracic aorta is usually involved

51. Most fatalities are due to rupture

52. Cystic medial necrosis is the characteristic histopathologic change

53. Aggressive antihypertensive therapy is indicated

For each of the following statements, choose whether it describes acute bacterial endocarditis, subacute bacterial endocarditis, both, or neither.

    A. Acute bacterial endocarditis
    B. Subacute bacterial endocarditis
    C. Both
    D. Neither

54. Produced by *Staphylococcus aureus* in most cases

55. Produced by streptococci in most cases

56. Characteristically occurs on an abnormal valve

57. Yields positive blood cultures in 90% of cases

58. Associated with changing cardiac murmurs

59. Associated with drug addiction

For each of the characteristics listed below, choose whether it describes rheumatic mitral valve disease, mitral valve prolapse (floppy valve syndrome), both, or neither.

    A. Rheumatic mitral valve disease
    B. Mitral valve prolapse (floppy valve syndrome)
    C. Both
    D. Neither

60. Occurs more commonly in women

61. Predisposes to bacterial endocarditis

62. Associated with commissural fusion of valve cusps

63. Associated with fibrosis and thickening of chordae tendineae

64. Associated with ventricular arrhythmias and sudden death

65. Eventually requires valve replacement in most cases

For each of the features listed below, choose whether it describes valvular heart disease producing regurgitation, stenosis, both of these, or neither of these.

    A. Valvular insufficiency
    B. Valvular stenosis
    C. Both
    D. Neither

66. Characterized by failure of the valve to open completely

67. Characterized by failure of the valve to close completely

68. Almost always due to abnormalities of the valve cusps alone

69. Produced by postinflammatory scarring (rheumatic heart disease)

70. Produced by infective endocarditis

71. Occasionally occurs in association with rheumatoid arthritis

72. Frequently produced by severe atherosclerosis

For each of the characteristics listed below, choose whether it describes subendocardial myocardial infarction, transmural myocardial infarction, both, or neither.

    A. Subendocardial infarction
    B. Transmural infarction
    C. Both
    D. Neither

73. Severe atherosclerosis of multiple extramyocardial coronary vessels is usually present

74. Stenosing atherosclerosis of penetrating intramyocardial arterial vessels is usually present

75. Involvement is limited to the left ventricle in most cases

76. Acute coronary thrombosis is present in most cases

77. Pericarditis usually develops as a consequence

78. It is frequently seen at autopsy in patients who suffer sudden cardiac death

For each of the following cardiac regions, choose whether it usually receives its blood supply from the left coronary artery, the right coronary artery, both, or neither.

    A. Left coronary artery
    B. Right coronary artery
    C. Both
    D. Neither

79. Interventricular septum

80. Anterior wall of the left ventricle

81. Posterior wall of the left ventricle

82. Mitral valve

83. Anterior wall of the right ventricle

84. Posterior wall of the right ventricle

85. Endothelium of the left lateral wall

For each of the following features, choose whether it is commonly associated with left-sided heart failure, with right-sided heart failure, both left and right heart failure, or neither.

    A. Left-sided heart failure
    B. Right-sided heart failure
    C. Both
    D. Neither

86. Caused by ischemic heart disease

87. Caused by valvular heart disease

88. Caused by chronic obstructive pulmonary disease

89. Produces pulmonary edema

90. Produces aldosterone-induced sodium retention

91. Produces prerenal azotemia

92. Produces centrilobular necrosis of liver

DIRECTIONS: Questions 93 to 128 are matching questions. For each numbered item, choose the most likely associated lettered item from those provided. Each numbered item has ONLY ONE answer. Within each group, each lettered item may be the answer to one, more than one, or none of the numbered items.

For each of the characteristics listed below, choose whether it corresponds to a transmural myocardial infarction less than 6 hours old, 6 to 24 hours old, 1 to 3 days old, 4 to 6 days old, or 7 to 14 days old.

    A. Less than 6 hours old
    B. 6 to 24 hours old
    C. 1 to 3 days old
    D. 4 to 6 days old
    E. 7 to 14 days old

93. Peak serum levels of myocardial lactate dehydrogenase

94. Peak tissue infiltration by neutrophils

95. Normal appearance of myocardium on gross examination

96. Earliest detection of increased creatine kinase serum levels

97. Prominent granulation tissue at the periphery of the infarct

98. Maximal coagulative necrosis

99. Beginning of electrocardiographic abnormalities

100. Maximal risk of cardiac rupture

For each of the features of vasculitis listed below, choose whether it is characteristic of polyarteritis nodosa, giant cell arteritis, Kawasaki's disease, Buerger's disease, or none of these.

    A. Polyarteritis nodosa
    B. Giant cell arteritis
    C. Kawasaki's disease
    D. Buerger's disease
    E. None of these

101. Young children and infants are most often affected

102. The disease is rare before age 50

103. Cigarette smoking is an etiologic factor

104. Cardiac involvement is very common

105. Kidney involvement is very common

106. Gangrene of the extremities is often produced

107. Lymph node enlargement is an associated finding

108. Response to steroids alone is excellent

For each of the conditions listed below, choose the type of pericardial effusion it is most likely to produce.

    A. Serous effusion
    B. Serosanguineous effusion
    C. Chylous effusion
    D. Cholesterol effusion
    E. Serosuppurative effusion

109. Cardiopulmonary resuscitation

110. Myxedema

111. Congestive heart failure

112. Nephrotic syndrome

113. Mediastinal tumor

For each of the statements listed below, choose whether it describes stable angina only, unstable angina only, Prinzmetal's angina only, both stable and unstable angina, both unstable and Prinzmetal's angina, or all of these.

    A. Stable angina only
    B. Unstable angina only
    C. Prinzmetal's angina only
    D. Stable and unstable angina
    E. Unstable and Prinzmetal's angina
    F. All of these

114. Associated with coronary atherosclerosis

115. Occurs at rest

116. Induced by exertion, relieved by rest

117. Most commonly accompanied by ST segment elevation on electrocardiogram

118. Most commonly accompanied by ST segment depression on electrocardiogram

119. Frequently causes reversible injury to myocardial cells

120. Associated with very high risk of myocardial infarction

Match each of the therapeutic alternatives for treatment of acute myocardial infarction listed below with the most important rationale for its use.

    A. Reduction of myocardial oxygen demand
    B. Prevention of coronary thrombosis
    C. Coronary thrombolysis
    D. Reduction of coronary vasospasms
    E. Relief of pain
    F. None of these

121. Phenobarbital

122. Verapamil

123. Streptokinase

124. Morphine

125. Enforced activity restriction

126. Propranolol

127. Lidocaine

128. Tissue plasminogen activator (TPA)

5

The Cardiovascular System

1. (**C**) Heart weight is the most accurate reflection of myocardial hypertrophy. It is independent of such superimposed factors as cardiac dilatation in the failing heart, the contractile state of the ventricles that could cause variations in the ventricular wall thickness, or the histologic picture of the left ventricular myocardium. Measurement of heart size by cardiac silhouette on chest x-ray is the least accurate way to assess myocardial hypertrophy; a markedly hypertrophied heart may have a normal cardiac silhouette size. Only when the hypertrophied heart begins to fail and undergo dilatation will the cardiac silhouette increase in size.

Although the weight of the heart varies with the stature of the individual, the range of normal heart weight for the average female is 250 to 300 gm and for the average male is 300 to 350 gm (*pp. 597, 616*).

2. (**E**) Acute myocardial infarctions are seldom without complications. In fact, the initial ischemic event proves fatal in approximately 25% of the victims. Of those who survive, only about 10 to 20% recover without complications. In 60% of complicated cases, left ventricular congestive failure and pulmonary edema develop, but frank cardiogenic shock occurs in only 10%. By far the most common complication of myocardial infarction is the appearance of cardiac arrhythmias (75 to 95% of complicated cases). It is believed that arrhythmias are responsible for most of the sudden deaths related to cardiac ischemia (*p. 613*).

3. (**E**) Hypertensive heart disease is the second most common cause of cardiac disease. The morbidity and mortality from hypertension and hypertensive heart disease have been declining, but hypertension remains a major health problem. Although this positive trend has been attributed to effective treatment methods, the decline in mortality actually began before such therapy

was widely used. About 30 to 50% of patients with untreated systemic hypertension now die of hypertensive heart disease. Heart failure accounts for about one-third of all deaths among hypertensives. Other common causes of death include stroke, hypertensive renal vascular disease, or vascular complications such as aneurysms. Rupture of a berry aneurysm, an uncommon cause of death in general, is frequently unrelated to systemic hypertension (*pp. 616, 1406–1408*).

4. (**D**) Epidemiologic studies have clearly defined a number of risk factors for myocardial infarction. Cigarette smoking increases the risk of myocardial infarction from 2 to 20 times over that of nonsmokers. If smoking is stopped, the increased risk disappears within a few years. Use of oral contraceptives (as formulated in the past) has been shown to carry a 4.5-fold increased risk of myocardial infarction, largely among smokers older than 35 years. Current formulations of "the pill" with lower estrogen content have reduced the risk. There is also a clear-cut association between systemic hypertension and susceptibility to ischemic heart disease and myocardial infarction. The higher the blood pressure, the greater the risk, with diastolic pressure being the most important predictive factor. Diastolic pressures greater than 105 mm Hg are associated with a fourfold increased risk of ischemic heart disease over that of individuals with diastolic pressures of 84 mm Hg or less.

Numerous prospective studies in well-defined population groups have identified hyperlipidemia as a major risk factor predisposing to ischemic heart disease. Of particular significance is the level of low-density lipoproteins, which contain about 70% of the total plasma cholesterol and are strongly correlated with atherosclerosis. In contrast, the serum levels of high-density lipoproteins are inversely related to risk of ischemic heart disease. Diabetes mellitus is a clear-cut risk factor for ischemic heart disease and is associated with an increase in atherosclerosis observed at autopsy and a twofold increase in the incidence of myocardial infarction as compared with nondiabetics.

The association between obesity and heart disease is not as clear-cut. Obesity predisposes to other conditions that are associated with an increased mortality due to myocardial infarction such as hyperlipoproteinemia, hypertension, and diabetes mellitus, but only a small increased risk can be ascribed directly to obesity alone (*pp. 557–562, 602*).

5. (D) The immediate consequences of acute cardiac ischemia are varied and include (1) reversible ischemic injury producing classic substernal chest pain known as angina pectoris, (2) sudden death without infarction believed in most cases to be related to ischemia-induced arrhythmias, (3) irreversible transmural myocardial damage (transmural infarction), and (4) less commonly, no clinical symptoms. Diabetes mellitus may be associated with asymptomatic ischemic heart disease, because diabetic neuropathy sometimes interferes with the sensory perception of ischemic pain.

Cardiac rupture does not occur as an immediate consequence of ischemic damage. It is an uncommon event that occurs many days (mean time 4 to 5 days) after an acute transmural infarction during the period of peak muscle necrosis, when weakening and thinning of the infarcted wall is most pronounced (*pp. 612–613*).

6. (B) In the vast majority of cases, sudden cardiac death occurs as a complication of ischemic heart disease, the ultimate event being a lethal arrhythmia. Less commonly it occurs as a consequence of marked aortic stenosis, hereditary or acquired conduction system abnormalities, or electrolyte derangements. However, it can be caused by lethal arrhythmias due to any cause, including myocarditis (*p. 615*).

7. (A) There are two basic aims of therapy of acute myocardial infarction: (1) acute intervention to improve immediate survival and to reduce or limit the size of the infarction and (2) long-term intervention to improve survival during the year or two after the acute infarction. Clinical studies have shown that the long-term prognosis is improved by treatment with drugs that act to prevent precipitation of myocardial ischemia. For example, beta-adrenergic blocking agents and calcium channel blocking agents (e.g., nifedipine, verapamil) decrease cardiac contractility and reduce oxygen demand. Antiplatelet drugs, such as aspirin, prevent the atheroma-induced aggregation of platelets that contributes to thrombosis and other events in myocardial ischemia dehiscence. When myocardial ischemia cannot be adequately controlled medically, surgical revascularization via coronary artery bypass is frequently successful.

Administration of tissue plasminogen activator (TPA) is only useful in the immediate postinfarction period (within 4 hours of onset) in an attempt to rescue the muscle at the edge of an infarct from irreversible injury.

Its beneficial effect results from immediate plasmin-mediated thrombolysis in the occluded vessels and restoration of perfusion. TPA is not useful for long-term therapy, however (*pp. 604–607, 613–614*).

8. (A) Chronic ischemic heart disease is characterized by insidious ischemic atrophy of the myocardium leading to heart failure. Histologically, small patchy foci of fibrosis are present amid atrophic myofibers in the left ventricle. Scars from previous infarcts may or may not be observed, even though moderate to severe stenosing atherosclerosis of the coronary arteries is invariably present. As more and more myofibers undergo ischemic atrophy, cardiac decompensation and heart failure ensue. Although some patients have anginal attacks or acute myocardial infarctions during the course of their disease, chronic ischemic heart disease may be entirely asymptomatic until heart failure becomes manifest. The mural endocardium is usually normal in this form of heart disease (*p. 614*).

9. (E) Hypertensive heart disease is characteristically insidious in its onset. It develops over a period during which the left ventricle undergoes hypertrophy in order to maintain a normal cardiac output in the presence of increased peripheral resistance. During this period of compensation, the patient is usually free of clinical symptoms. Myocardial hypertrophy (characteristically concentric in configuration) leads to a significant increase in heart weight and myocardial oxygen demand. During the compensated phase of hypertensive heart disease, however, the size of the heart as measured by chest x-ray is not significantly increased. Only when the heart can no longer compensate and dilatation of the failing heart ensues does the cardiac silhouette on chest x-ray show a significant increase. Characteristic electrocardiographic changes are usually present in hypertensive heart disease, even during the asymptomatic phase, and may aid in the diagnosis (*pp. 615–617*).

10. (D) The microscopic changes of myocardial hypertrophy and hypertensive heart disease are subtle and require close attention to the cytologic features of the myofibers. Characteristic features of hypertrophied myofibers include (1) increased cell diameter, (2) increased nuclear size, and (3) nuclear hyperchromatism. The intramyocardial arterioles, like arterioles elsewhere in the body, are thickened as a result of the hypertension, but there is no other alteration of the myocardial vascular bed. Although the myocardial oxygen demand is increased, there is no detectable change in the number or distribution of capillaries in the hypertensive heart (*p. 616*).

11. (B) A number of cardiac changes are associated with aging, although their causes remain largely unknown. Such senile changes include calcific aortic stenosis, a fibrotic and calcific deformity of the aortic valve in the elderly that in most cases is related to neither a congenitally deformed valve nor a healed infective endocarditis.

Equally obscure in its etiology is calcification of the mitral annulus or deposition of amyloid in the geriatric heart. Brown atrophy refers to the organ shrinkage (atrophy) and lipofuscin accumulation that are sometimes observed in the heart and/or liver of elderly patients.

Mitral stenosis is usually the result of injury from rheumatic heart disease but may also be produced by healed infective endocarditis. Unlike aortic stenosis, it does not occur simply as an aging phenomenon *(pp. 626–627, 632, 636, 638)*.

12. (D) Diseased heart valves frequently are surgically excised and replaced by mechanical or porcine bioprosthetic valves. Although valvular heart disease produces significant morbidity and mortality, prosthetic valves used in treatment are also associated with numerous complications and considerable risks. Minor risks include hemolytic anemia and paravalvular leaks. Hemolytic anemia develops from the mechanical destruction of erythrocytes passing through the prosthesis, especially one that is degraded from wear. Partial separation of the suture line anchoring the valve (dehiscence) occurs uncommonly. The paravalvular leaks that result are usually insignificant but may cause hemolysis as blood is forced through the narrow channel of the dehiscence. Mechanical malfunction of the valve can result from dehiscence.

The major problems associated with prosthetic valves are infection, thromboembolism, and valve deterioration with mechanical dysfunction. Thrombus formation on the valve or its sewing ring is universal, but thrombus-related complications are more common with mechanical than bioprosthetic valves. Thrombi may give rise to emboli (most often to the brain, producing stroke or death), become infected to produce infective endocarditis, or interfere mechanically with valve function. Infective endocarditis develops in about 6% of patients within 5 years of valve replacement when the prosthesis becomes seeded by blood-borne bacteria (most often at the suture line). Prosthesis-associated infective endocarditis is a serious complication and can be fatal. Deterioration with valve dysfunction can occur with mechanical valves but is most common with bioprostheses. About 20 to 30% of porcine valves require replacement within 10 years because of sterile tissue degeneration.

Although arrhythmias occasionally occur in the postoperative period, they are not commonly associated with prosthetic valves installed by experienced cardiac surgeons *(pp. 639–640)*.

13. (A) Sterile thrombotic vegetations are the hallmark of nonbacterial thrombotic endocarditis (NBTE). They may occur on either normal or abnormal valves, involve either side of the heart, and tend to be small (1 to 5 mm). NBTE occurs in various clinical conditions, many of which are associated with a hypercoagulable state (e.g., underlying adenocarcinoma). Because NBTE is often associated with chronic debilitating disease such as malignancy, renal failure, or chronic sepsis, it has been called marantic (i.e., "wasting") endocarditis, but it can also occur in young and well-nourished persons. Iatrogenic endocardial trauma is a well-known predisposing factor. Other specific conditions that produce bland (devoid of organisms or pus) valvular vegetations include rheumatic fever and systemic lupus erythematosus (SLE). In SLE, endocardial involvement is known as Libman-Sacks disease. The major significance of all sterile vegetations is their embolic potential.

Mitral valve prolapse is a valvular abnormality that is associated with an increased risk of infectious endocarditis but has no independent association with NBTE *(pp. 628, 636–638)*.

14. (A) Although aortic stenosis may occur in rheumatic heart disease, either alone or in combination with mitral involvement, most isolated calcific aortic stenoses are nonrheumatic in origin. In the vast majority of cases of isolated aortic stenosis, the lesion is an age-related degenerative phenomenon. It can involve normal valves, but congenitally deformed (e.g., bicuspid) valves represent a significant risk factor. Concentric left ventricular hypertrophy occurs with obstruction to left ventricular outflow but is usually asymptomatic for many years. Once symptoms occur, the prognosis is poor unless treated by surgical valve replacement. Without treatment, heart failure and death usually ensue within 2 to 3 years *(pp. 626–627)*.

15. (C) The conduction system of the heart is composed of specialized cardiac muscle fibers called Purkinje's cells that conduct action impulses faster than contractile myofibers. The conduction system regulates the rate and rhythm of the heart. The impulse originates in the sinoatrial node in the posterior wall of the right atrium beside the opening of the superior vena cava. It travels through the atrioventricular (AV) bundle to the AV node, located where the median wall of the right atrium joins the interventricular septum. From the AV node, the impulse is propagated along the interventricular septum toward the apex through the bundle of His. At the apex, the bundle of His splits to form the right and left bundle branches that carry the impulse laterally to the two ventricles *(p. 598)*.

16. (D) A multitude of microorganisms may cause infectious endocarditis, including viruses, chlamydia, bacteria, fungi, and metazoans. Viruses are the most common cause of myocarditis, producing more than half of all cases. Coxsackie viruses A and B, echo viruses, poliovirus, and influenza virus are the most frequently encountered viral agents. Among the causative bacterial agents are diphtheria bacillus, meningococcus, and leptospira. Although Chagas' disease is uncommon in the United States, *Trypanosoma cruzi* is a common cause of myocarditis in endemic regions (Mexico, Central America, and South America). Staphylococci, although a common cause of endocarditis, rarely cause myocarditis *(pp. 633, 640–641)*.

17. **(B)** Hypertrophic cardiomyopathy, also known as idiopathic hypertrophic subaortic stenosis or asymmetric septal hypertrophy, is characterized by cardiac enlargement and myocardial hypertrophy. The hypertrophy may be either symmetrical or asymmetric with disproportionate thickening of the septal wall. Microscopically, a characteristic pattern of myofiber disarray (random rather than parallel orientation) is seen in the involved portions of the myocardium. The thickened wall causes a reduction in the volume of the left ventricular cavity in 90% of the cases and a dilated left atrium in virtually every case. When the subaortic region of the septal wall is markedly involved, outflow obstruction that mimics aortic valvular stenosis may occur. However, the aortic valve is characteristically normal in this condition and does not contribute to the outflow obstruction *(pp. 644–646)*.

18. **(C)** Toxic injury to heart muscle is known to be produced by numerous chemical agents, including some that are commonly used in the treatment of malignant tumors. Cyclophosphamide and doxorubicin (Adriamycin), as well as daunorubicin, are common chemotherapeutic agents that have known cardiac toxicity. Neither prednisone nor bleomycin, however, is associated with cardiac toxicity *(pp. 647–648)*.

19. **(A)** Cor pulmonale, or pulmonary heart disease, refers to right ventricular enlargement secondary to hypertension in the pulmonary vascular tree caused by disorders of lung structure or function. Pulmonary hypertension may result from primary (idiopathic) disease in the pulmonary vasculature or from pulmonary parenchymal disease with secondary vascular changes (e.g., emphysema). Occasionally, pulmonary hypertension may be produced by inadequate function of the chest bellows (e.g., pickwickian syndrome) or inadequate ventilatory drive from the respiratory centers in the brain. In addition, acute cor pulmonale may develop from massive pulmonary embolization.

By definition, cor pulmonale is limited to right heart overload caused by lung-related disease and excludes right ventricular enlargement caused by left heart disease or congenital heart disease (e.g., patent ductus arteriosus) *(pp. 617–618)*.

20. **(B)** Cardiac muscle is a highly specialized form of striated muscle that can easily be distinguished from skeletal muscle on the basis of several unique histologic features. Cardiac muscle has a characteristic branching pattern of myofibers that are joined to one another by specialized structures known as intercalated disks. This branching pattern contrasts with the regular parallel alignment of skeletal muscle cells, which connect not to each other but rather to the connective tissue of the muscle sheath or its tendinous insertion. Also unique to cardiac muscle is the central location of the nuclei within the muscle fibers. In skeletal muscle, the nuclei occupy a peripheral position. These differences notwithstanding, both types of striated muscle are characterized

histologically by so-called cross-striations of the cell cytoplasm, an illusion created by the alignment of the A band and I band of the myofibrils across the short axis of the cell. Striated muscle, in fact, is named for this feature. Longitudinal striations are characteristic of smooth, rather than striated, muscle *(pp. 598, 1363)*.

21. **(B)** Cardiac myxomas are connective tissue tumors of the endocardium. They are the most common primary tumor of the heart. Myxomas usually have the gross appearance of a soft, translucent pedunculated mass. They may arise in any chamber, but 90% occur in the atria. When they occur in the left atrium (the favored location), they can be associated with intermittent ball valve obstruction of the mitral valve orifice and produce syncopal attacks.

Cardiac myxomas are benign tumors in all age-groups. Their major morbidity and mortality is associated with ball valve obstruction, which may lead to acute cardiac insufficiency or even sudden death. Fragmentation and embolization of papillary tumors is also encountered *(pp. 652–653)*.

22. **(E)** Ischemic heart disease is exacerbated by processes that create an imbalance between myocardial oxygen supply and myocardial oxygen demand. A diminished oxygen-carrying capacity of the blood (anemia) reduces myocardial oxygen supply. Increased muscle mass (myocardial hypertrophy), increased contractile activity (tachycardia), or increased cardiac output states (pregnancy) increases myocardial oxygen demand. All of these factors may be superimposed on coronary atherosclerosis and contribute significantly to the production of myocardial ischemia *(p. 601)*.

23. **(E)** Two criteria must be met in order to make the diagnosis of hypertensive heart disease: a prior history of hypertension and left ventricular hypertrophy as an isolated finding. The diagnosis of hypertensive heart disease cannot be made in the presence of other cardiovascular abnormalities, which can themselves lead to increased left ventricular pressure or volume overload with subsequent compensatory hypertrophy (e.g., diseases of the aorta, such as coarctation or Takayasu's arteritis; valvular disease, such as aortic stenosis; or myocardial disease, such as hypertrophic cardiomyopathy). In Takayasu's arteritis ("pulseless disease"), a granulomatous vasculitis of unknown etiology that produces fibrous thickening of the aortic arch and stenosis of aortic tributaries, systemic hypertension may be produced the primary effect on the aorta or the secondary effect of renal arterial stenosis. The diagnosis of hypertensive heart disease refers exclusively to cardiac hypertrophy without accompanying lesions that might account for it (i.e., resulting from primary systemic hypertension) *(pp. 576, 615)*.

24. **(A)** For several anatomic and physiologic reasons, the subendocardial region is the area of the heart at highest risk of myocardial infarction. It has a higher

metabolic demand (oxygen requirement) than the outer zone of the myocardium, and it is less well perfused because contraction exerts a greater compressive force on its vascular bed. In addition, the collateral vascular supply to this region is less abundant than that in peripheral zones of the myocardium. However, atherosclerosis of intramyocardial arteries is virtually never encountered in any zone of the cardiac wall and is not a contributing factor to subendocardial ischemia *(p. 608)*.

25. (E) Infective endocarditis is a hazardous disease associated with numerous grave complications. Primary among these are cardiac complications, embolic infarction, metastatic infection, and glomerulonephritis. Fragmentation and embolization of septic vegetations can produce ischemic death of the tissue in the embolized site and/or establish metastatic abscesses. When the valves of the left heart are involved (most common pattern), embolization and/or abscess formation may involve almost any organ including the heart, kidneys, spleen, brain, and meninges. Lung abscesses may occur with right-sided bacterial endocarditis, the form often associated with intravenous drug abuse. Immunologic responses to the infecting organism may lead to immune complex formation and subsequently to glomerulonephritis or vasculitis. Local complications of infectious endocarditis involve valvular dysfunction. Rarely, large vegetations cause stenosis or occlusion of the valve orifice. More commonly, tissue destruction from invasive organisms causes valvular incompetence. Acute valvular insufficiency, especially of the aortic valve, is life threatening and requires emergent surgical intervention (valve replacement) *(p. 636)*.

26. (E) About 10% of transmural myocardial infarctions are not associated with atherosclerotic thrombosis of the coronary arteries. In these cases, other mechanisms of coronary injury and/or thrombosis are often implicated in the pathogenesis. Cocaine abuse with or without underlying coronary atherosclerosis induces myocardial infarction by mechanisms believed to be related to vasospasm and superimposed thrombosis. Arteritis involving the coronary arteries (e.g., polyarteritis nodosa, Kawasaki's disease, or infectious arteritis) or direct mechanical trauma can cause local injury and thrombosis. Another mechanism of occlusion is embolism. Emboli may originate from mitral or aortic valvular vegetations in either infective endocarditis or nonbacterial thrombotic endocarditis, left atrial or ventricular mural thrombi, or even fragments of a papillary myxoma. Paradoxical emboli from the venous system or the right heart can occur if an abnormal communication between the right and left heart is present (e.g. patent foramen ovale) *(pp. 604, 607)*.

27. (A) The consequences of necrotic muscle rupture after transmural myocardial infarction (median time to rupture: 4 to 5 days) depend on the site of involvement. Rupture of the left ventricular free wall results in hemopericardium and acute cardiac tamponade (almost always fatal). Rupture of the interventricular septum produces a left-to-right shunt. Because the function of the mitral valve depends on the anchorage of its free margins to the ventricular wall (via chordae tendinae) and the coordinated contraction of the papillary muscles during systole, papillary muscle rupture causes acute mitral valvular insufficiency. In contrast, aortic valve function is not dependent on muscle contraction or tethering and is not made insufficient by muscle rupture *(p. 609)*.

28. (True); 29. (False); 30. (True); 31. (True); 32. (True)

(28) Ischemic heart disease (IHD) is the leading cause of death in the United States and other industrialized nations. In the United States, about 550,000 deaths due to IHD occur annually, many more than all forms of cancer collectively.

(29) The vast majority of cases of IHD are associated with severe, widespread atherosclerosis of the coronary arteries, underscoring the primary importance of coronary atherosclerosis in the pathogenesis of myocardial infarction (MI).

(30) Although the present mortality rate from IHD is still very high, it represents a decline in recent years due, in part, to improved therapy of IHD (mainly MI). An equally important factor contributing to the declining death rate is improved life-styles that lessen the incidence of IHD.

(31) Except for those having some disorder predisposing to atherosclerosis (e.g., diabetes or hyperlipidemia), females of reproductive age are at significantly lower risk of dying from IHD than their male counterparts. After age 45, the difference in risk diminishes considerably.

(32) A number of variables are believed to influence the risk and outcome of MI. Coincident with the current interest in physical fitness, a number of studies have shown that regular exercise reduces the rate of fatal MI *(pp. 601–605)*.

33. (False); 34. (False); 35. (True); 36. (True); 37. (False); 38. (True); 39. (True); 40. (False); 41. (True); 42. (True); 43. (True); 44. (False)

(33) Rheumatic fever is an inflammatory disease process that is caused not by infection by group A beta-hemolytic streptococci but rather by the immunologic response to that organism. Thus, tissue damage in this disease is not the direct result of streptococcal sepsis but is produced by immunologically mediated injury most likely occurring as the result of cross-reactivity between streptococcal antigens and native tissue antigens.

(34) Although the heart is the tissue most commonly damaged by this process, the large joints may also be affected, producing a migratory polyarthritis known as rheumatic arthritis (not rheumatoid arthritis). Rheumatic arthritis is a transitory process and always resolves without sequelae. Rheumatoid arthritis, on the other hand, is a chronic systemic inflammatory disease of unknown cause that produces progressive crippling deformity of involved joints. There is no known etiologic connection between the two diseases, despite the similarity of their names.

(35) The most significant consequence of rheumatic fever is injury to the cardiac tissues. Although injury may be produced in any layer of the heart from epicardium to endocardium, rheumatic valvulitis produces the most significant late complications. Injured valves undergo progressive fibrous scarring and permanent deformity.

(36) Although acute rheumatic fever is principally a disease of children, it does occur in adults and usually follows a pharyngeal infection with group A beta-hemolytic streptococci. (37) The latent period between the streptococcal pharyngitis and the onset of acute rheumatic fever is 1 to 5 weeks. At the time of the rheumatic attack, throat cultures are usually negative. Evidence of immunologic response to streptococcal antigens in the form of antistreptolysin O, antihyaluronidase, antistreptokinase, or anti-NADase antibodies is present in 90 to 95% of patients, however.

(38) Prompt antibiotic therapy of streptococcal pharyngitis reduces the incidence of injurious immune responses and is the major factor responsible for the declining incidence of acute rheumatic fever.

(39) Streptococcal sepsis occurring through other portals of entry such as the skin (impetigo) is usually not followed by rheumatic fever. Streptococcal skin infections, like streptococcal infections elsewhere in the body, tend to induce an immune response that causes immune complex-mediated glomerulonephritis. In fact, acute rheumatic fever and acute poststreptococcal glomerulonephritis rarely occur together and do so only coincidentally. It is believed that the nephritogenic strains of streptococci lack the antigens to which the cross-reacting antibodies of rheumatic fever are directed.

(40) There is a strong correlation between the severity and duration of the initial streptococcal pharyngitis and the likelihood of developing subsequent rheumatic fever. (41) Furthermore, an individual who has once had an initial attack of rheumatic fever is more vulnerable to recurrence of the disease with subsequent bouts of streptococcal pharyngitis. If the initial attack of rheumatic fever produces carditis, subsequent attacks usually produce increasingly severe recurrences of this lesion. Even in the absence of reactivation, however, rheumatic carditis generally produces postinflammatory fibrocalcific valvular deformity as a late consequence. (42) In the absence of cardiac involvement, however, the patient often recovers completely from rheumatic fever and is spared recurrences or chronic sequelae. (43) In order to prevent recurrent attacks to which the rheumatic patient is more prone, long-term prophylactic antistreptococcal therapy is required.

(44) There is evidence that genetic factors, probably related to immune response genes to streptococcal antigens, do influence individual susceptibility to rheumatic fever. However, there is no sexual predominance in this disease, nor is there a characteristic HLA profile in susceptible individuals (pp. 629–633).

45. (True); 46. (False); 47. (False); 48. (True)

(45) Involvement of the heart is one of the major histologic concomitants of the carcinoid syndrome. This syndrome is produced by carcinoid tumors (argentaffinomas) that release various bioactive products into the bloodstream. These substances include serotonin, kallikrein, histamine, and prostaglandins that produce the principal manifestations of the syndrome: (1) vasomotor disturbances (flushing of the skin), (2) intestinal hypermotility (diarrhea, cramps, and vomiting), and (3) bronchoconstriction (asthma-like symptoms of dyspnea and wheezing). The cardiac involvement of the carcinoid syndrome, like the syndrome itself, is unlikely to develop in association with intestinal carcinoid tumors unless liver metastases are present. Tumor products can then bypass the rapid polypeptide deamination that occurs in the liver, reach the systemic circulation, and produce the carcinoid syndrome and carcinoid heart disease. (46) The characteristic cardiac lesion associated with the syndrome occurs mainly on the right side of the heart and (47) consists of sclerotic, endocardial plaques that, unlike atherosclerotic plaques, do not contain elastic fibers. (48) Characteristically, the plaques occur on the pulmonary valve, although the tricuspid valve and mural endocardium may be involved. The affected valve leaflets become thickened and fused, producing valvular insufficiency. Although the pathogenesis of these lesions is still uncertain, it is believed that they are most likely due to elevated blood levels of serotonin and/or bradykinin (p. 639).

49. (D); 50. (B); 51. (C); 52. (D); 53. (D)

(49) The three major types of aortic aneurysms are atherosclerotic, syphilitic, and dissecting aneurysms. Only the latter fails in most cases to produce the marked dilatation of the aorta that is the hallmark of atherosclerotic and syphilitic aneurysms. (50) Syphilitic aneurysms almost always involve the thoracic aorta, usually the ascending and transverse portions of the arch. Atherosclerotic aneurysms, in contrast, usually occur in the distal abdominal aorta, although they may occasionally involve the descending portion of the aortic arch. (51) Rupture of the dilated, weakened wall of an atherosclerotic or syphilitic aneurysm is a catastrophic, all too common event that constitutes the major cause of mortality associated with these lesions. Death due to congestive heart failure is also common with syphilitic aneurysms that lead to dilatation and incompetency of the aortic valve or narrowing of the coronary ostia.

(52) All aortic aneurysms are caused by processes that destroy the structural integrity of the arterial wall. In aortic atherosclerosis, the aortic wall is eventually weakened by the progressive tissue destruction and replacement by plaque. Syphilis causes an obliterative endarteritis of the vasa vasorum of the aorta and ischemic destruction of the aortic wall with fibrous scarring of the

media. Cystic medial necrosis is the underlying defect in dissecting aortic aneurysms. This lesion is characterized by accumulations of pools of basophilic mucoid material within the media and elastic tissue. The resultant mural weakening allows blood to dissect into the wall at a point of intimal rupture. Both intimal tears and extension of dissecting hemorrhage within the vessel wall once a tear has occurred are believed to be consequences of hypertension. **(53)** Thus, aggressive antihypertensive therapy is often effective in limiting the extent of dissection in these aneurysms *(pp. 579–584)*.

54. (A); 55. (B); 56. (B); 57. (C); 58. (A); 59. (A)

(54) Bacterial infective endocarditis (IE) is a life-threatening condition whose incidence has not diminished, despite the efforts of modern medicine. Acute bacterial endocarditis, the form associated with abrupt onset and rapid valvular destruction, often occurs on normal cardiac valves and is most commonly caused by *Staphylococcus aureus*. **(55, 56)** Subacute bacterial endocarditis, in contrast, characteristically occurs on abnormal valves, either congenitally deformed valves or rheumatic valves. This form of infective endocarditis is often insidious in onset, and the most common causative organisms tend to be of relatively low virulence. Overall, about 65% of cases are caused by various species of streptococci. **(57)** In both acute and subacute infective endocarditis, the causative agent can in 90% of cases be identified from blood cultures when repeated sufficiently often.

(58) Changing cardiac murmurs are associated with acute infective endocarditis. The murmurs represent valvular function and flow abnormalities produced by the characteristically bulky vegetations. They change suddenly when vegetations fragment and embolize.

(59) The acute form of infective endocarditis is frequently associated with drug addiction. The cardiac lesions in drug addiction are distinctive, however, because they tend to affect normal, right-sided heart valves, especially the tricuspid valve *(pp. 633–636)*.

60. (C); 61. (C); 62. (A); 63. (C); 64. (B); 65. (A)

(60) There is no sexual predominance in rheumatic carditis. Once the disorder occurs, however, women are more prone to the subsequent development of mitral stenosis than men. Mitral valve prolapse is primarily a disorder of women.

(61) Both rheumatic mitral valve disease and mitral valve prolapse predispose to bacterial endocarditis and require antibiotic prophylaxis for procedures known to induce bacteremias (e.g., dental extractions).

(62) One of the most characteristic gross pathologic features of rheumatic mitral valve disease is fibrous bridging across the valvular commissures (commissural fusion), producing the characteristic "fish-mouth" stenotic deformity. In mitral valve prolapse, individual leaflets are enlarged and may show myxoid degenerative changes that become fibrotic at a later stage, but the commissures are not affected. **(63)** Fibrosis and thickening of chordae tendineae may occur in either

disorder and are present in virtually every case of rheumatic mitral valve disease.

(64) Although myocarditis occurring during an acute attack of rheumatic fever may cause fatal arrhythmias, rheumatic mitral valve disease, the product of postinflammatory scarring, is only associated with rhythm disorders late in the clinical course. Mitral valve prolapse, in contrast, is occasionally associated with ventricular arrhythmias, particularly ventricular tachycardia and fibrillation, and even sudden death.

(65) Mitral stenosis from rheumatic valve disease is one of the most significant causes of late morbidity and mortality in rheumatic patients; thus most patients eventually require valve replacement. Although severe isolated mitral regurgitation may complicate mitral valve prolapse and require valvular replacement, overall this is quite uncommon. However, because isolated mitral regurgitation severe enough to require valvular replacement is itself uncommon, mitral valve prolapse has become the most common cause of this problem in some major medical centers *(pp. 629–633)*.

66. (B); 67. (A); 68. (B); 69. (C); 70. (A); 71. (A); 72. (D)

Valvular heart disease encompasses a number of disorders whose primary features are cardiac valvular damage and dysfunction. Although the causes are numerous and often produce fairly distinctive morphologic changes in the valves, the functional deficits produced tend to fall into only two categories: (1) valvular insufficiency and (2) valvular stenosis. In certain conditions, both insufficiency and stenosis may be present.

(66) Valvular stenosis is characterized by a failure of the valve to open completely, impeding flow through the valve. **(67)** Valvular insufficiency implies a failure of the valve to close completely, producing regurgitant flow.

(68) Although valvular insufficiency may result from damage to either valve cusps or supporting structures (such as papillary muscles, annular rings, or chordae tendineae), valvular stenosis is almost always due to pathologic changes in the valve cusps.

(69) Both types of valvular dysfunction may occur in valves damaged by rheumatic heart disease, which characteristically produces fibrosis, distortion, and dysfunction of the valve cusps and of the supporting structures (chordae tendineae).

(70) Infectious endocarditis produces destructive lesions of the valves and supporting structures that can cause perforation of the valve leaflet, erosion of the free margins of the valve, or both. These anatomic changes destroy the competency of the valve and produce valvular insufficiency.

(71) Cardiac involvement by rheumatoid arthritis is associated with valvular insufficiency. In this condition, rheumatoid granulomas form in the mitral and aortic valve rings and in the myocardium. The granulomas cause fibrosis, thickening, and calcification of the affected valve leaflets and the attached chordae tendineae, leading to valvular incompetence and regurgitation.

(72) Although atherosclerotic lesions may be found on heart valves, they are usually of no functional significance *(pp. 626–636, 1351)*.

73. (C); 74. (D); 75. (C); 76. (B); 77. (B); 78. (D)

According to the extent of the ischemic damage, acute myocardial infarction (MI) may be divided into two basic patterns: subendocardial infarction or transmural infarction. Subendocardial infarction typically appears as multifocal areas of necrosis confined to the inner one-third to one-half of the left ventricular wall. Transmural infarction is ischemic necrosis involving the complete or nearly complete thickness of the ventricular wall and is at least 2.5 cm in greatest dimension. The patterns may occasionally overlap, and in some cases transmural infarcts begin with subendocardial necrosis that is extended by increasing severity or duration of ischemia.

(73) Regardless of the pattern, MI is associated with severe multivessel stenotic atherosclerotic disease in the great majority of cases. (74) The atherosclerotic lesions of the coronary vessels are virtually always confined to the extramyocardial arterial segments. Intramyocardial arterial vessels are free of atherosclerotic changes in all forms of ischemic heart disease.

(75) Almost all subendocardial and transmural infarctions are limited to the left ventricular wall in most cases. In only 15 to 30% of transmural infarction involving the posterior wall and posterior septum is the adjacent right ventricular wall involved. Isolated infarction of the right ventricle is extremely rare.

(76) The reported incidence of coronary thrombosis at autopsy in patients dying of transmural infarction differs from the incidence of thrombosis observed by angiography within hours of onset of an MI. At autopsy, less than 50% of cases may show coronary thrombosis, whereas angiography reveals thrombosis in 90% of cases within 4 hours and in 60% within 12 to 24 hours after onset of symptoms. Thus, spontaneous lysis of thrombi apparently occurs with passage of time, but it is clear that the vast majority of transmural infarctions are associated with acute coronary thrombosis. Subendocardial infarction, in contrast, is associated with occlusive thrombus at autopsy in only about 20% of cases. Although angiographic studies show a higher incidence, documented coincidence of coronary thrombosis and subendocardial infarction is relatively uncommon, suggesting the possibility that other mechanisms may be more important in the pathogenesis (e.g., increased oxygen demand, vasospasm, or platelet aggregation).

(77) Postinfarction pericarditis is a well-recognized complication of transmural MI. A fibrinous or fibrinohemorrhagic exudate usually appears from 1 to 3 days after the myocardial infarction and often produces an audible friction rub. This complication, as well as ventricular aneurysm and myocardial rupture, is generally associated only with transmural necrosis and rarely follows subendocardial infarction.

(78) Because morphologic evidence of myocardial necrosis is not present for hours after irreversible injury has occurred, diagnosis of acute MI is rarely possible in patients who suffer sudden cardiac death (death within 1 hour of a cardiac event). Nevertheless, ischemic heart disease is implicated as the major cause of sudden cardiac death, because severe stenosing coronary atherosclerosis is present in 75 to 95% of victims. More uncommonly, myocarditis, mitral valve prolapse, hypertrophic cardiomyopathy, or other disorders are found at autopsy. Whatever the underlying disease, almost all cases of sudden cardiac death are believed to be related to arrhythmias *(pp. 607–614)*.

79. (C); 80. (A); 81. (B); 82. (D); 83. (C); 84. (B); 85. (D)

The most common pattern of coronary artery distribution is a right dominant pattern, in which the right coronary artery supplies the posterior descending arterial system. Thus the right coronary artery normally supplies (79, 81, 84) the posterior wall of both the right and left ventricles, the posterior half of the interventricular septum, and (83) the anterolateral wall of the right ventricle. (80) The left coronary artery normally supplies the anterior wall of the left ventricle, part of the anterior wall of the right ventricle, and the anterior half of the interventricular septum.

(82 and 85) The mitral valve is a thin, endothelium-covered, avascular structure that, like the endothelial lining of the chambers, receives its oxygen supply directly from the blood within the lumen and does not require coronary arterial supply *(pp. 597–598)*.

86. (A); 87. (A); 88. (B); 89. (A); 90. (C); 91. (C); 92. (C)

The right side of the heart receiving the systemic venous return and supplying the low-pressure pulmonary vascular system and the left side of the heart receiving the pulmonary venous return and supplying the high-pressure systemic arterial system compose two separate anatomic and functional systems. Failure of one of these systems can be related to either decreased myocardial contractility and/or an increased workload imposed on it.

(86) Because the left ventricle contains the bulk of the cardiac muscle, does the greatest amount of work, and has the highest oxygen demand, ischemic heart disease primarily affects the left ventricular function and is most frequently associated with left-sided heart failure. (87) Valvular heart disease most commonly involves the mitral and aortic valves and is usually associated with left-sided heart failure.

(88) Chronic obstructive pulmonary disease causes secondary abnormalities in the pulmonary vasculature that impose an increased workload on the right side of the heart and may cause right-sided heart failure.

(89) Pulmonary edema is most commonly the result of left heart failure and increased back pressure in the pulmonary venous system.

(90) Aldosterone-induced sodium retention is produced by both left-sided and right-sided heart failure. Left-sided failure leads to decreased cardiac output and a reduction in renal perfusion, whereas right-sided

failure leads to congestion and hypoxia of the kidneys from increased venous pressure. In both of these conditions, the angiotensin-aldosterone system is activated, leading to sodium and fluid retention. (91) The decreased renal blood flow and renal hypoxia induced by either left-sided or right-sided heart failure can, in addition, lead to impaired excretion of nitrogenous waste products and produce prerenal azotemia.

(92) Centrilobular necrosis of the liver can result from either passive congestion in the centrilobular area or ischemia associated with reduced arterial flow. Thus centrilobular necrosis is a common concomitant of both left-sided and right-sided heart failure *(pp. 598–601)*.

93. (C); 94. (C); 95. (A); 96. (A); 97. (E); 98. (C); 99. (A); 100. (D)

The histopathologic changes associated with an acute myocardial infarction evolve in a relatively predictable progression. This reproducible sequence of histologic changes makes it possible to estimate the age of the infarction. (95) During the first few hours after an ischemic event, the myocardium appears grossly and histologically normal. Coagulative necrosis cannot be seen by routine histologic staining or by histochemical stains for about 3 to 6 hours. (94 and 98) Histologically, coagulative necrosis of the myocardium and neutrophilic infiltration of the infarcted area are maximal 24 to 48 hours after the ischemic event. (97) Toward the end of the first week, the formation of granulation tissue begins, and by 10 days, the fibrovascular response is prominent around the periphery of the infarcted area.

(99) Clinically, the diagnosis of acute myocardial infarction can best be made on the basis of electrocardiographic changes and temporal patterns of specific serum enzyme elevations. Electrocardiographic changes occur in most cases and are present almost immediately after the ischemic event. Unfortunately, they may be nondiagnostic in as many as 25% of patients. (93) Alterations of serum enzyme levels are the most sensitive and reliable indicators of myocardial infarction. The myocardial isozyme of lactate dehydrogenase is apparent in the serum about 12 hours after infarction but reaches peak levels in 48 to 72 hours. The elevation in this isozyme is found to be about 90% sensitive and 95% specific for acute myocardial infarction. It usually persists for as long as 6 days after the ischemic event. (96) The myocardial isozyme of creatine phosphokinase (CPK-MB) appears in the serum within 4 to 8 hours after myocardial damage and reaches its peak approximately 19 hours after infarction.

(100) After transmural infarction, the dead muscle undergoes progressive myocytolysis and loses its structural integrity. At 4 to 5 days, when the ischemic focus is maximally soft, scar formation is just beginning and lends no structural support to the tissue. Myocardial rupture occurs most frequently during this period *(pp. 608–613)*.

101. (C); 102. (B); 103. (D); 104. (C); 105. (A); 106. (D); 107. (C); 108. (B)

(101, 104, 107) Although the vasculitides are a diverse group of disorders producing vascular inflammation and necrosis, they tend to fall into a set of distinctive clinicopathologic syndromes. Kawasaki's disease, for example, is a distinctive disorder of young children and infants manifested by fever, conjunctival and oral erythema and erosion, skin rash, and enlargement of lymph nodes. A severe vasculitis primarily involving the heart (coronary arteries) is the major pathologic feature and major cause of mortality. The finding of reverse transcriptase in Kawasaki's disease has raised the possibility of a retroviral cause *(p. 577)*.

(102 and 108) Giant cell arteritis, in contrast, is a condition that rarely occurs before the age of 50 (average age 70) and most commonly involves the temporal artery. The disease may be difficult to diagnose and can cause visual impairment if untreated, but the therapeutic response to steroids is excellent *(pp. 574–576)*.

(103 and 106) Buerger's disease (thromboangiitis obliterans) is a distinctive vasculitic syndrome, strongly related to cigarette smoking, that causes thrombosis and occlusion of the intermediate and small arteries and veins of the extremities. Vascular insufficiency that often leads to severe pain and gangrene of the extremities is produced *(p. 577)*.

(105) Polyarteritis nodosa is the prototypic systemic vasculitis. It may affect any artery of medium or small size in any organ or system of the body. In contrast to the other disorders mentioned above, the kidneys are commonly (85%) involved by polyarteritis nodosa. In fact, kidney involvement with renal failure is the most common cause of death in this disorder. This disease most often affects young adults and can be effectively treated in 80% of cases by corticosteroids and cyclophosphamide administration (supportive evidence of an immunologic origin for this disorder) *(pp. 571–573)*.

109. (B); 110. (D); 111. (A); 112. (A); 113. (C)

The character of a pericardial effusion is often an indication of its cause. (109) Cardiopulmonary resuscitation produces cardiac trauma and acute inflammation that characteristically produce a serosanguineous effusion. (110) Myxedema, which commonly but not invariably produces hypercholesterolemia, is the most common form of nonidiopathic cholesterol pericardial effusion.

(111) Congestive heart failure with its increased hydrostatic pressure is the most common cause of a serous pericardial effusion. (112) Serous pericardial effusion may also be caused by hypoproteinemic states and decreased serum oncotic pressure. Hypoproteinemia may be produced by increased renal losses (e.g., the nephrotic syndrome), decreased hepatic production (e.g., cirrhosis), or decreased protein intake (e.g., malnutrition). (113) Mediastinal tumor with lymphatic infiltration and blockage characteristically causes a chylous effusion in the pericardium *(pp. 649–651)*.

114. (F); 115. (E); 116. (A); 117. (C); 118. (D); 119. (F); 120. (B)

(114, 115, 116) All forms of angina pectoris are associated with coronary atherosclerosis. Stable (typical) angina is severe chest pain caused by increased oxygen demand (e.g., exercise) in the presence of restricted arterial flow (atherosclerotic narrowing of the coronary arteries). It is characteristically induced by physical exertion or emotional excitement and relieved by relaxation. In contrast to stable angina, unstable angina and Prinzmetal's angina often occur at rest. Unstable or crescendo angina refers to a deteriorating pattern of previously stable angina, precipitated by less exertion, occurring with greater frequency, and lasting for longer periods. Prinzmetal's variant angina refers to chest pain that occurs at rest and is caused by coronary vasospasm. However, Prinzmetal's angina is usually associated with coronary atherosclerosis, and its pathogenesis is thought to be related to atherosclerosis-induced hypercontractility of segments of the coronary trunks.

(**117 and 118**) Most commonly, only Prinzmetal's angina is associated with ST segment elevations on the electrocardiogram. Stable angina and unstable angina typically produce ST segment depressions corresponding to subendocardial ischemia in the left ventricle.

(**119**) All forms of anginal pain are caused by myocardial ischemia, which falls short of producing infarction. Thus the myocardial injury that occurs during a transient anginal attack is usually reversible. The myocardial cells will recover if the balance of oxygen supply and demand are restored relatively quickly.

(**120**) The development of unstable angina, characterized by either prolonged pain, onset of pain at rest in a patient with stable angina, or an increased intensity of exertional anginal pain, is an ominous sign portending myocardial infarction and has thus been dubbed "preinfarction angina" *(p. 604).*

121. (A); 122. (D); 123. (C); 124. (E); 125. (A); 126. (A); 127. (F); 128. (C)

(**121**) Phenobarbital or diazepam is often used in the initial management of acute myocardial infarction to sedate the patient, relieve anxiety, and thereby reduce stress-related increase in cardiac workload.

(**122**) Verapamil is a calcium channel blocker that produces vasodilatation and is especially useful in reducing the vasospastic component of an acute ischemic event. It also has negative inotropic and chronotropic effects on the heart, which help to reduce myocardial work.

(**123**) Streptokinase is used primarily for its fibrinolytic effects. It may be infused directly into the coronary arteries or into the systemic circulation to lyse coronary thrombi.

(**124**) Although morphine has sedative and sympatholytic effects that may be beneficial in initial treatment, the most important reason for its use is for prompt relief of the severe pain of acute myocardial infarction.

(**125**) Restriction of the patient's physical activities is of primary importance in reducing the work of the heart and minimizing its oxygen demand.

(**126**) Propranolol is a beta-adrenergic blocking agent that reduces heart rate, contractility, and blood pressure. All of these effects tend to reduce oxygen consumption by the myocardium.

(**127**) Lidocaine is a local anesthetic that stabilizes neuronal membranes and prevents the initiation and conduction of nerve impulses. The drug also increases the electrical stimulation threshold of the myocardium during diastole. It is sometimes used intravenously in the management of acute myocardial infarction to control life-threatening arrhythmias of ventricular origin.

(**128**) Tissue plasminogen activator is a fibrinolytic agent that is effective in producing coronary thrombolysis and restoring coronary patency if administered within 4 hours of the onset of infarction *(pp. 613–614).*

6

The Respiratory System

DIRECTIONS: For Questions 1 to 12, choose the ONE BEST answer to each question.

1. Clara cells are specialized secretory cells that:

   A. Secrete mucus
   B. Produce surfactant
   C. Produce immunoglobulins
   D. Make bronchiolar lining protein
   E. Possess cilia

2. All of the following commonly contribute to postoperative atelectasis after uncomplicated abdominal surgery EXCEPT:

   A. Adult respiratory distress syndrome
   B. Diaphragmatic elevation
   C. Voluntary suppression of coughing
   D. Excessive bronchial secretions
   E. Limitation of respiratory movements

3. Diffuse alveolar damage (adult respiratory distress syndrome) is the major pattern of pulmonary damage produced by all of the following EXCEPT:

   A. Oxygen toxicity
   B. Narcotic overdose
   C. Septic shock
   D. Cardiopulmonary bypass surgery
   E. Pneumothorax

4. All of the following features are commonly associated with chronic bronchitis EXCEPT:

   A. Hypertrophy of bronchial mucous glands
   B. Productive cough
   C. Severe dyspnea
   D. Increased airways resistance
   E. Frequent infections

5. Complications of necrotizing bronchopneumonia include all of the following EXCEPT:

   A. Chronic bronchitis
   B. Bronchiectasis

C. Pleural fibrosis
D. Metastatic abscess formation
E. Permanent lobar solidification

6. All of the following factors commonly predispose to bacterial pneumonias EXCEPT:

   A. Viral respiratory tract infections
   B. Cigarette smoking
   C. Congestive heart failure
   D. Bacterial urinary tract infection
   E. General anesthesia

7. Aspiration of gastric contents can produce any of the following types of pulmonary injury EXCEPT:

   A. Adult respiratory distress syndrome
   B. Lipoid pneumonia
   C. Lung abscess
   D. Empyema
   E. Pulmonary alveolar proteinosis

8. Known causes of diffuse interstitial fibrosis include all of the following EXCEPT:

   A. Sarcoidosis
   B. Asbestos
   C. Rheumatoid arthritis
   D. Cigarette smoke
   E. Bleomycin

9. Eosinophilic infiltrates characterize all of the following disorders EXCEPT:

   A. Pneumocystis infection
   B. Löeffler's syndrome
   C. Allergic bronchopulmonary aspergillosis
   D. Bronchial asthma
   E. Pigeon breeder's lung

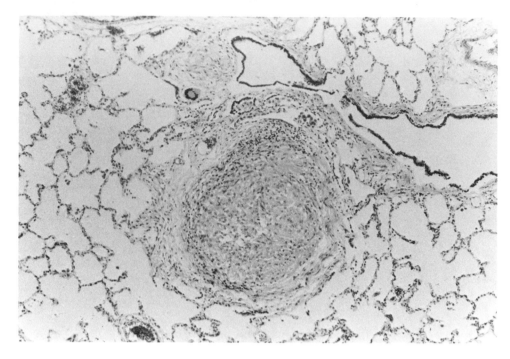

Figure 6–1

10. All of the following statements about diffuse alveolar damage (adult respiratory distress syndrome) are true EXCEPT:

    A. Endothelial injury is the initial pathogenetic event

    B. Type I pneumocytes sustain greater injury than type II cells

    C. Interstitial infiltrates on chest x-ray usually precede the onset of dyspnea

    D. The overall mortality rate is about 50%

    E. It is the underlying cause of most diffuse interstitial fibrotic lung disease

11. Cigarette smoke contributes to the pathogenesis of emphysema by all of the following mechanisms EXCEPT:

    A. Attracts neutrophils into the lung

    B. Stimulates release of neutrophil elastase

    C. Inhibits the ability of pulmonary leukocytes to clear bacteria

    D. Directly inhibits alpha$_1$-antitrypsin

    E. Stimulates macrophage elastase activity

12. The type of pulmonary lesion pictured in Figure 6–1 is produced by all of the following diseases EXCEPT:

    A. Chronic berylliosis

    B. Silicosis

    C. Sarcoidosis

    D. Histoplasmosis

    E. Tuberculosis

DIRECTIONS: For Questions 13 to 19, ONE or MORE of the completions given correctly finishes the incomplete statement. Choose:

    A—if only *1, 2, and 3* are correct

    B—if only *1 and 3* are correct

    C—if only *2 and 4* are correct

    D—if only *4* is correct

    E—if *all* are correct

13. Primary pulmonary hypertension is a disease process that:

    1. Is strongly associated with cigarette smoking

    2. Is often associated with Raynaud's phenomenon

    3. Is usually associated with chronic obstructive lung disease

    4. Produces atherosclerosis of the pulmonary arteries

    A. 1,2,3   B. 1,3   C. 2,4   D. 4 Only   E. All

14. An air bronchogram or a chest x-ray of a 15-year-old girl who has suffered from repeated pulmonary infections all her life shows bilateral bronchiectasis. Which of the following disorders is this patient likely to have?

    1. Cystic fibrosis

    2. IgA immunodeficiency

    3. Kartagener's syndrome

    4. Congenital bronchiectasis

    A. 1,2,3   B. 1,3   C. 2,4   D. 4 Only   E. All

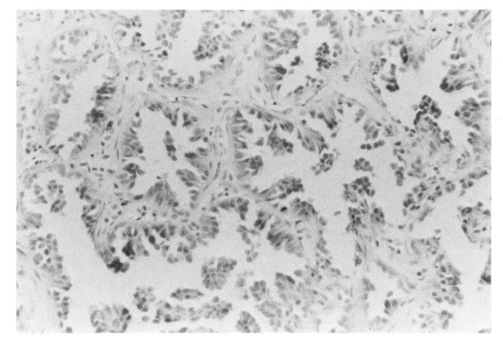

Figure 6–2

15. Which of the following problems are likely to afflict patients with lymphoma who are being treated with systemic chemotherapy?

1. *Pneumocystis carinii* infection
2. Drug-induced diffuse alveolar damage
3. Cytomegalovirus infection
4. Lymphomatous infiltrates

    A. 1,2,3 B. 1,3 C. 2,4 D. 4 Only E. All

16. Vasculitis in the lungs commonly occurs in:

1. Wegener's granulomatosis
2. Polyarterits nodosa
3. The Churg-Strauss syndrome
4. Systemic lupus erythematosus

    A. 1,2,3 B. 1,3 C. 2,4 D. 4 Only E. All

17. Mesothelioma is an uncommon tumor that:

1. Often resembles an adenocarcinoma histologically
2. Often resembles a sarcoma histologically

3. Is causally related to asbestos exposure
4. Is causally related to cigarette smoke

    A. 1,2,3 B. 1,3 C. 2,4 D. 4 Only E. All

18. Chronic obstructive pulmonary disease is an unremitting form of respiratory disease that:

1. Limits lung expansion
2. Includes centrilobular emphysema
3. Includes diffuse interstitial fibrosis
4. Produces difficulty in deflating the lung

    A. 1,2,3 B. 1,3 C. 2,4 D. 4 Only E. All

19. The lesion pictured in Figure 6–2 is a tumor that:

1. Does not destroy alveolar architecture
2. Mimics bronchopneumonia on chest x-ray
3. Frequently contains Clara cells
4. Has a better prognosis than other lung cancers

    A. 1,2,3 B. 1,3 C. 2,4 D. 4 Only E. All

DIRECTIONS: For Questions 20 to 38, you are to decide whether EACH choice is TRUE or FALSE.

For each of the following statements about pulmonary emboli, choose whether it is TRUE or FALSE.

20. They are associated with the use of birth control pills

21. The most common source is pelvic vein thrombi

22. They are usually readily apparent on chest x-ray

23. They commonly resolve without treatment

24. Infarction of the lung rarely occurs when the bronchial arterial supply is adequate

25. The mortality rate with treatment is about 10%

26. Unresolved pulmonary emboli eventually lead to diffuse interstitial fibrosis (honeycomb lung)

For each of the following statements about bronchial asthma, choose whether it is TRUE or FALSE.

27. Most bronchial asthma is mediated by an immune response producing IgE

28. In nearly all patients with asthma, the airways are hyperreactive to bronchoconstrictor agents

29. Infection-induced asthma is usually caused by gram-positive cocci

30. Aspirin-sensitive asthma is caused by the formation of immune complexes

31. Curschmann's spirals are a characteristic histologic finding

For each of the following statements about pulmonary tuberculosis, choose whether it is TRUE or FALSE.

32. The primary focus of infection is most commonly located in the apex of the upper lobe

33. Pneumonia occurs with initial infection in immunodeficient individuals

34. Most initial infections produce fever and cough

35. Reactivation of the primary infection occurs eventually in most untreated individuals

36. Miliary dissemination throughout the body is likely to occur if a tuberculous lesion extends into a pulmonary artery

37. With the most severe tuberculous infections, granulomas frequently fail to form

38. Most patients newly developing a floridly positive purified protein derivative (PPD) skin test require antituberculous chemotherapy

DIRECTIONS: For Questions 39 to 51, the set of lettered headings is followed by a list of numbered words or phrases. For each numbered word or phrase choose:

    A—if the item is associated with (A) only
    B—if the item is associated with (B) only
    C—if the item is associated with *both* (A) and (B)
    D—if the item is associated with *neither* (A) nor (B)

39. Bronchiectasis in adults is most often associated with:
    A. Bronchial obstruction
    B. Bronchial infection
    C. Both
    D. Neither

For each of the characteristics listed below, choose whether it describes bronchogenic cysts, pulmonary cysts, both, or neither.

    A. Bronchogenic cysts
    B. Pulmonary cysts
    C. Both
    D. Neither

40. Usually occur singly

41. Usually occur in a peripheral location

42. Rarely communicate with a main bronchus

43. Frequently become infected

44. Occasionally contain adenocarcinoma

For each of the characteristics listed below, choose whether it describes Goodpasture's syndrome, idiopathic pulmonary hemosiderosis, both, or neither.

    A. Goodpasture's syndrome
    B. Idiopathic pulmonary hemosiderosis
    C. Both
    D. Neither

45. Striking male predominance

46. Associated with interstitial nephritis

47. Usually occurs in children

48. Characterized by necrotizing hemorrhagic interstitial pneumonitis

49. Characterized by pulmonary vasculitis

50. Caused by anti–basement membrane antibodies

51. Often improves without treatment

DIRECTIONS: Questions 52 to 83 are matching questions. For each numbered item, choose the most likely associated item from those provided. Each numbered item has ONLY ONE answer. Within each group, each lettered item may be the answer to one, more than one, or none of the numbered items.

For each of the characteristics listed below, choose whether it describes bronchi, bronchioles, alveoli, all of these, or none of these.

    A. Bronchi
    B. Bronchioles
    C. Alveoli
    D. All of the above
    E. None of the above

52. Contain pores of Kohn

53. Contain goblet cells

54. Contain Clara cells

55. Coated by surfactant

56. Rich in secretory immunoglobulin

57. Contain macrophages in their lumina

58. Contain mucous glands

59. Contain neuroendocrine cells

60. Contain squamous cells

61. Contain mast cells

For each of the characteristics listed below, choose whether it describes centriacinar (centrilobular) emphysema, panaciner (panlobular) emphysema, irregular emphysema, interstitial emphysema, or none of these.

    A. Centriacinar (centrilobular) emphysema
    B. Panacinar (panlobular) emphysema
    C. Irregular emphysema
    D. Interstitial emphysema
    E. None of these

62. Associated with alpha$_1$-antitrypsin deficiency

63. Occurs most commonly in cigarette smokers

64. Occurs in residual lung after lobectomy

65. Occurs in children with whooping cough

66. Does not produce bullae

For each of the microorganisms listed below, choose the pattern of pulmonary injury with which it is most

commonly associated: diffuse alveolar damage, lobar pneumonia, necrotizing bronchopneumonia, lung abscess, or none of these.

    A. Diffuse alveolar damage
    B. Lobar pneumonia
    C. Necrotizing bronchopneumonia
    D. Lung abscess
    E. None of these

67. Cytomegalovirus

68. *Staphylococcus aureus*

69. *Streptococcus pneumoniae* (pneumococcus)

70. Bacteroides

71. Microfilariae

72. Thermophilic bacteria

73. *Mycobacterium tuberculosis*

74. *Mycoplasma pneumoniae*

75. *Klebsiella pneumoniae*

76. *Legionella*

For each of the characteristics listed below, choose which type of bronchogenic carcinoma it describes: squamous cell carcinoma, adenocarcinoma, small (oat) cell carcinoma, or none of these.

    A. Squamous cell carcinoma
    B. Adenocarcinoma
    C. Small (oat) cell carcinoma
    D. None of the above

77. Most common histologic type of lung cancer

78. Occurs with equal frequency in males and females

79. Usually occurs in the periphery of the lung

80. Etiologically unrelated to cigarette smoking

81. Elaborates parathyroid hormone more frequently than any other lung cancer

82. Produces the syndrome of inappropriate antidiuretic hormone secretion more frequently than any other lung cancer

83. Is not usually treated by surgery

The Respiratory System

1. (D) Clara cells are specialized secretory cells found only in bronchioles. They secrete a protein, poor in mucus, that covers the bronchiolar surface. The proteinaceous secretion coats the ciliated cells that make up most of the bronchiolar surface area. Clara cells themselves have no cilia. Because they lack mucin, bronchiolar secretions differ from those of bronchi, which are largely composed of mucous substances produced by epithelial goblet cells and mucosal mucous glands. Bronchiolar secretions are also distinct from those of the alveoli; they lack the surfactant that is the distinctive product of the alveolar type II pneumocytes. Although bronchiolar secretions are characteristically rich in immunoglobulins, these are not produced by the Clara cells. Like immunoglobulins produced elsewhere in the body, those found in the bronchiolar secretions are made by immunocompetent cells of the B-lymphocyte series. These immunocompetent cells reside in or beneath the bronchiolar epithelium and contribute their products to the water-protein layer coating the bronchiolar surface *(pp. 756–757).*

2. (A) Atelectasis is a collapse or an incomplete expansion of alveoli and is characterized by areas of relatively airless pulmonary parenchyma. It may occur in normal lung tissue or as part of a pathologic process in the lung. In a patient who has had an abdominal operation, atelectasis is frequently multifactorial. Unless the surgery is complicated by factors that cause lung injury (e.g., shock, infection, aspiration), it occurs in otherwise normal lungs. The compressive form of atelectasis may result from elevated diaphragms secondary to abdominal distention. Compressive atelectasis also occurs in this setting because of patients' voluntary suppression of coughing or limitation of respiratory movements because of pain. Furthermore, with increased bronchial secretions elicited by general anesthetics, the obstructive form of atelectasis also occurs in these patients.

Although the adult respiratory distress syndrome (adult hyaline membrane disease) produces atelectasis through damage to pneumocytes and loss of surfactant, uncomplicated abdominal surgery is not associated with this life-threatening disorder *(pp. 758–759, 760–761).*

3. (E) Diffuse alveolar damage is the pathologic equivalent of the adult respiratory distress syndrome. It is a pattern of pulmonary injury characterized by congestion, interstitial and intra-alveolar edema and inflammation, fibrin deposition, and focal hemorrhage. Necrosis of alveolar epithelial cells results in the formation of hyaline membranes in the airspaces. Diffuse alveolar damage is characteristic of injury caused by (1) oxygen toxicity; (2) narcotic overdose; (3) shock associated with sepsis, trauma, hemorrhagic pancreatitis, burns, or complicated surgery, especially cardiac surgery involving extracorporeal cardiac bypass pumps; (4) inhalation of toxins and irritant gases; (5) aspiration of gastric contents; (6) hypersensitivity reactions to organic solvents and drugs; and (7) diffuse pulmonary infections, most commonly viral.

Pneumothorax (filling of the pleural cavity with air) results in compressive atelectasis of the involved lung but not diffuse alveolar damage. Infectious, toxic, or oxidant injury to the alveolar endothelium and epithelium causes diffuse alveolar damage, whereas compressive atelectasis simply causes collapse of normal lung tissue *(pp. 760–761).*

4. (C) Chronic bronchitis is defined clinically as a condition causing persistent cough with sputum production for at least 3 months in at least 2 consecutive years. Histologically, the condition is characterized by hypertrophy of the tracheal and bronchial submucosal glands and goblet cell hyperplasia of the bronchial epithelium. One of the earliest manifestations of the disease is an alteration in the resistance of the small airways measurable by a closing volume test. Such tests have shown that small airway dysfunction is present in young smokers before the development of clinical symptoms of respiratory obstruction. Chronic bronchitis predisposes to frequent pulmonary infections that in turn play a secondary role in maintaining or exacerbating the condition. In contrast to patients with pulmonary emphysema, patients with chronic bronchitis do not suffer from severe dyspnea. In long-standing cases of chronic bronchitis, dyspnea on exertion eventually develops but is never as marked as in patients with other forms of chronic obstructive pulmonary disease *(pp. 766, 771–773).*

5. (A) Necrotizing organisms are by definition capable of tissue destruction. They elaborate extracellular enzymes, which allow them to penetrate and destroy normal structures. Additional tissue injury is produced by the liberation of lysosomal enzymes from neutrophils attracted to the site of infection. Thus, the consequences of necrotizing bronchopneumonia can be quite severe. The process may permanently damage airways and result in a postinfective bronchiectasis. Spread to the pleural cavities with resultant empyema formation may organize to form a ring of pleural fibrosis around the involved lung. Penetration of venous structures and lymphatics by the organism leads to systemic bacteremia and metastatic abscess formation. Organization of the exudate and scarring of the damaged lung may lead to permanent solidification of the lung parenchyma. Chronic bronchitis, however, is not a consequence of bronchopneumonia. It is caused by chronic irritation of airways by inhaled substances (usually cigarette smoke), with microbiologic infections playing only a secondary role in its pathogenesis *(pp. 772, 780–783).*

6. (D) Conditions that predispose to bacterial pneumonias are those that impair the natural defense mechanisms of the lung or the resistance of the host in general. Injury to the mucociliary apparatus is one of the most common predisposing factors, because it is produced by both viral respiratory tract infections and cigarette smoke. Another of the common predispositions to bronchopneumonia is pulmonary congestion and edema occurring in patients with congestive heart failure, although the exact mechanism by which this interferes with pulmonary bacterial clearance is not known. A third important predisposing factor is the loss or suppression of the cough reflex occurring from general anesthesia, coma, neuromuscular disorders, drugs, or chest pain.

Bacterial infections elsewhere in the body such as the urinary tract do not usually lead to bacterial bronchopneumonia unless some other predisposing factor is present. If, for instance, a bacteremia from a urinary tract infection occurs in a patient with pulmonary edema or bronchial obstruction with accumulation of secretions, the development of bronchopneumonia would be likely *(p. 780).*

7. (E) Diverse types of pulmonary injury may result from aspiration of regurgitated gastric contents. The specific pattern of injury depends on the nature of the aspirated material. Aspiration of hydrochloric acid produces a pattern of diffuse alveolar damage and results in the clinical syndrome of adult respiratory distress. If the regurgitated material has a high lipid content (e.g., mineral oil or ice cream), alveolar macrophages ingesting the lipids fill the alveolar spaces. The resultant pattern of foamy macrophages and acute inflammation in alveolar spaces is known as lipoid pneumonia. Aspiration of infected material is most commonly associated with acute alcoholism, coma, anesthesia, sinusitis, gingival dental sepsis, and debilitation; lung abscess formation may result. Anaerobic organisms normally found in the oral cavity (*Bacteroides, Fusobacterium,* and *Peptococcus* species) are the most common causative agents. Likewise, aspiration of bacteria-laden material may result in an infection that extends to the pleural cavity, resulting in empyema.

Pulmonary alveolar proteinosis is unrelated to aspiration injury. Its cause is unknown, but it develops in association with dust or chemical inhalation, immunosuppression, and hematologic malignancies with opportunistic infection. The "protein" in pulmonary alveolar proteinosis is the turbid fluid that characteristically fills the alveolar spaces in this disease. The fluid is endogenously rather than exogenously derived (aspirated) and is rich in surfactant thought to accumulate because of increased synthesis by type II pneumocytes or decreased macrophage clearance. Pulmonary alveolar proteinosis does not progress to chronic fibrosis *(pp. 760, 780, 785, 795, 796).*

8. (D) The condition known as diffuse interstitial fibrosis of the lung includes a heterogeneous group of diseases, all of which lead to increased interstitial collagen deposition in the alveolar walls. Although the causes are diverse, the disorders tend to produce similar clinical signs, symptoms, x-ray alterations, and pathophysiologic changes that justify their consideration as a group. Among the known causes of diffuse interstitial fibrosis of the lung are sarcoidosis, asbestosis, collagen vascular diseases such as rheumatoid arthritis, and diffuse alveolar damage (end stage) due to any cause, including bleomycin toxicity. Although cigarette smoke is associated with a multitude of pulmonary diseases, including chronic bronchitis, emphysema, and bronchogenic carcinoma, it is not known to be associated with diffuse interstitial fibrosis *(pp. 789–791).*

9. (A) A number of pathologic entities of the lungs are characterized primarily by infiltration with eosinophils and are often accompanied by eosinophilia in the blood. These disorders run the gamut from benign transitory disease to chronic debilitating conditions. Whatever their clinical course or primary cause, these disorders all are believed to be immunologically mediated. Löeffler's syndrome is a transient benign condition causing simple interstitial eosinophilia in the lungs and is thought to result from an allergic reaction (type I immune response) to parasitic agents (commonly to *Ascaris* and *Strongyloides*). Allergic bronchopulmonary aspergillosis is an example of a chronic pulmonary eosinophilic syndrome; it is caused by hypersensitivity to *Aspergillus* antigens. Bronchial asthma is a classic example of a type I immunologic response in the lung—usually to environmental antigens—causing bronchoconstriction. In bronchial asthma, the walls of the affected airways are infiltrated by eosinophils (see Questions 27 to 31.) Pigeon breeder's lung is an example of a hypersensitivity pneumonitis caused by an allergic response to inhaled proteins from serum, excreta, or feathers of birds. In the acute phase of the disease, pigeon breeder's lung, like other forms of hypersensitivity pulmonary disease, is characterized pathologically by inflammatory infiltrates that include numerous eosinophils.

Although pulmonary eosinophilia is associated with a number of parasitic, fungal, and bacterial infections in the lungs, it is not produced by the protozoan *Pneumocystis carinii*. This particular protozoan characteristically produces a pattern of diffuse alveolar damage (with diffuse interstitial inflammation) in the lung *(pp. 784, 790, 793)*.

10. (C) Although many diverse conditions may produce diffuse alveolar damage (DAD), the initial and basic lesion in all of them is endothelial injury. Alveolar epithelial injury follows. Of the two epithelial cell types, the type I pneumocyte is the more sensitive to injury and sustains the greater degree of damage in DAD. Because they are more hardy and replicate more readily, type II pneumocytes replace the destroyed type I cells during the reparative phases of DAD. Although the process does not necessarily progress in all patients and may be successfully treated with reversal of the underlying disease process and respiratory support therapy, the overall mortality for this syndrome is still about 50%. Many cases evolve to chronic disease, however, and result in diffuse interstitial fibrosis of the lung. In fact, diffuse alveolar damage is the underlying cause of most interstitial fibrotic lung diseases. One of the clinical features peculiar to diffuse alveolar damage is the onset of rather profound symptoms with severe dyspnea and tachypnea before any evidence of pulmonary pathology is seen on chest x-ray. Thus, early in the course of the disease, patients may have acute respiratory distress with a normal chest x-ray *(pp. 760–761)*.

11. (C) Emphysema is a chronic obstructive lung disease characterized by the destruction of alveolar walls. The damage is caused by enzymatic digestion of alveolar structural elements, principally elastic tissue. Neutrophils and macrophages produce elastases that initiate the injury. These cells are attracted to the lungs and stimulated to release their elastases by cigarette smoke. Neutrophil chemotaxis is either induced directly by nicotine or indirectly via the release of neutrophil chemotactic factors from macrophages or activation of the alternate complement pathway. Counterbalancing antielastase activity is normally provided by alpha₁-antitrypsin. However, oxidants in cigarette smoke and free radicals produced by neutrophils reduce alpha₁-antitrypsin activity. Although cigarette smoke does compromise the ability of pulmonary leukocytes to clear bacteria and thus increases susceptibility to infection, infection is not known to contribute to the pathogenesis of emphysema. However, infection does contribute to the pathogenesis of another obstructive lung disease of smokers, chronic bronchitis (see Question 4 and *pp. 769, 772*).

12. (B) Figure 6–1 shows a noncaseating pulmonary granuloma. Granulomas in the lungs are caused by either fungal (e.g., histoplasmosis), mycobacterial (e.g., tuberculosis), or bacterial (brucellosis) infection; hypersensitivity or foreign body responses to inhaled dusts (organic or inorganic); or idiopathic hypersensitivity responses (sarcoidosis, Wegener's granulomatosis). Although fungal and mycobacterial granulomas are often associated with central necrosis, it should be remembered that all large caseating granulomas come from small noncaseating granulomas. Thus the absence of caseation by no means rules out infectious causes.

Silicosis does not produce granulomas but rather collagenous pulmonary nodules that may coalesce to form large calcified fibrous scars. These collagenous nodules are the result of macrophage-particle interactions possibly involving elaboration of fibroblast growth factors *(pp. 476–479, 787, 793, 796)*.

13. (C) Primary pulmonary hypertension is a disease process characterized by increased resistance in the pulmonary vascular tree in the absence of any known cause of increased pulmonary pressure (chronic lung disease, recurrent pulmonary emboli, or antecedent heart disease). The disease occurs most commonly in young women. It is often associated with Raynaud's phenomenon, which lends support to the concept that primary pulmonary hypertension is a form of autoimmune collagen vascular disease. Both Raynaud's phenomenon and pulmonary hypertension occur in such disorders as scleroderma, systemic lupus erythematosus, and rheumatoid arthritis. At present, the underlying cause of primary pulmonary hypertension remains unknown. Yet, by definition, it is not associated with any form of chronic obstructive or interstitial lung disease, which itself is known to produce (secondary) pulmonary hypertension. Whether primary or secondary, however, pulmonary hypertension produces identical changes in the pulmonary vascular tree. The increased pressures in the pulmonary arteries produce atheromatous lesions that, although not as severe, are indistinguishable from those of systemic atherosclerosis. Smaller arterial branches and arterioles show intimal thickening, medial hypertrophy, and varying amounts of intramural and adventitial fibrosis *(p. 764)*.

14. (A) Brochiectasis is permanent dilatation of bronchi or bronchioles produced by necrotizing infection in these airways. In children and young adults, bronchiectasis is usually the result of a congenital or hereditary condition, because bronchiectasis following necrotizing pneumonias complicating childhood diseases such as measles, whooping cough, and influenza is no longer common in the United States. Therefore, cystic fibrosis, immunodeficiency states, immotile cilia syndromes (e.g., Kartagener's syndrome), and congenital bronchiectasis all are associated with bronchiectasis in the pediatric and young adult age-group. These conditions are associated with bronchial mucus plugging (obstruction), increased susceptibility to bronchial infection, or both. In cystic fibrosis, the characteristic thick tenacious bronchial secretions obstruct bronchi and frequently become infected with necrotizing bacterial organisms. With IgA immunodeficiency, the lung is robbed of one of its most important natural defense mechanisms against microbial invasion. Thus, heightened susceptibility to repeated bacterial infection results and is associated with localized or diffuse bronchiectasis. The immotile cilia syndromes result from structurally abnormal, dyskinetic, or akinetic cilia. In Kartagener's syndrome, this defect occurs in association with infertility and situs inversus.

Congenital bronchiectasis is caused by a defect in the development of bronchi. Although it is certainly a cause of bronchiectasis in the young, it usually affects either a lobe or an entire lung but is not usually diffuse (bilateral) (*pp. 777–778*).

15. (E) Patients who have lymphoma and are being treated with systemic chemotherapy and are immunosuppressed may develop various life-threatening pulmonary diseases that require rapid diagnosis (often by open lung biopsy) and treatment. Infection by either common pathogens or opportunistic organisms is frequent in immunosuppressed patients such as these. *Pneumocystic carinii*, a ubiquitous protozoan that rarely if ever infests normal individuals, is a relatively common cause of pneumonia. Viral (e.g., cytomegalovirus) pneumonias are also common.

Noninfectious causes of pulmonary disease in patients who have lymphoma and are undergoing treatment include chemotherapeutic drug-related injury and involvement of the lung by tumor. Numerous chemotherapeutic drugs are associated with the production of diffuse alveolar damage in the lung. This produces a radiologic picture of diffuse pulmonary infiltrates that is often indistinguishable from viral or *Pneumocystis* pneumonia. The correct diagnosis is of emergent importance in cases such as the one described. Antibiotics have no effect on drug reactions or lymphomatous infiltrates. Conversely, additional chemotherapy (and further immunosuppression) is contraindicated in the case of infection or drug reaction but is required if the infiltrate is of lymphomatous origin (*pp. 783–784, 790*).

16. (B) Vasculitis in the lungs, although uncommon, occurs in certain well-defined syndromes. Wegener's granulomatosis and the Churg-Strauss syndrome (allergic granulomatosis and angiitis) are two conditions that are characterized primarily by pulmonary vasculitis. Wegener's granulomatosis produces the classic triad of (1) necrotizing granulomas of the upper and lower respiratory tract, (2) focal necrotizing vasculitis of the lungs, and (3) necrotizing glomerulitis. Unlike Wegener's granulomatosis, the Churg-Strauss syndrome lacks respiratory tract granulomas and glomerulonephritis. The Churg-Strauss syndrome is strongly associated with bronchial asthma and eosinophilia and only rarely involves the kidneys.

Polyarteritis nodosa and systemic lupus erythematosus may indeed involve the lungs and usually produce interstitial pneumonitis, but these entities rarely if ever produce pulmonary vasculitis. In fact, their sparing of pulmonary vessels helps to differentiate them diagnostically from the Churg-Strauss syndrome and Wegener's granulomatosis (*pp. 201, 572–574*).

17. (A) Mesotheliomas are uncommon tumors that arise from either the viscera or the parietal pleura. They can present diagnostic difficulties because they manifest several different histologic patterns. The tubular pattern resembles adenocarcinoma histologically and can be difficult to differentiate from a peripheral bronchogenic adenocarcinoma that has secondarily involved the pleura. In addition, mesotheliomas may exhibit a spindle cell growth pattern and resemble a sarcoma. Mesotheliomas are causally related to heavy asbestos exposure, and the lifetime risk of developing this tumor in heavily exposed individuals is as high as 7 to 10%. Cigarette smoking does not seem to be causally related to mesothelioma, because asbestos workers who smoke appear to be at no greater risk than their nonsmoking cohorts. However, asbestos workers who smoke are at much greater risk of developing bronchogenic carcinoma than nonsmoking asbestos workers (*pp. 481, 807*).

18. (C) All diffuse pulmonary disease can be divided into two categories by the predominant pattern of physiologic dysfunction: obstructive disease and restrictive disease. Obstructive disease is characterized predominantly by an obstruction to flow of air through the airways. Chronic obstructive pulmonary disease comprises the recurrent and unremitting forms of obstructive disease: emphysema, chronic bronchitis, bronchial asthma, and bronchiectasis. Restrictive disease refers to decreased ability to expand the lungs, not because the airways are blocked but because the plasticity of the alveolar walls is reduced by interstitial disease (e.g., diffuse interstitial fibrosis) or because the chest wall cannot be moved normally. Although many diseases have overlapping features, obstructive and restrictive categorization of pulmonary dysfunction is helpful in assessing pulmonary function tests and radiographic abnormalities in patients with chronic pulmonary disease (*pp. 765–766*).

19. (E) Figure 6–2 shows a bronchoalveolar carcinoma. Although clearly malignant tumors, they are distinctive because they do not destroy alveolar architecture but rather use the alveolar wall as a scaffold for growth. This growth pattern gives them the appearance of bronchopneumonia rather than a tumor on chest x-ray and on gross examination of the resected lung. Bronchoalveolar carcinomas originate from terminal airways and contain mucin-producing bronchiolar cells and/or Clara cells. Rarely, type II pneumocytes are also present. These tumors are also distinctive among other forms of brochogenic carcinoma in their tendency to metastasize late and their overall better prognosis (25% 5-year survival rate for bronchoalveolar carcinoma versus 9% for other forms of lung cancer). In addition, association with cigarette smoking is less well defined for bronchoalveolar carcinoma than for other primary lung cancers *(p. 802)*.

20. (True); 21. (False); 22. (False); 23. (True); 24. (True); 25. (True); 26. (False)

Pulmonary emboli are by far the most common cause of thrombotic occlusion of the pulmonary artery. In situ thrombosis is rare. **(20)** Pulmonary embolism usually occurs in patients suffering from some underlying disease (e.g., cardiac disease or cancer) or in those immobilized for long periods. However, young women who use oral contraceptive steroids, who are nearing parturition, or who have just given birth are also at increased risk of pulmonary embolism. **(21)** The most common source of emboli is the deep veins of the lower extremities.

(22) Unfortunately, pulmonary emboli are quite elusive on chest x-ray. If infarction has occurred, a wedge-shaped infiltrate may appear on the chest x-ray 12 to 36 hours later. In the absence of infarction, however, the chest x-ray of a patient with pulmonary embolism may be entirely normal. **(23)** Fortunately, emboli often resolve completely after the initial acute insult without medical treatment. The embolus initially contracts like all thrombi and is subsequently reduced in size by the serum thrombolytic activity. Total lysis of the clot usually ensues.

(24) Because of its dual blood supply, the lung undergoes infarction from pulmonary emboli only if the bronchial arterial supply is also compromised. Thus, pulmonary infarction tends to occur in elderly patients with severe systemic atherosclerosis. Overall, less than 10% of pulmonary emboli actually cause infarction.

(25) Although pulmonary embolus is a common and potentially lethal disorder causing more than 50,000 deaths in the United States each year, the overall mortality rate in patients treated for pulmonary embolism is about 10%. In the presence of an underlying predisposing disease process, however, patients who have suffered one pulmonary embolus have a 30% chance of developing a second.

(26) Unresolved multiple small pulmonary emboli may eventually lead to pulmonary hypertension and pulmonary vascular sclerosis with cor pulmonale but do not cause interstitial fibrosis in the lungs *(pp. 762–764)*.

27. (True); 28. (True); 29. (True); 30. (False); 31. (True)

Bronchial asthma is a chronic obstructive pulmonary disease characterized by irritability of the tracheobronchial tree, producing paroxysmal episodes of bronchospasm with severe dyspnea. Asthma has been divided into three basic types according to the precipitating factor and the pathogenetic mechanism: (1) extrinsic or atopic asthma triggered by environmental antigens (e.g., dust, pollen, foods); (2) intrinsic or idiosyncratic asthma precipitated by respiratory tract infection but not clearly associated with a hypersensitivity immune response; and (3) mixed-pattern asthma, which has some properties of both the intrinsic and extrinsic types. **(27)** Most bronchial asthma is the extrinsic type, which is mediated by an immune response to an environmental antigen that leads to the production of IgE. On exposure to the antigen, presensitized IgE-coated mast cells and basophils release a host of chemical mediators that cause bronchoconstriction, increase venular permeability, and increase bronchial secretions. **(28)** No matter what the type of asthma—extrinsic, intrinsic, or mixed—the airways are hyperreactive to bronchoconstrictor agents. Indeed, the hyperreactivity of the airways to nonspecific irritants and bronchoconstrictor agents is an important feature of asthma of any type.

(29) Although hypersensitivity to microbial antigens may possibly play a part in triggering the intrinsic type of asthma produced by some respiratory tract infections, the organism involved is usually a virus. Gram-positive cocci are more commonly associated with bronchopneumonia than with bronchial asthma.

(30) Aspirin-sensitive asthma, in contrast to other types of asthma, is thought to be related to aspirin's inhibition of the cyclooxygenase pathway of arachidonic acid metabolism without affecting the lipooxygenase route. Thus, the elaboration of the bronchoconstrictor leukotriences is favored, and asthma ensues. The pathogenetic mechanism of aspirin-sensitive asthma does not appear to involve an immunologic response of any sort; no antibodies or immune complexes are formed.

(31) Histologically, the most striking feature in bronchial asthma is the occlusion of bronchi and bronchioles by thick mucus plugs that contain whorls of shed epithelium known as Curschmann's spirals. Within the bronchiole are also numerous eosinophils that contain characteristic inclusions known as Charcot-Leyden crystals *(pp. 773–776)*.

32. (False); 33. (True); 34. (False); 35. (False); 36. (False); 37. (True); 38. (True)

The lungs are by far the most common site of infection by *Mycobacterium tuberculosis*. **(32)** The initial pulmonary infection has a characteristic pattern of involvement. This pattern, called the Ghon complex, consists of a focus of caseating granuloma formation in the pulmonary parenchyma plus involvement of the lymph nodes draining that area. The location of the parenchymal focus is characteristically either just above or just below the interlobar fissure between the upper and lower lobes. This is the region of the lung in which air flow is the greatest and, consequently, where the greatest number of organisms is likely to be carried. The apices of the lungs are the sites of highest oxygen tension, and it is here that a secondary focus of reactivated tuberculosis is most likely to occur. (33) In the absence of normal immunologic responses to the organism, however, this common pattern of involvement is not likely. Instead, the organism tends to produce a diffuse necrotizing bronchopneumonia.

(34) Most primary tuberculosis is asymptomatic. It is only in the secondary form of the disease (chronic pulmonary tuberculosis) that symptoms are usually produced. (35) Most cases of secondary pulmonary tuberculosis develop from reactivation of an old, sometimes subclinical primary infection. Fortunately, however, reactivation occurs in no more than 5 to 10% of cases of untreated primary infection.

(36) Once reactivation has occurred, the subsequent course of the disease is somewhat unpredictable. Widespread hematogenous dissemination may occur with the erosion of caseous lesions into vascular structures. With erosion into the pulmonary artery, miliary spread throughout the lungs occurs. Systemic dissemination, however, occurs with erosion into a pulmonary vein.

(37) In addition to the unpredictable pattern of spread of the disease, the pattern of host response may be unpredictable. Although granuloma formation is usually the hallmark of host response to the mycobacteria, in the most severe tuberculous infections this response can be overwhelmed, and granulomas may fail to form altogether. (38) Because the consequences of secondary pulmonary tuberculosis may be severe, eradication of the primary disease is warranted. Any patient who has recently developed a floridly positive skin test to purified protein derivative (indicating recent infection) requires antituberculous chemotherapy for at least 1 year (*pp. 786–789*).

39. (C) Bronchiectasis is a condition characterized by abnormal dilatation of bronchi and bronchioles and manifested clinically by cough, fever, and production of copious amounts of foul-smelling, purulent sputum. In adults, this condition is most often the result of both bronchial obstruction and secondary necrotizing bronchial infection. Common causes of obstruction are tumor, foreign bodies, and occasionally mucus impaction. Once obstructed, the bronchus becomes filled with mucus, which may become infected. Infection then produces bronchial wall inflammation, weakening, and dilatation. In addition, endobronchial obliteration may result from inflammation, organization, and scarring. Luminal obliteration, in turn, causes further obstruction and bronchiectasis, perpetuating a vicious cycle (*pp. 777–778*).

40. (A); 41. (B); 42. (B); 43. (C); 44. (D)
Congenital cysts of the lungs are of two basic types: bronchogenic and pulmonary. The two types have numerous contrasting features. (40) Bronchogenic cysts usually occur singly and are generally central in location, although they may occur anywhere in the lung. (41) Pulmonary cysts are generally multiple, often bilateral, and usually peripheral in location. (42) Unlike bronchogenic cysts, pulmonary cysts rarely communicate with a main bronchus. (43) Because they are basically sacs filled with proteinaceous secretion, both types of cysts are prime sites for the development of infection, which may lead to abscess formation. (44) Although the cysts are lined by a glandular type of epithelium, neither of these two types of congenital cysts is associated with neoplastic transformation (*p. 758*).

45. (A); 46. (D); 47. (B); 48. (C); 49. (D); 50. (A); 51. (B)
Both Goodpasture's syndrome and idiopathic pulmonary hemosiderosis are two distinctive pulmonary interstitial diseases that produce intrapulmonary hemorrhage as their major manifestation. (45 and 46) Goodpasture's syndrome is characterized by the simultaneous development of a necrotizing hemorrhagic interstitial pneumonitis and rapidly progressing glomerulonephritis (not interstitial nephritis). The syndrome has a striking predominance among males usually in the second or third decade of life. (50) Although the underlying cause is still unknown, it is clear that Goodpasture's syndrome is mediated by the production of antibodies directed against the capillary basement membrane in glomeruli and alveolar septae.

(47) Idiopathic pulmonary hemosiderosis is an uncommon pulmonary hemorrhagic syndrome of unknown cause and pathogenesis. Unlike Goodpasture's syndrome, it has no striking male sexual predominance and tends to occur in children and younger adults.

(48) Although both of these disorders are characterized by necrotizing hemorrhagic interstitial pneumonitis, (49) neither produces vasculitis. Vasculitis-associated hemorrhage constitutes a separate and distinctive category of pulmonary hemorrhagic syndromes, which includes polyarteritis nodosa and Wegener's granulomatosis.

(51) In contrast to Goodpasture's syndrome, which is a devastating disease process requiring treatment with immunosuppressant chemotherapy and plasma exchange, idiopathic pulmonary hemosiderosis often improves without treatment. The course of idiopathic pulmonary hemosiderosis in any given patient is unpredictable. Some patients develop progressive disease with interstitial fibrosis, and others die suddenly of massive pulmonary hemorrhage (*pp. 794–795*).

52. (C); 53. (A); 54. (B); 55. (C); 56. (B); 57. (C); 58. (A); 59. (A); 60. (E); 61. (D)
(53, 58, 59) The distinctive histologic features of different components of the pulmonary parenchyma correspond to their physiologic roles. The bronchi are characterized by their submucoal mucus-secreting glands, mucosal goblet cells, mural cartilage, and con-

tent of mucosal neuroendocrine cells. The mucus produced by submucosal glands and goblet cells coats the bronchial surface, entraps inhaled particles, and is swept toward the oropharynx by ciliary action, where it is swallowed or expectorated. This mucociliary transport is the major defense mechanism of the tracheobronchial tree. Mural cartilages prevent total luminal occlusion when the smooth muscle of the wall is constricted. Neuroendocrine cells produce serotonin, calcitonin, and bombesin (gastrin-releasing hormone) and can give rise to neuroendocrine tumors (bronchial carcinoids).

(**54 and 56**) In contrast to bronchi, bronchioles are devoid of goblet cells and mucous glands. They are normally coated with a watery proteinaceous material that is made by mucosal Clara cells and that is rich in secretory immunoglobulin contributed by mucosal B lymphocytes and plasma cells. Bronchioles contain no cartilage and are capable of complete luminal occlusion on constriction of their mural smooth muscle (e.g., in an asthmatic attack).

(**52, 55, 57**) Alveoli are unique in the production of surfactant by type II pneumocytes in their walls. Surfactant is critical for maintaining low surface tension in the alveoli and, hence, lung compliance. Adjacent alveoli are interconnected by mural passages known as pores of Kohn. They provide a pathway by which bacteria and exudate can spread through neighboring alveoli during the course of bronchopneumonia. Within their lumina, alveoli normally contain macrophages that are the basis for alveolar defense against inhaled bacteria and small particulate matter.

(**60 and 61**) Mast cells are ubiquitous in the lungs; they are found in the walls of bronchi, bronchioles, and alveoli. Thus, mast cells can participate in hypersensitivity responses at any level of the pulmonary tree. In contrast, squamous cells are never present in normal lungs. When found, they represent a metaplastic response to injury. Metaplastic squamous cells may evolve to become dysplasic or neoplastic with continued injury (e.g., cigarette smoking). Thus, squamous cell carcinoma is the most common type of lung cancer, even though normal lungs contain no squamous mucosa (*pp. 756–757, 799–800*).

62. (**B**); 63. (**A**); 64. (**E**); 65. (**D**); 66. (**D**)

Emphysema is a chronic obstructive pulmonary disease defined by the American Thoracic Society as "abnormal permanent enlargement of the air spaces distal to the terminal bronchioles, accompanied by destruction of their walls." Some types of emphysema have been defined on the basis of their particular pathologic and clinical patterns. (**62**) One of the most clinically distinctive types is panacinar (panlobular) emphysema. This type is associated with alpha$_1$-antitrypsin deficiency and is characterized pathologically by uniform enlargement of the acini from the level of the respiratory bronchioles to the terminal alveolar sacs. (**63**) Centriacinar (centrilobular) emphysema, in contrast, is the type that occurs most commonly in cigarette smokers. As its name implies, centriacinar emphysema is characterized by en-

largement of the central or proximal structures of the acini (the respiratory bronchioles) with sparing of the distal alveoli.

(**64**) Although hyperinflation of the residual lung occurs after surgical removal of the lobe, the process does not involve any pulmonary parenchymal destruction and cannot be classified as an emphysematous process even though it is known by the unfortunate term of "compensatory emphysema." Enlargement of airspaces without destruction of their walls is properly called overinflation. (**65**) Likewise, it should be recognized that interstitial emphysema is a process wholly separate from and unrelated to pulmonary emphysema as defined above. Interstitial emphysema refers to the entrance of air into the connective tissue stroma of the lungs, mediastinum, or subcutaneous tissue, most commonly resulting from tears in the alveolar walls. Alveolar tears usually occur when pressures in the alveolar sacs are sharply increased by a combination of coughing plus some bronchiolar obstruction such as occurs in children with whooping cough. (**66**) Thus, because it is not a form of pulmonary emphysema or chronic obstructive pulmonary disease, interstitial edema is not associated with bullous disease. Any of the subtypes of pulmonary emphysema may form bullae or blebs when extensive alveolar destruction has occurred. The class of emphysema most commonly associated with bulla formation is irregular emphysema, a type almost invariably associated with pulmonary scarring (*pp. 766–771*).

67. (**A**); 68. (**C**); 69. (**B**); 70. (**D**); 71. (**E**); 72. (**E**); 73. (**E**); 74. (**A**); 75. (**C**); 76. (**C**)

Although not totally predictable in every case, specific microorganisms tend to produce characteristic patterns of pulmonary injury. (**67 and 74**) Diffuse alveolar damage is a pattern of injury most commonly encountered in viral and mycoplasmal pneumonias. (**69**) Bronchopneumonia involving an entire lobe (lobar pneumonia) is most commonly caused by *Streptococcus pneumoniae* (pneumococcus) but may be caused by other nonnecrotizing bacteria. (**68, 75, 76**) Necrotizing bronchopneumonia is characteristic of such virulent organisms as *Staphylococcus aureus*, *Klebsiella pneumoniae*, and *Legionella* species. Although any necrotizing bronchopneumonia may evolve to abscess formation, this is a relatively infrequent complication. (**70**) *Bacteroides* species and other anaerobic organisms are more commonly associated with lung abscess formation than with any other pattern of pulmonary injury. Pulmonary abscesses from anaerobic organisms are usually the result of aspiration.

(**72**) Thermophilic bacteria, such as those that infect heated water reservoirs in humidifiers or air-conditioners, are of low virulence and do not cause direct pulmonary injury. Instead, thermophilic bacteria elicit a hypersensitivity immune response (both type I and type IV immune reactions). The hypersensitivity pneumonitis that results is characterized by an interstitial inflammatory infiltrate of mononuclear cells and eosinophils and scattered, noncaseated granulomas. (**73**) *My-*

cobacterium tuberculosis is an organism of low virulence. In an immunocompetent host, it elicits a type IV immune response, producing granulomas that are the hallmark of this type of infection.

(71) Microfilariae produce a distinctive reaction in the lungs characterized by patchy interstitial and intraalveolar inflammatory infiltrates composed predominantly of eosinophils. Thus the disease is known as tropical pulmonary eosinophilia *(pp. 337, 342, 348–349, 375, 417–418, 793).*

77. (A); 78. (B); 79. (B); 80. (D); 81. (A); 82. (C); 83. (C)

In industrialized nations, bronchogenic carcinoma is the most common visceral malignancy and accounts for the greatest number of cancer deaths. (77) Among the histologic types of lung cancer, squamous cell carcinoma is the most common, accounting for 35 to 50% of all bronchogenic malignancies. Although there are no squamous cells in a normal lung, squamous cell carcinoma tends to arise from the large airways, which have undergone squamous metaplasia, have become dysplastic, and have finally evolved to frank neoplasia.

(78) Unlike squamous cell carcinoma or small cell carcinoma, which both occur more frequently in men, adenocarcinoma of the lung occurs with equal frequency in males and females. (79) Because adenocarcinoma usually occurs in a peripheral location, it differs even further from squamous and small cell carcinomas, which tend to occur centrally in the lung. (80) Although adenocarcinoma is less frequently associated with a history of cigarette smoking than squamous cell or oat cell carcinomas, none of the major forms of bronchogenic carcinoma can be said to be etiologically unrelated to cigarette smoking.

(81) Bronchogenic carcinomas occasionally produce and secrete hormones that are not responsive to normal feedback regulatory mechanisms. One of the most characteristic ectopic hormonal syndromes associated with a specific tumor type is the production of parathyroid hormone by squamous cell carcinoma of the lung. The other major histologic types of bronchogenic carcinoma rarely, if ever, produce parathyroid hormone. (82) Small cell carcinoma of the lung, in contrast, is the most common type of malignancy to be associated with the syndrome of inappropriate antidiuretic hormone production.

(83) Small cell carcinoma of the lung is the only type of lung tumor for which surgical resection is ineffective. This type of lung cancer is more often treated with radiotherapy and chemotherapy, but the mean survival time for treated small cell carcinoma is only about 1 year. For the other histologic types, early diagnosis with lobectomy or pneumonectomy presents the best chance for cure of the disease. Unfortunately, most bronchogenic carcinoma is discovered in clinically advanced (unresectable) stages, accounting for the overall poor prognosis of the disease *(pp. 295, 798–802).*

7

The Hematopoietic and Lymphoid Systems

DIRECTIONS: For Questions 1 to 6, choose the ONE BEST answer to each question.

1. Manifestations of hereditary spherocytosis include all of the following EXCEPT:

A. Mild jaundice
B. Hemoglobinuria
C. Splenomegaly
D. Cholelithiasis
E. Reduced plasma haptoglobin levels

2. Features of megaloblastic anemia include all of the following EXCEPT:

A. Hypersegmented neutrophils
B. Giant platelets
C. Increased intramedullary hemolysis
D. Increased extramedullary hemolysis
E. Epithelial atypia of the gastric mucosa

3. Characteristics of a normal spleen include all of the following EXCEPT:

A. Involvement in immune responses
B. Destruction of abnormal erythrocytes
C. Storage of erythrocytes
D. Production of erythrocytes
E. Storage of platelets

4. All of the following are known causes of aplastic anemia EXCEPT:

A. Whole-body irradiation
B. Infectious mononucleosis
C. Paroxysmal nocturnal hemoglobinuria
D. Chloramphenicol
E. Metastatic carcinoma

5. All of the following statements about disseminated intravascular coagulation are true EXCEPT:

A. The disorder is characterized by widespread thromboses
B. The disorder is characterized by widespread hemorrhages
C. It most often presents as a primary (idiopathic) condition
D. The brain is the organ most often involved
E. The disorder is associated with mucin-secreting adenocarcinomas

6. Multiple myeloma is associated with all of the following features EXCEPT:

A. Hypercalcemia
B. Renal failure
C. Amyloidosis
D. Increased susceptibility to viral infections
E. Rouleau formation on peripheral smear

DIRECTIONS: For Questions 7 to 18, ONE or MORE of the completions given correctly finishes the incomplete statement. Choose:

A—if only *1, 2, and 3* are correct
B—if only *1 and 3* are correct
C—if only *2 and 4* are correct
D—if only *4* is correct
E—if all are correct

7. Osmotic fragility characterizes the erythrocytes in:

1. Fanconi's syndrome
2. Sickle cell anemia
3. Glucose-6-phosphate dehydrogenase deficiency
4. Hereditary spherocytosis

A. 1,2,3   B. 1,3   C. 2,4   D. 4 Only   E. All

8. Hematologic disorders occurring mainly in populations in the Middle East (Mediterranean region) include:

1. Glucose-6-phosphate dehydrogenase deficiency
2. Thalassemia major
3. Alpha-chain disease
4. Factor IX deficiency (Christmas disease)

A. 1,2,3   B. 1,3   C. 2,4   D. 4 Only   E. All

9. Microangiopathic hemolytic anemia is encountered in:

1. Thrombotic thrombocytopenic purpura
2. The hemolytic-uremic syndrome
3. Malignant hypertension
4. Prosthetic heart valves

A. 1,2,3   B. 1,3   C. 2,4   D. 4 Only   E. All

10. Iron deficiency anemia is correctly described as:

1. Associated with colon cancer
2. Associated with lung cancer
3. Commonly occurring after gastrectomy
4. Commonly producing leukopenia

A. 1,2,3   B. 1,3   C. 2,4   D. 4 Only   E. All

11. Polycythemia vera is a proliferative disorder of stem cells that:

1. Is an X-linked recessive condition
2. Is associated with high levels of erythropoietin
3. Produces abnormalities in the red cell series only
4. Predisposes to myelofibrosis

A. 1,2,3   B. 1,3   C. 2,4   D. 4 Only   E. All

12. Viral hepatitis predisposes to which of the following hematologic disorders?

1. Idiopathic thrombocytopenic purpura
2. Aplastic anemia
3. Erythropoietic depression
4. Autoimmune hemolytic anemia

A. 1,2,3   B. 1,3   C. 2,4   D. 4 Only   E. All

13. Increased blood viscosity (hyperviscosity syndrome) is a major complication of which of the following disorders?

1. Polycythemia vera
2. IgA myeloma
3. Sickle cell anemia
4. Waldenström's macroglobulinemia

A. 1,2,3   B. 1,3   C. 2,4   D. 4 Only   E. All

14. Nodular lymphomas are correctly described as:

1. Associated with a predictable chromosomal translocation
2. Having a better prognosis than diffuse lymphomas
3. Characterized by cells with irregular nuclear contours
4. Always composed of B lymphocytes

A. 1,2,3   B. 1,3   C. 2,4   D. 4 Only   E. All

15. Which of the following features are characteristic of myeloid metaplasia with myelofibrosis?

1. Giant platelets
2. Teardrop-shaped red blood cells
3. Elevated leukocyte alkaline phosphatase levels
4. Massive splenomegaly

A. 1,2,3   B. 1,3   C. 2,4   D. 4 Only   E. All

16. Transformation to acute leukemia occurs as a complication of:

1. Paroxysmal nocturnal hemoglobinuria
2. Myeloid metaplasia with myelofibrosis
3. Aplastic anemia
4. Polycythemia vera

A. 1,2,3   B. 1,3   C. 2,4   D. 4 Only   E. All

17. Low-grade lymphomas include:

1. Follicular mixed-cell lymphoma
2. Lymphoblastic lymphoma
3. Small lymphocytic lymphoma
4. Diffuse large cell lymphoma

A. 1,2,3   B. 1,3   C. 2,4   D. 4 Only   E. All

18. Chronic myelogenous leukemia is characterized by:

1. Lack of alkaline phosphatase in circulating granulocytes
2. Giant splenomegaly
3. Transition to acute leukemia
4. Philadelphia chromosomes in stem cells

A. 1,2,3   B. 1,3   C. 2,4   D. 4 Only   E. All

DIRECTIONS: For Questions 19 to 25, you are to decide whether EACH choice is TRUE or FALSE.

For each of the following statements about Hodgkin's disease, choose whether it is TRUE or FALSE.

19. Reed-Sternberg cells are the malignant component of the tumor

20. Mixed cellularity is the most common subtype

21. All subtypes of Hodgkin's disease spread by contiguity from one lymph node group to another

22. A leukemic phase is common in the lymphocyte-predominant subtype

23. The subtype of Hodgkin's disease is the most important prognostic indicator

24. In young adults, infectious mononucleosis poses an increased risk of developing Hodgkin's disease

25. Patients successfully treated for Hodgkin's disease have an increased risk of developing a non-Hodgkin's lymphoma

DIRECTIONS: For Questions 26 to 55, the set of lettered headings is followed by a list of numbered words or phrases. For each numbered word or phrase choose:
A—if the item is associated with (A) only
B—if the item is associated with (B) only
C—if the item is associated with *both* (A) and (B)
D—if the item is associated with *neither* (A) nor (B)

For each of the features listed below, choose whether it is characteristic of warm antibody autoimmune hemolytic anemia (AHA), cold agglutinin AHA, both, or neither.

    A. Warm antibody AHA
    B. Cold agglutinin AHA
    C. Both
    D. Neither

26. Antibodies to red blood cells are usually monoclonal IgG

27. Antibodies to red blood cells are usually monoclonal IgM

28. The disorder is often caused by drugs

29. The disorder occurs in association with lymphoma

30. Splenomegaly is commonly produced

31. Complement-mediated intravascular hemolysis is commonly produced

For each of the statements listed below, choose whether it describes acute lymphocytic leukemia, acute myelogenous leukemia, both, or neither.

    A. Acute lymphocytic leukemia
    B. Acute myelogenous leukemia
    C. Both
    D. Neither

32. The disease most commonly occurs in the elderly

33. Leukemic cells usually contain the enzyme terminal deoxynucleotidyl transferase

34. Leukemic cells commonly contain Auer rods

35. Patients with the Philadelphia chromosome have a poor prognosis

36. Leukemic cells suppress normal hematopoiesis

37. Patients treated for Hodgkin's disease with chemotherapy and irradiation are at increased risk

38. Prominent lymphadenopathy is characteristically present

39. Bleeding of the gums from thrombocytopenia is common

40. Infiltration of the gums by leukemic cells is common

41. Soft tissue chloromas are characteristic

42. Bone pain is a common symptom

43. Intensive chemotherapy cures about 50% of patients

For each of the features listed below, choose whether it describes idiopathic thrombocytopenic purpura, thrombotic thrombocytopenic purpura, both, or neither.

    A. Idiopathic thrombocytopenic purpura
    B. Thrombotic thrombocytopenic purpura

C. Both
D. Neither

44. Produces an abnormal bleeding time

45. Produces splenomegaly

46. Associated with antiplatelet antibodies

47. Caused by activation of the coagulation system

48. Associated with microangiopathic hemolytic anemia

49. Associated with systemic lupus erythematosus

50. Has a high mortality rate

For each of the statements below, choose whether it describes acute lymphocytic leukemia, chronic lymphocytic leukemia, both, or neither.

A. Acute lymphocytic leukemia
B. Chronic lymphocytic leukemia
C. Both
D. Neither

51. The disease is often asymptomatic

52. The malignancy is usually of B-cell origin

53. Hyperdiploidy is a favorable prognostic feature

54. Prognosis correlates with clinical state of disease

55. Most cells express immunoglobulin light chains

DIRECTIONS: Questions 56 to 94 are matching questions. For each numbered item, choose the most likely associated lettered item from those provided. Each numbered item has ONLY ONE answer. Within each group, each lettered item may be the answer to one, more than one, or none of the numbered items.

For each of the following features of hemolytic anemia, choose whether it is characteristic of beta-thalassemia, paroxysmal nocturnal hemoglobinuria, sickle cell anemia, glucose-6-phosphate dehydrogenase deficiency, or none of these.

A. Beta-thalassemia
B. Paroxysmal nocturnal hemoglobinuria
C. Sickle cell anemia
D. Glucose-6-phosphate dehydrogenase deficiency
E. None of these

56. Antimalarial drugs cause hemolytic crises

57. Splenic hypofunction predisposes to infections

58. Ingestion of fava beans causes hemolytic crises

59. Heinz bodies appear within red blood cells

60. Hypoxia causes hemolytic crises

61. Platelets are abnormal

62. Granulocytes are abnormal

63. Transformation to acute myelogenous leukemia occasionally occurs

64. Usually leads to death before age 20

65. Red blood cell precursors are characteristically destroyed within the marrow

66. Expansion of the erythron within the bone marrow is not a feature of the disease

67. Autoantibodies to red blood cells contribute to the hemolysis

For each of the conditions or situations associated with hemorrhagic diatheses listed below, choose whether the major cause is vascular fragility, thrombocytopenia, defective platelet function, a clotting factor defect, or disseminated intravascular coagulation.

A. Vascular fragility
B. Thrombocytopenia
C. Defective platelet function
D. Clotting factor defect
E. Disseminated intravascular coagulation

68. Cushing's syndrome

69. Uremia

70. Von Willebrand's disease

71. Massive transfusions

72. Henoch-Schönlein purpura

73. Rickettsial infection

74. Promyelocytic (M3) leukemia

75. Scurvy

76. Folate deficiency

77. Acquired immunodeficiency syndrome

For each of the drugs and chemicals listed below, choose whether the hematologic defect with which it is associated is autoimmune hemolytic anemia, aplastic anemia, neutropenia, all of these, or none of these.

    A. Drug-related autoimmune hemolytic anemia
    B. Drug-related aplastic anemia
    C. Drug-related neutropenia
    D. All of these
    E. None of these

78. Penicillin

79. Alpha-methyldopa

80. Thiouracil

81. Quinidine

82. Benzene

83. Aminopyrine

84. Phenacetin

For each of the diseases listed below, choose whether it is characterized by increased circulating numbers of neutrophils, lymphocytes, eosinophils, or none of these.

    A. Elevated neutrophil count
    B. Elevated lymphocyte count
    C. Elevated eosinophil count
    D. None of these

85. Tuberculosis

86. Bronchial asthma

87. Infectious mononucleosis

88. Myocardial infarction

89. Eosinophilic granuloma

For each of the features listed below, choose whether it is characteristic of acute disseminated Langerhans cell histiocytosis (Letterer-Siwe syndrome), multifocal Langerhans cell histiocytosis (Hand-Schüller-Christian disease), unifocal Langerhans cell histiocytosis (eosinophilic granuloma), all of these, or none of these.

    A. Acute disseminated Langerhans cell histiocytosis (Letterer-Siwe syndrome)
    B. Multifocal Langerhans cell histiocytosis (Hand-Schüller-Christian disease)
    C. Unifocal Langerhans cell histiocytosis (eosinophilic granuloma)
    D. All of these
    E. None of these

90. Diabetes insipidus is a classic manifestation

91. The disease commonly occurs before the age of 3 years

92. The mortality rate is 100% in untreated disease

93. Infiltrating histiocytes contain pentalaminar inclusion bodies

94. Skin rash is characteristically absent

The Hematopoietic and Lymphoid Systems

1. (B) Hereditary spherocytosis is an autosomal dominant disorder characterized by a structural defect in the skeleton of the red blood cell membrane. The abnormality is related to a deficiency of spectrin, the major protein in the cell membrane-associated filamentous network responsible for maintenance of cell shape. The defect results in spherically shaped cells that are less deformable and hence more vulnerable to splenic sequestration and destruction than normal erythrocytes. The premature destruction of red blood cells produces a chronic hemolytic anemia with accumulation of hemoglobin breakdown products and a concomitant increase in erythropoiesis in the bone marrow. The extravascular hemolysis produces a mild jaundice with unconjugated hyperbilirubinemia. Moderate splenic enlargement resulting from the congestion of the cords of Billroth is characteristic of hereditary spherocytosis. Pigment (bilirubin) gallstones are also found in many patients.

Haptoglobin, a serum glycoprotein whose physiologic function is to bind free hemoglobin in the serum and prevent its urinary loss, is characteristically reduced in hereditary spherocytosis because some hemoglobin invariably escapes from the phagocytic cells in the spleen. In contrast to intravascular hemolytic processes, the amount of hemoglobin released into the serum is small, and haptoglobin is reduced but not depleted. Depletion of haptoglobin and subsequent excretion of hemoglobin through the kidneys (hemoglobinuria) are characteristic of most forms of intravascular hemolysis but in general do not occur in hereditary spherocytosis (*pp. 663–665*).

2. (B) Megaloblastic anemias resulting from either vitamin B_{12} or folate deficiency are characterized by defective DNA synthesis in all hematopoietic cells. This defective synthesis leads to the production of abnormal erythrocytes and leukocytes and a decrease in the production of all cell lines. Asynchrony between the nuclear and cytoplasmic maturation develops during hematopoiesis, resulting in macrocytic erythrocytes, giant neutrophils with hypersegmented nuclei, and large bizarre megakaryocytes. Defective erythropoiesis leads to increased intramedullary hemolysis of the abnormal precursors. Increased extramedullary hemolysis of defective red blood cells occurs as well, augmented by a poorly characterized plasma factor produced in this disease. Although the impact on the hematopoietic system is most profound, the acquired defect in DNA synthesis affects all rapidly proliferating cells in the body. Therefore, the intestinal mucosa (especially the gastric epithelium) also suffers from nuclear-cytoplasmic asynchrony and develops megaloblastic cytologic changes.

Although giant megakaryocytes are observed in megaloblastic anemia as mentioned, giant platelets are not a feature of this disease. Instead, giant platelets usually occur either in the absence of the spleen or in myeloproliferative disorders such as myeloid metaplasia (*pp. 679–681*).

3. (D) The normal spleen is the filter for the bloodstream and has both immunologic and hematologic functions. It is the "lymph node" of the circulatory system—that is, it traps circulating antigens in the periarteriolar lymphoid sheaths, where they come in contact with effector lymphocytes. The spleen also traps defective and obsolete circulating erythrocytes. Half of the normal daily effete erythrocyte clearance occurs in the spleen, and in disease states, virtually all of the destruction of structurally abnormal (e.g., spherocytes) or antibody-coated red blood cells occurs there. The spleen also functions as a reservoir pool and storage site for erythrocytes and platelets. Normally, stored elements can be extruded on demand. In disease states with splenomegaly and hypersplenism, the spleen traps and hoards blood cells of all types, leading to peripheral cytopenias.

Although the spleen functions as a hematopoietic organ in fetal life and in disease states that compromise or replace bone marrow, hematopoiesis does not normally take place in the spleen (*pp. 747–749*).

4. (E) Aplastic anemia is a condition caused by hematopoietic stem cell injury and characterized by bone marrow failure involving all cell lines. Although the condition may occasionally be primary and idiopathic or hereditary (Fanconi's anemia), it most often occurs as a result of stem cell injury from a variety of chemical agents, physical agents, infections, or other stem cell disorders. Whole-body irradiation is the prototypic cause of injury by physical agents. Infections that are known to induce aplastic anemia are largely, if not exclusively, viral in origin and include infectious mononucleosis, dengue fever, and viral hepatitis. Paroxysmal nocturnal hemoglobinuria is a disorder of stem cells that causes a hemolytic anemia and sometimes evolves into aplastic anemia. Chloramphenicol is one of a long list of drugs that can cause aplastic anemia but is curiously the only one that is known to do so in either a dose-related or an idiosyncratic manner. Although the exact mechanism of injury is unknown and may differ somewhat in all these settings, recent evidence suggests that the stem cell suppression may be immunologically mediated (by suppressor T cells) in some cases. Whatever the cause, aplastic anemia can be effectively treated by bone marrow transplantation.

Metastatic carcinoma in the bone marrow may produce pancytopenia but is considered a form of myelophthisic anemia rather than aplastic anemia. Myelophthisic anemias are produced by space-occupying lesions that destroy significant amounts of normal marrow and, in contrast to aplastic anemias, are not associated with stem cell defects (*pp. 688–691*).

5. (C) Disseminated intravascular coagulation (DIC) is an acquired thrombohemorrhagic disorder characterized by activation of the coagulation cascades. The result is widespread thrombosis and hemorrhage (a consequence of depletion of the elements required for homeostasis). Although any organ can be affected, the brain is most often involved. DIC occurs in association with several disorders, especially sepsis, major trauma, obstetric conditions, and malignancy. Mucin-secreting adenocarcinomas are frequently associated with DIC, because they release various thromboplastic substances including tissue factors, proteolytic enzymes, and mucin, all of which are thrombogenic. It is important to recognize that DIC is, in fact, always secondary to some other underlying condition and does not occur as a primary idiopathic process (*pp. 698–701*).

6. (D) Multiple myeloma is a neoplastic proliferation of plasma cells that are differentiated enough to secrete immunoglobulins or their components. These tumors have numerous distinctive manifestations resulting from their patterns of growth and secretory activity. Typically, multiple myeloma forms osteolytic lesions in bones that have a characteristic "punched-out" appearance on radiographs. The bony destruction frequently leads to hypercalcemia. Renal failure is common in patients with multiple myeloma and is a frequent cause of death in this disease. The most significant factor leading to renal failure is the toxic effect of filtered immunoglobin light chains (Bence Jones proteins) on the renal tubular epithelium, although infiltration of the interstitium by tumor cells also occurs. Amyloidosis of immunologic origin occurs in about 10% of patients with multiple myeloma and may also contribute to renal failure. Coating of erythrocytes with circulating immunoglobulins causes a rouleau formation characteristically seen on peripheral smear.

Although susceptibility to infection is a common complication of multiple myeloma and the leading cause of death, it is due to the severe depression of normal immunoglobulin production in this disease. Cellular immunity, however, is relatively unaffected. Therefore, increased susceptibility to viral infections is not prominent, whereas recurrent infections with encapsulated bacteria pose a major clinical problem (*pp. 739–743*).

7. (D) Osmotic fragility is a property of the red blood cells in hereditary spherocytosis and forms the basis of a common laboratory test used in confirming the diagnosis of this disease (see Question 1).

In the hereditary form of aplastic anemia, known as Fanconi's anemia, red blood cell production is drastically reduced, but the structural properties of the erythrocytes in this disease are not known to be abnormal. In sickle cell anemia, erythrocytes characteristically undergo structural deformation in environments of lowered oxygen tension but are not osmotically fragile. Therefore, common diagnostic tests for sickle cell anemia are based on mixing a blood sample with an oxygen-consuming reagent such as metabisulfite to induce sickling. Red blood cells in glucose-6-phosphate dehydrogenase deficiency are characterized by their sensitivity to oxidative injury and undergo hemolysis when exposed to oxidant drugs; however, they are not osmotically fragile (*pp. 665–666, 688–689*).

8. (A) A number of hematologic disorders occur largely in populations in the Mediterranean area or in patients of Middle Eastern extraction. Principal among these are two hereditary hemolytic anemias: a severe form of glucose-6-phosphate dehydrogenase (G6PD) deficiency and beta-thalassemia (thalassemia major). The Mediterranean form of G6PD deficiency is characterized by impaired synthesis of this enzyme. The resultant abnormalities in glutathione metabolism impair the ability of the red blood cells to protect themselves against oxidative injuries and lead to hemolysis. Beta-thalassemia is a defect in the production of beta-globin chains that in combination with alpha chains make up the major adult human hemoglobin. The inability to produce normal hemoglobin leads to a severe, transfusion-dependent anemia.

Alpha-chain disease is a third disorder that occurs most commonly in Mediterranean populations. It is a form of IgA-producing monoclonal gammopathy characterized by massive infiltration of the intestinal mucosa with lymphocytes, plasmacytes, and histiocytes. The infiltrate also produces a severe malabsorption syndrome, a prominent feature of this disorder. Furthermore, transformation into an immunoblastic sarcoma of B cells occasionally occurs.

Christmas disease or hemophilia B is a rare but severe coagulopathy resulting from a deficiency of factor IX. This disease has no increased incidence among Mediterranean populations *(pp. 665–666, 673–675, 698, 744).*

9. **(E)** Hemolysis due to narrowing or obstruction in the microvasculature is called microangiopathic hemolytic anemia. The disorder is always secondary to some vascular lesion that physically traumatizes and fragments red blood cells. Microangiopathic hemolytic anemia is encountered in thrombotic thrombocytopenic purpura, a disorder characterized by widespread platelet microthrombi in arterioles, capillaries, and venules (see Questions 44 to 50). In the hemolytic-uremic syndrome, glomerular capillaries and afferent arterioles are occluded by microthrombi that constitute the source of red blood cell injury. In malignant hypertension, red blood cells are damaged while passing through the markedly narrowed arterioles. Prosthetic heart valves occasionally create turbulent blood flow and abnormal pressure gradients, which lead to red blood cell injury *(p. 678).*

10. **(B)** Although dietary deficiency is the most common cause of iron deficiency anemia worldwide, chronic blood loss is by far the most common cause of this disorder in the Western world. Chronic blood loss often occurs in benign or malignant diseases of the gastrointestinal tract, causing bleeding into the lumen and subsequent loss of blood in the stool. In fact, patients with colon cancer may first present to the clinician with symptoms of iron deficiency anemia. With the exception of malignancies of the gastrointestinal tract, female genital tract, and urinary tract, hemorrhage produced by other malignancies usually occurs within the tissues and does not lead to iron loss. Gastrectomy is commonly associated with iron deficiency anemia, because gastric acid is important to iron absorption. Furthermore, gastrectomy reduces transit time through the duodenum, the principal site of iron absorption. Unlike anemias resulting from folate or vitamin B_{12} deficiency, iron deficiency anemia affects only red cell hemoglobin production and does not produce abnormalities in any of the other hematopoietic cell lines. Leukopenia, therefore, is not a feature of iron deficiency anemia *(pp. 661–662, 686–688).*

11. **(D)** Polycythemia vera is a proliferative disorder of hematopoietic stem cells in which erythropoietin-hypersensitive erythrocyte precursors predominate. It characteristically produces a striking elevation in the total red blood cell mass, composed mostly of progeny of the abnormal erythrocyte stem cells. The abnormal erythrocytosis suppresses erythropoietin production, and normal red blood cell proliferation requiring higher levels of erythropoietin is diminished. Although the predominant manifestation of polycythemia vera is excessive proliferation of the erythroid series, the granulocytic and megakaryocytic cell lines are also affected to a lesser degree. In fact, the concomitant elevation in the granulocyte and platelet count is supportive evidence that polycythemia vera is a disorder of pluripotent myeloid stem cells. Although more common in males than in females and in whites than in blacks, polycythemia vera has no well-defined mode of genetic transmission. The disease has a variable course, but 15 to 20% of patients develop myelofibrosis after an average period of 10 years. Less commonly, terminal transformation to acute myeloblastic leukemia occurs *(p. 736).*

12. **(A)** Viral hepatitis predisposes to a number of hematologic disorders, some of which have more severe consequences than the hepatitis itself. Idiopathic thrombocytopenic purpura, aplastic anemia, and a depression of red blood cell production all are associated with viral hepatitis. Idiopathic thrombocytopenic purpura occurring in association with viral hepatitis is an acute self-limited form of this disease. In contrast, aplastic anemia occurring in association with viral hepatitis has an extremely grave prognosis. The anemia associated with diffuse liver diseases of any form, including those of viral cause, is attributed to bone marrow failure, but the exact pathogenetic mechanisms are still obscure. Although cold agglutinin autoimmune hemolytic anemia (AHA) or cold hemolysin AHA occasionally occurs after a viral infection such as infectious mononucleosis or influenza, AHA is not associated with infections by the hepatotropic viruses *(pp. 678, 689–691, 693–694).*

13. **(E)** Increased serum viscosity causes circulatory impairment, particularly in the central nervous system and retina, yielding symptoms such as headache, dizziness, or visual impairment. A hyperviscosity syndrome is a common consequence of hematologic disorders that significantly increase either numbers of cellular elements or serum protein levels. Thus, hyperviscosity frequently complicates plasma cell dyscrasias and monoclonal gammopathies such as IgA myeloma and Waldenström's macroglobulinemia. It is also responsible for the major symptomatic manifestations of polycythemia vera. In sickle cell anemia, increased blood viscosity is caused by the inelasticity of sickled red blood cells. Hyperviscosity in turn contributes to the relative hypoxia that favors further sickling of red blood cells upstream, eventually leading to complete vascular occlusion and infarction *(pp. 668, 736, 744).*

14. **(E)** Irrespective of their specific cellular subtype, non-Hodgkin's lymphomas with nodular growth patterns

have several notable similarities. They are always composed of neoplastic B cells, and their nodularity is a recapitulation of lymphoid follicle formation. The cells of nodular lymphomas typically have cleaved or folded nuclear contours, another reflection of their B-cell lineage. (B lymphocytes inside normal germinal [follicular] centers have similar nuclear irregularities.) In about 85% of cases, tumor cells in low-grade nodular lymphomas contain a characteristic chromosomal abnormality (a t[14;18] translocation).

Clinically, nodular lymphomas are indolent tumors and have a much better prognosis than their diffuse counterpart. Unlike diffuse lymphomas, nodular lymphomas are extremely rare in individuals younger than 20 years and occur with equal frequency in males and females. *(pp. 712–713).*

15. (E) Myeloid metaplasia with myelofibrosis is a myeloproliferative syndrome characterized by fibrous replacement of the bone marrow and extramedullary hematopoiesis. The spleen is the major site of the extramedullary hematopoiesis (myeloid metaplasia) and is usually enormously enlarged, weighing as much as 4000 gm. The blood elements produced in this disease have numerous abnormalities. Particularly characteristic are teardrop-shaped erythrocytes and giant platelets. Because myeloblasts, myelocytes, and metamyelocytes typically constitute a small fraction of the white blood cell population on the peripheral smear in myelofibrosis, the disease can sometimes be difficult to differentiate from chronic myelogenous leukemia. In myeloid metaplasia, however, leukocyte alkaline phosphatase levels are often elevated, whereas in chronic myelogenous leukemia they are characteristically low *(pp. 737–739).*

16. (E) Paroxysmal nocturnal hemoglobinuria (see Questions 56 and 67), myeloid metaplasia with myelofibrosis (see Question 15), aplastic anemia (see Question 4), and polycythemia vera (see Question 11) all are myeloid stem cell disorders. Although their etiologies and manifestations are completely different, they have one unfortunate feature in common—predisposition to leukemia. In each disease, a small but well-defined proportion of cases is complicated by transformation to acute leukemia *(pp. 676, 689, 736, 738–739).*

17. (B) The Working Formulation for Clinical Usage is a widely used classification of lymphomas based on survival statistics. It has three grades: low, intermediate, and high; average 5-year survival rates are 50 to 70%, 35 to 45%, and 23 to 32%, respectively. Each grade includes several morphologically defined categories. Lymphomas with the most favorable prognosis (low grade) include small lymphocytic lymphoma, follicular small cleaved cell lymphoma, and follicular mixed-cell lymphoma. Diffuse large cell lymphoma is one of four intermediate-grade lymphomas (the other are follicular large cell, diffuse small cleaved cell, and diffuse mixed small and large cell lymphomas). Lymphoblastic lymphoma is one of three high-grade tumors (the others are large cell immunoblastic lymphoma and small non-

cleaved lymphoma including Burkitt's lymphoma). Although it may not seem like it, the Working Formulation actually represents a simplified approach to this complex group of malignancies and to their even more complex and numerous previous classification schemes *(pp. 711–716).*

18. (E) Chronic myelogenous leukemia (CML) is one of four chronic myeloproliferative disorders that represent clonal neoplastic proliferations of multipotent myeloid stem cells. The other three diseases in this category are polycythemia vera, essential thrombocythemia, and myeloid metaplasia with myelofibrosis. CML is unique among these diseases because affected stem cells and their progeny have a characteristic chromosomal abnormality, the Philadelphia (Ph[1]) chromosome. Although the abnormal stem cells give rise to erythroid, granulocytic, and megakaryocytic precursors, the granulocytic series predominates in CML. In contrast to the situation in acute myelogenous leukemia, granulocyte maturation is not blocked, and a vast number of mature leukemic cells fill the bone marrow and peripheral blood. Although they look identical to normal neutrophils, leukemic neutrophils of CML can be distinguished by their almost total lack of alkaline phosphatase. Another characteristic feature of CML is extreme splenomegaly. Chemotherapy is unsatisfactory in CML and does not alter the median survival time. The inevitable course of the disease is terminal transition to an acute leukemic phase known as blast crisis *(pp. 728–729).*

19. (True);   20. (False);   21. (True);   22. (False); 23. (False); 24. (True); 25. (True)

Hodgkin's disease has long been classified separately from the non-Hodgkin's lymphomas on the basis of its numerous unique features. **(19)** Hodgkin's disease is characterized by a proliferation of giant neoplastic cells of probable lymphoid lineage known as Reed-Sternberg (RS) cells. The RS cell is the only malignant element in Hodgkin's disease. In each of the histologic subtypes of Hodgkin's disease, RS cells are associated with a variable number of other leukocytes, but these so-called background cells are reactive rather than neoplastic in character.

(20) The most common subtype of Hodgkin's disease is nodular sclerosis, representing about 40% of cases. Mixed cellularity, lymphocyte-predominant, and lymphocyte-depleted subtypes of Hodgkin's disease follow in descending order of frequency.

(21) No matter what the subtype, Hodgkin's disease almost always spreads by contiguity from one chain of lymph nodes to the adjacent group, a feature rarely associated with non-Hodgkin's lymphoma.

(22) In further contrast to most non-Hodgkin's lymphomas, Hodgkin's disease (of any type) rarely manifests a leukemic state.

(23) Although the subtypes of Hodgkin's disease, based on the relative numbers of RS cells and background cells, are associated with differences in clinical behavior, they are far less important than clinical staging as indicators of prognosis.

(24) Although the pathogenesis of Hodgkin's disease is still obscure, it has been suggested that it may represent a consequence of delayed infection with a common viral agent. Usually cited in support of this hypothesis is the resemblance of the RS cell to a virally transformed cell and the increased incidence (two- to three-fold) of Hodgkin's disease in young adults with infectious mononucleosis.

(25) Although the modern aggressive modes of therapy have largely obliterated the prognostic differences between the various subtypes of Hodgkin's disease and significantly improved survival, it appears that this has not happened without a cost. Long-term survivors of combined chemotherapy and radiotherapy have a significantly increased risk of developing a non-Hodgkin's lymphoma or an acute leukemia *(pp. 717–722)*.

26. (D); 27. (B); 28. (A); 29. (C); 30. (A); 31. (D)

Autoimmune hemolytic anemias are characterized by the production of anti–red blood cell antibodies that either directly cause hemolysis or indirectly lead to increased red blood cell destruction. The type of antibody produced determines to a large extent the character of the resultant disorder and forms the basis of the classification of the immunohemolytic disorders.

(26 and 27) In cold agglutinin autoimmune hemolytic anemia (AHA), the antibodies produced are primarily monoclonal IgM. Although the antibodies in warm antibody AHA are usually IgG, they do not appear to be of monoclonal origin.

(28) Warm antibody AHA often occurs in association with drugs. The drug (e.g., penicillin, quinidine, or phenacetin) acts as a hapten in inducing an immune response to red blood cells or may directly initiate the production of antibodies that are directed against intrinsic red blood cell antigens like the Rh blood group antigens (e.g., alpha-methyldopa). (29) In contrast to drug-associated AHA, lymphoma-associated AHA may be of either the warm antibody or cold agglutinin type.

(30) In warm antibody AHA, antibody-coated red blood cells or red blood cells coated with drug-induced immune complexes are susceptible to splenic sequestration and destruction. Thus, splenomegaly is a common feature of warm antibody AHA. In cold agglutinin AHA, the liver sequesters most of the affected red blood cells, and splenomegaly is uncommon. The reason for this phenomenon is poorly understood.

(31) The hemolysis in both warm antibody AHA and cold agglutinin AHA is extravascular (i.e., mainly in the spleen). Only in cold hemolysin AHA, a third major class of autoimmune hemolytic anemia, does intravascular hemolysis occur. In this disorder, autoantibodies bind to red blood cells at low temperature and induce complement-mediated hemolysis when the temperature is elevated *(pp. 677–679)*.

32. (D); 33. (A); 34. (B); 35. (C); 36. (C); 37. (B); 38. (A); 39. (C); 40. (B); 41. (B); 42. (C); 43. (A)

Acute leukemias are dramatic neoplastic proliferations of white blood cell precursors that do not undergo normal maturation (i.e., are arrested at early stages of maturation). They are characterized by dramatically increased numbers of circulating immature white cells (blasts). Although they have many common features, acute leukemias of lymphocytic origin differ from those of granulocytic origin in both pathologic and clinical behavior.

(32, 39, 42) A common feature of acute lymphocytic leukemia (ALL) and acute myelogenous leukemia (AML) is their predominance in the young. ALL is the most frequent type of leukemia in children under 15 years of age, whereas AML occurs mainly in young adults (the 15 to 39 year age-group). Another feature common to both forms of acute leukemia is the suppression of normal hematopoiesis, probably by a combination of bone marrow replacement by neoplastic cells and tumor induced humoral inhibition. The result is anemia and thrombocytopenia with abnormal bleeding (e.g., gingival bleeding, petechiae, epistaxis). The marrow expansion in both ALL and AML leads to subperiosteal bone infiltration, bone resorption, and bone pain.

(33 and 34) By routine histologic examination, ALL and AML may be difficult to distinguish from one another, since both are composed of a uniform population of undifferentiated blast elements. However, special enzymatic and histochemical marker studies are beneficial in determining the cell of origin in acute leukemias. For example, the enzyme terminal deoxynucleotidyl transferase (TdT), a DNA polymerase, is present in 95% of cases of ALL but in less than 5% of AML. Distinguishing intracytoplasmic features of AML cells (myeloblasts) include azurophilic granules and, in some cases, distinctive red-staining needle-like structures known as Auer rods. Lymphoblasts contain neither cytoplasmic granules nor Auer rods.

(36) The Philadelphia chromosome, a reciprocal translocation from a long arm of chromosome 22 to chromosome 9, is a characteristic feature of chronic myelogenous leukemia (CML), present in about 95% of cases. It occurs uncommonly in acute leukemia. When present in either ALL (5% of childhood cases; 15% of adult cases) or AML (3% of cases), it is associated with poor prognosis. In contrast, the absence of the Philadelphia chromosome in CML is associated with a poor prognosis.

(37) Patients treated with chemotherapy and radiotherapy for Hodgkin's disease are at increased risk of developing AML and non-Hodgkin's lymphomas. ALL, however, does not occur with increased frequency in these patients (see Question 25).

(38, 40, 41) Clinical features are often helpful in differentiating ALL from AML. Generalized lymphadenopathy, splenomegaly, and hepatomegaly are characteristic of ALL but are not prominent in AML. Distinctive clinical features of AML include infiltration of gums (in M4 and M5 AML) and of soft tissues (in M1 and M3 AML) by tumor cells. Tumorous accumulations of AML cells in soft tissues often have a greenish color and are known as chloromas.

(43) The response to treatment is markedly different in ALL and AML. The ability to achieve complete remission in 90% and 5-year survival in 60% (most are cured) of children with ALL represents a triumph of

modern chemotherapy. Current treatment modalities for AML, in contrast, achieve long-term disease-free survival in only 10 to 15% of cases (*pp. 723–728*).

44. (C); 45. (D); 46. (A); 47. (D); 48. (B); 49. (A); 50. (B)

(**44 and 47**) Both idiopathic thrombocytopenic purpura (ITP) and thrombotic thrombocytopenic purpura (TTP) are hemorrhagic disorders related to reduced platelet numbers (hence increased bleeding time). The coagulation system is unaffected in these disorders (hence prothrombin time and partial thromboplastin time are usually normal).

(**45, 46, 49**) ITP is an autoimmune thrombocytopenia associated with antiplatelet antibodies. Although it usually appears as a primary disease, it sometimes occurs in association with another autoimmune disease such as systemic lupus erythematosus. Antibody-coated platelets are destroyed in the spleen, but the spleen remains normal in size. In the bone marrow, megakaryocytes are usually increased to compensate for the peripheral destruction of platelets. The disease can be effectively treated by steroids and/or splenectomy.

(**45, 48, 50**) TTP is a platelet consumption syndrome of unknown cause characterized by widespread platelet thrombi throughout the body, causing a microangiopathic hemolytic anemia. Although suspected to be immunologically mediated, there are no antiplatelet antibodies or immunologically mediated splenic platelet destruction. The immunologic injury may be primarily endothelial, predisposing to secondary platelet aggregation. This rare disorder is life threatening and uniformly fatal unless treated aggressively with corticosteroids, platelet aggregation inhibitors, and exchange transfusions. Even with treatment, many patients succumb (*pp. 693–695*).

51. (B); 52. (C); 53. (A); 54. (A); 55. (B)

(**51**) Only chronic leukemias with their insidious set and indolent course may be for a time asymptomatic; acute leukemias are characteristically abrupt in onset and highly symptomatic (fatigue, fever/infection, bleeding). This is the case whether the leukemia is lymphoid or myeloid in origin.

(**52, 53, 54, 55**) The vast majority of lymphocytic leukemias, both acute and chronic, are composed of transformed B cells. T-cell leukemias are rare. In ALL, the prognosis correlates with cytogenic factors such as the cell surface markers reflecting the degree of differentiation (maturation) of the B cells. For example, early precursor B-cell ALL has the most favorable prognosis. Hyperdiploidy in the range of 51 to 60 chromosomes is also associated with a good prognosis. There is no staging system for acute leukemia. In CLL, on the other hand, stage is the most important determinant of prognosis, and cytogenic factors are of undetermined significance. Most CLL cells express surface immunoglobulin (monoclonal kappa or lambda light chains) and are more mature than ALL cells but are unable to differentiate into plasma cells (*pp. 724, 729–730*).

56. (D); 57. (C); 58. (D); 59. (D); 60. (C); 61. (B); 62. (B); 63. (B); 64. (A); 65. (A); 66. (D); 67. (E)

Beta-thalassemia, paroxysmal nocturnal hemoglobinuria (PNH), sickle cell anemia, and glucose-6-phosphate dehydrogenase (G6PD) deficiency all are major forms of hemolytic anemias. The unique pathogenetic defect in each disorder produces characteristic features.

(**56**) G6PD deficiency produces derangements in the hexose monophosphate shunt and glutathione metabolism. Because glutathione is essential to red blood cell protection against oxidant injury, oxidant substances such as the antimalarial drugs trigger red blood cell injury and hemolysis in affected individuals. (**58**) Unique to this disorder are the hemolytic crises induced by ingestion of fava beans, which in some individuals are metabolized to a highly oxidant derivative. (**59**) Heinz bodies (precipitates of denatured hemoglobin) form within the red blood cells of G6PD-deficient individuals when oxidation of the sulfhydryl group of globin chains occurs. Heinz bodies contribute to the demise of the red blood cell in two ways: (1) They render the red cell membrane to which they are attached less deformable and more prone to sequestration in the spleen, and (2) when they are "pitted" from the cell by splenic macrophages, the resultant loss of cell membrane produces spherocytes that are themselves more susceptible to splenic sequestration. (**66**) Unlike the other forms of hemolytic anemias that produce chronic red blood cell destruction, G6PD deficiency produces intermittent bouts of acute hemolysis. It does not, therefore, lead to prolonged stimulation of erythropoietic production with expansion of the erythron in the bone marrow.

(**57**) Sickle cell anemia classically produces a unique if somewhat poorly understood depression of splenic function, even while the spleen is enlarged early in the course of the disease. The resultant splenic hypofunction predisposes to blood-borne infections, especially to those caused by *Salmonella* and pneumococci. Later in the course of the disease, the spleen may actually undergo autoinfarction as a result of repeated bouts of sickling in the sinuses, leading to thrombosis, hypoxic injury, and resultant scarring. Predisposition to bacterial infection is a major consequence of splenectomy (functional or otherwise) in any individual. (**60**) Because it is the deoxygenated form of sickle hemoglobin that undergoes polymerization and causes red blood cell deformation, hypoxia is the major stimulus to sickling and hemolytic crises.

(**61 and 62**) In contrast to thalassemia, sickle cell anemia, and G6PD deficiency, all of which affect red blood cell function only, PNH produces functional abnormalities in all hematopoietic cell lines. PNH is a disorder of myeloid stem cells characterized by a cell membrane defect that renders red blood cells as well as platelets and granulocytes more sensitive to lysis by complement. The striking predisposition to intravascular thromboses and infection is evidence of additional platelet and granulocyte abnormalities in individuals with PNH. (**63**) Supportive evidence that this unique form of hemolytic anemia is a stem cell disorder is its occasional transformation into other myeloid stem cell diseases such as acute myelogenous leukemia or aplastic anemia.

(64) Although the other forms of hemolytic anemia can be severe and debilitating, beta-thalassemia clearly has the worst prognosis. The disease produces such a profound, transfusion-dependent anemia that most patients die at an early age. Even with medical therapy, the average age at death is 17 years. (65) In this disorder, caused by a defect in the synthesis of beta-globin chains, red blood cell precursors are characteristically destroyed within the marrow. This occurs because the free alpha-globin chains form unstable intracellular aggregates that are injurious to the red blood cell precursors. In severely affected patients, it is estimated that 70 to 85% of the marrow normoblasts are destroyed in situ. This contrasts with the other forms of hemolytic anemia discussed earlier, in which red blood cell destruction is primarily extramedullary.

(67) All four of these diseases are the result of an intrinsic defect in the red blood cell. In contrast to autoimmune hemolytic anemias, which represent acquired defects of red blood cells and are often associated with autoantibodies to erythrocytes, these disorders are not associated with immunologically mediated red blood cell destruction (*pp. 665–675, 676–677*).

68. (A); 69. (C); 70. (D); 71. (B); 72. (A); 73. (A); 74. (E); 75. (A); 76. (B); 77. (B)

(68) Hemorrhagic disorders occur when an abnormality of vessel walls, platelets, coagulation factors, or a combination of these is present. In Cushing's syndrome, vascular fragility predisposing to skin hemorrhages results from the protein wasting effect of excessive corticosteroids.

(69) The hemorrhagic diathesis in uremia represents an acquired defect of platelet function. It is thought to occur as a consequence of impaired platelet membrane interaction with normal von Willebrand's factor.

(70) In von Willebrand's disease, on the other hand, the von Willebrand's factor (vWF) component of the factor VIII-vWF complex is qualitatively or quantitatively defective. Von Willebrand's factor is a series of polypeptide multimers of various sizes that are linked to the procoagulant protein of factor VIII, the enzymatic portion of the molecule responsible for the activation of factor X in the intrinsic coagulation pathway. The major function of vWF is facilitation of platelet adhesion to subendothelial collagen. Thus, a prolonged bleeding time (a measure of platelet function) and a marked tendency toward spontaneous bleeding occur in von Willbrand's disease.

(71) Because blood stored for longer than 24 hours is virtually depleted of platelets, massive transfusions can produce a hemorrhagic diathesis simply by diluting platelets to thrombocytopenic levels. In the presence of a normal bone marrow, the effect is transient.

(72) Widespread weakening of vascular walls with resultant hemorrhage is a common feature of hypersensitivity vasculitides. Henoch-Schönlein purpura is a prototypic example of immune complex-mediated vascular damage with a resultant hemorrhagic diathesis.

(73) Direct damage to the vascular wall occurs in certain infections caused by organisms that have the ability to invade vessels. Rickettsial infections, for example, classically cause vascular damage and a hemorrhagic diathesis.

(74) Disseminated intravascular coagulation is a well-known complication of promyelogenous leukemia (M3 subclass of AML). In this disorder, the release of procoagulant substances from the granules of the neoplastic promyelocytes activates the coagulation cascade, producing disseminated coagulation and an attendant hemorrhagic diathesis.

(75) Because vitamin C is required for cross-linking and other events in normal collagen metabolism, scurvy causes structural weakness of collagen in connective tissues and blood vessel walls (see Chapter 3, Question 9). Abnormal bleeding is the result of vascular fragility.

(76) Folate deficiency causes a megaloblastic anemia with defective production of all hematopoietic elements (see Chapter 3, Questions 49 and 50). Ineffective megakaryopoiesis results in thrombocytopenia and abnormal bleeding.

(77) Thrombocytopenia is also one of the most common hematologic manifestations of the acquired immunodeficiency syndrome (AIDS). It is thought to result from immune complex-mediated injury (*pp. 695–698, 726*).

78. (A); 79. (A); 80. (C); 81. (A); 82. (B); 83. (C); 84. (A)

Drugs and chemicals cause numerous hematologic problems. Although drug-related hematologic disorders are seldom completely predictable, many are repeatedly associated with particular drugs or drug classes. These hematologic effects are often among the most important complications of drug therapy.

(78) Penicillin is the prototype drug, which acts antigenically as a hapten. It combines with the red blood cell membrane, induces antibody production to the drug erythrocyte antigen complex, and produces a warm antibody autoimmune hemolytic anemia.

(79) Alpha-methyldopa is also a prototype drug associated with autoimmune hemolytic anemia, but in contrast to penicillin, it directly initiates the production of antibodies against intrinsic red blood cell antigens.

(80) Thiouracil is one of a small number of drugs that are often associated with agranulocytosis, probably on the basis of decreased production and/or increased destruction of neutrophils. Thiouracil may also cause an immunologically mediated destruction of mature neutrophils.

(81) Quinidine is another prototype drug responsible for the genesis of autoimmune hemolytic anemia. In contrast to both penicillin and alpha-methyldopa, the drug serves as a hapten that binds to a plasma protein; the drug-protein complex, in turn, evokes antibody production. It is the attachment of the resultant complement-fixing immune complexes to the red blood cell

membrane that is responsible for the red blood cell destruction. (84) Phenacetin is another drug associated with the induction of autoimmune hemolytic anemia by this same mechanism. (82) Benzene is a well-known cause of acquired aplastic anemia. It is one of a number of toxic drugs that cause myeloid stem cell damage in a dose-related manner.

(83) Along with thiouracil and certain sulfonamides, aminopyrine is one of the drugs associated with immunologically mediated agranulocytosis (*pp. 677–678, 688–689, 704*).

85. (B); 86. (C); 87. (B); 88. (A); 89. (D)

Reactive proliferations of white blood cells represent a normal host response to inflammatory stimuli. The relative degree of stimulation of each of the white blood cell series varies with the underlying cause. Certain inflammatory conditions classically stimulate one of the white blood cell lines much more than the others, a feature that can be helpful in diagnosis.

(**85 and 87**) An elevated lymphocyte count (lymphocytosis) is usually immunologic in origin. It often accompanies chronic inflammatory states with sustained immunologic stimulation such as tuberculosis. Lymphocytosis is also common in viral infections such as infectious mononucleosis, in which the primary host response is immunologic, and little acute inflammation is produced.

(86) Bronchial asthma is a prototypic example of a type I immune response with production of IgE that affixes to mast cells and stimulates mast cell degranulation on exposure to the inciting antigen (see Chapter 6, Question 27). Mast cells then release their eosinophil chemotactic factor, and an eosinophilic leukocytosis occurs.

(88) Elevated neutrophil counts (polymorphonuclear leukocytosis) characteristically occur in association with acute inflammatory states such as those produced by bacterial infection or tissue necrosis. The muscle necrosis that accompanies acute myocardial infarction classically produces this response.

(89) Eosinophilic granuloma is a proliferative disorder of histiocytes. Its cause is unknown. Eosinophils are a variable though frequently prominent feature of the parenchymal lesions that usually involve the bone marrow. However, systemic elevation of eosinophils does not usually occur, and the standard hematologic tests tend to be nondiagnostic in this disease (*pp. 705–706*).

90. (B); 91. (A); 92. (A); 93. (D); 94. (C)

(**91 and 92**) Proliferative disorders of Langerhans cells (antigen-presenting dendritic histiocytes) vary widely in their clinical and pathologic behavior. The Letterer-Siwe syndrome, also known as acute disseminated Langerhans cell histiocytosis, is an acute systemic proliferation of Langerhans cells that has an aggressive clinical course. It typically occurs in infants and young children before the age of 3 and is sometimes present at birth. Although the course of the condition is variable (from 6 months to 2 years), it is uniformly fatal, and in general, the younger the age of the patient, the more rapid the course of the disease. However, intensive chemotherapy has dramatically altered the outlook for this disease. The 5-year survival is 90% for patients without visceral involvement and 40 to 50% for those with organ dysfunction.

(90) In contrast to the devastating diffuse disease of the Letterer-Siwe syndrome, multifocal Langerhans cell histiocytosis (formerly known as Hand-Schüller-Christian disease) is relatively benign. The lesions spontaneously resolve in half the cases, and in the other half, they are cured by chemotherapy. Multifocal Langerhans cell histiocytosis is characterized by histiocytic infiltrates in multiple tissues and is typically accompanied by a diffuse skin eruption. The classic triad of organ involvement in this disease is (1) infiltration of the posterior pituitary stalk or hypothalamus leading to diabetes insipidus, (2) orbital involvement with exophthalmos, and (3) calvarial bone defects. However, only a minority of patients have the complete triad.

(93) In all of these syndromes of Langerhans cell proliferation, the cells contain unique rod-shaped cytoplasmic inclusions called pentalaminar bodies or HX bodies, which can be seen by electron microscopic examination.

(94) In the Letterer-Siwe syndrome, a diffuse macropapular, eczematous, or purpuric skin rash is often present as mentioned earlier, and a seborrhea-like skin eruption is typically present in Hand-Schüller-Christian disease. Only in unifocal Langerhans cell histiocytosis (eosinophilic granuloma) is involvement limited to the marrow cavity of the bone; skin (and other systemic) involvement is characteristically absent (*pp. 745–747*).

The Gastrointestinal Tract

DIRECTIONS: For Questions 1 to 12, choose the ONE BEST answer to each question.

1. Hiatal hernia is associated with all of the following pathologic lesions EXCEPT:

A. Esophageal webs
B. Acute esophagitis
C. Barrett's esophagus
D. Esophageal scarring
E. Esophageal tears

2. Abnormalities associated with achalasia include all of the following EXCEPT:

A. Incomplete relaxation of the lower esophageal sphincter
B. Lack of peristalsis in the esophagus
C. Loss of myenteric ganglion cells in the esophagus
D. Increased basal tone of the lower esophageal sphincter
E. Stenotic muscle hypertrophy of the lower esophageal sphincter

3. Cancer patients receiving medical treatment often develop esophagitis from all of the following EXCEPT:

A. Antibiotic toxicity
B. Viral infection
C. Chemotherapeutic agent toxicity
D. Radiation damage
E. Fungal infection

4. Esophageal disorders that are associated with pulmonary aspiration include all of the following EXCEPT:

A. Esophageal diverticula
B. Achalasia
C. Esophageal scleroderma
D. Viral esophagitis
E. Esophageal carcinoma

5. The acute gastric ulcerations known as Cushing's ulcers occur in patients who:

A. Ingest exogenous corticosteroids
B. Have severe sepsis
C. Have brain tumors
D. Have extensive burns
E. Have Cushing's syndrome

6. Mucosal ulceration is a characteristic histologic feature of all of the following causes of enterocolitis EXCEPT:

A. *Entamoeba histolytica* infection
B. Radiation to the bowel
C. *Campylobacter jejuni* infection
D. *Yersinia enterocolitica* infection
E. Rotavirus infection

7. All of the following statements about congenital megacolon (Hirschsprung's disease) are true EXCEPT:

A. Both Meissner's and Auerbach's plexuses fail to develop
B. Involvement of the entire colon is rare
C. The incidence is higher in patients with Down's syndrome
D. Massive dilatation of the affected bowel segment is characteristic
E. Surgical excision of the affected segment is curative

8. In the United States, the most likely cause of the form of enterocolitis pictured in Figure 8–1 is:

A. Ingestion of the infectious agent from an exogenous source
B. Reactivation of previous enteric infection

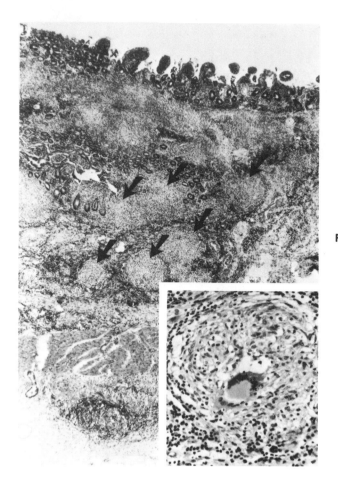

Figure 8–1

C. Blood-borne spread from another focus of infection in the body
D. Swallowing of organisms coughed up from a pulmonary source of infection
E. None of these

9. All of the following statements about small bowel neoplasms are true EXCEPT:

A. They account for less than 10% of all gastrointestinal tumors
B. Malignant tumors are more prevalent than benign tumors
C. Adenomatous polyps are the most common type of benign tumor
D. Large adenomas of the small bowel often undergo malignant transformation
E. Malignant lymphoma occurs more frequently than adenocarcinoma

10. All of the following statements about celiac sprue are true EXCEPT:

A. It is associated with specific histocompatibility antigen (HLA) profiles
B. The disorder is cured by a gluten-free diet

C. The disease is characterized histologically by diffuse flattening of mucosal villi
D. The distal (ileal) portion of the small bowel is the predominant site of injury
E. The disease is associated with an increased incidence of primary gastrointestinal lymphoma

11. Characteristic gross features of a benign (peptic) gastric ulcer include all of the following EXCEPT:

A. Location on the lesser curvature
B. Small size (less than 3 cm)
C. Heaped-up margins
D. Smooth base
E. Radial arrangement (puckering) of surrounding mucosal folds

12. The lesion pictured in Figure 8–2 is correctly described as:

A. A hamartoma
B. Occurring in long-standing inflammatory bowel disease
C. Associated with orofacial melanotic pigmentation
D. Associated with multiple osteomas
E. Having high potential for malignant transformation

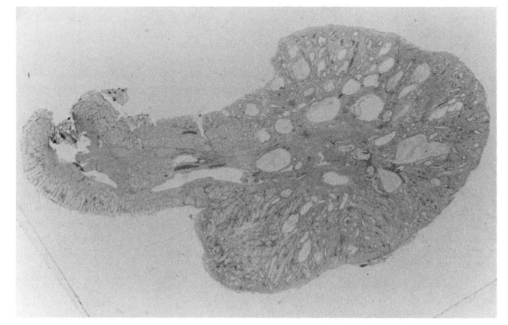

Figure 8–2

DIRECTIONS: For Questions 13 to 26, ONE or MORE of the completions given correctly finishes the incomplete statement. Choose:

A—if only *1, 2, and 3* are correct
B—if only *1 and 3* are correct
C—if only *2 and 4* are correct
D—if only *4* is correct
E—if all of these are correct

13. The lower esophageal sphincter is known to:

1. Require vagal innervation for relaxation
2. Prevent reflux of gastric contents
3. Relax in response to the swallowing reflex
4. Relax in response to gastrin

A. 1,2,3   B. 1,3   C. 2,4   D. 4 Only   E. All

14. Esophageal webs are correctly described as:

1. Morphologically identical to lower esophageal rings
2. Occurring almost exclusively in men
3. Frequently associated with hypochlorhydria
4. Composed of constricting bands of subepithelial fibrosis (scar)

A. 1,2,3   B. 1,3   C. 2,4   D. 4 Only   E. All

15. Which of the following factors are causally related to the development of reflux esophagitis?

1. Lower esophageal sphincter incompetence
2. Bile content of refluxed material
3. Esophageal motility dysfunction
4. Acid and pepsin content of refluxed material

A. 1,2,3   B. 1,3   C. 2,4   D. 4 Only   E. All

16. Which of the following characteristics are likely to be found in association with Barrett's esophagus?

1. Pseudomembrane formation
2. Metaplastic gastric parietal cells
3. Nuclear inclusion bodies
4. Adenocarcinoma of the esophagus

A. 1,2,3   B. 1,3   C. 2,4   D. 4 Only   E. All

17. Which of the following factors stimulate gastric acid secretion?

1. Gastric distention
2. Digested proteins in the small bowel
3. Histamine
4. Damage to the gastric mucosal barrier

A. 1,2,3   B. 1,3   C. 2,4   D. 4 Only   E. All

18. Which of the statements listed below describe angiodysplasia of the colon?

1. Multiple small arterial aneurysms are present in the submucosa
2. The sigmoid colon is most frequently involved
3. The disorder represents a congenital defect in the vascular media
4. Angiography is required for clinical diagnosis

A. 1,2,3   B. 1,3   C. 2,4   D. 4 Only   E. All

19. Melanosis coli is correctly described as:

1. Virtually always asymptomatic
2. Involving the small bowel in about 50% of cases
3. Associated with chronic laxative abuse
4. Associated with cutaneous malignant melanoma

    A. 1,2,3 B. 1,3 C. 2,4 D. 4 Only E. All

20. Antibiotic-associated pseudomembranous colitis is an inflammatory disorder that is:

1. Particularly related to clindamycin administration
2. Grossly similar to ischemic colitis
3. Curable with vancomycin therapy
4. Caused by mucosal invasion by *Clostridium difficile*

    A. 1,2,3 B. 1,3 C. 2,4 D. 4 Only E. All

21. Acute appendicitis is correctly characterized as:

1. Mainly a disease of adolescents
2. Most commonly confused clinically with mesenteric lymphadenitis
3. Accompanied by luminal obstruction in most cases
4. Diagnosed histologically by massive lymphoid hyperplasia in the submucosa

    A. 1,2,3 B. 1,3 C. 2,4 D. 4 Only E. All

22. Histologic changes commonly seen in reflux esophagitis include:

1. Elongated mucosal papillae
2. Hyperplasia of the mucosal basal zone
3. Intraepithelial eosinophils
4. Submucosal varices

    A. 1,2,3 B. 1,3 C. 2,4 D. 4 Only E. All

23. Primary gastric lymphoma is accurately described as:

1. The most common gastrointestinal lymphoma
2. Almost always a B-cell tumor
3. Having a better prognosis than other gastrointestinal lymphomas
4. Usually arising in the perigastric lymph nodes

    A. 1,2,3 B. 1,3 C. 2,4 D. 4 Only E. All

24. Acquired disaccharidase deficiency

1. Is caused by a hypersensitivity immune response to milk (lactose)
2. Produces a malabsorption syndrome
3. Characteristically shows mucosal eosinophilic abscesses on biopsy
4. Is treated by dietary restriction

    A. 1,2,3 B. 1,3 C. 2,4 D. 4 Only E. All

25. The lesion pictured in Figure 8–3 is a defect that:

1. Occurs most often in children
2. Depends on peristalsis for development
3. Causes intestinal obstruction
4. Causes intestinal infarction

    A. 1,2,3 B. 1,3 C. 2,4 D. 4 Only E. All

26. Figure 8–4 illustrates a lesion that:

1. Characteristically produces watery diarrhea
2. Is often associated with concomitant autoimmune disease
3. Frequently shows no mucosal abnormality on colonoscopy
4. Rarely occurs in children

    A. 1,2,3 B. 1,3 C. 2,4 D. 4 Only E. All

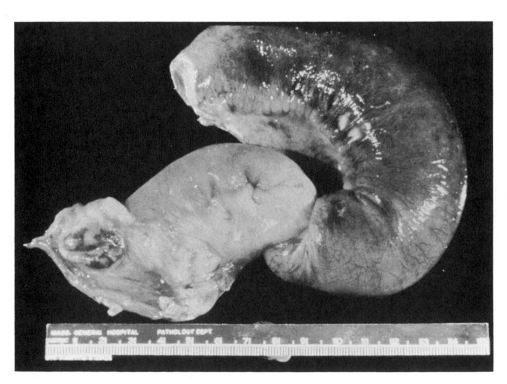

Figure 8–3

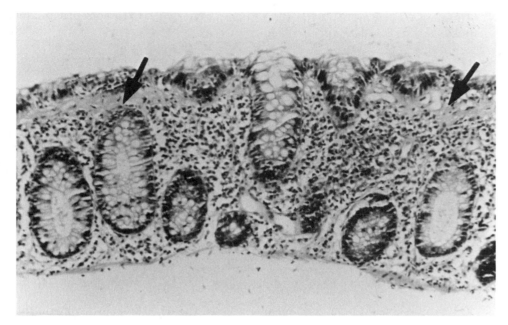

Figure 8-4

DIRECTIONS: For Questions 27 to 66, you are to decide whether EACH choice is TRUE or FALSE.

For each of the following statements about the normal esophagus, choose whether it is TRUE or FALSE.

27. The mucosa is composed of squamous epithelium that does not keratinize

28. The serosal surface is lined by a single layer of mesothelial cells

29. The wall of the upper third of the esophagus is composed of striated muscle

30. Esophageal sphincters are composed of hypertrophied segments of muscularis mucosae

31. The lumen narrows at the level of the bifurcation of the trachea

For each of the following statements about esophageal varices, choose whether it is TRUE or FALSE.

32. They occur in most patients with alcoholic cirrhosis

33. They are rarely produced by biliary cirrhosis

34. They are a common cause of epigastric pain in alcoholic patients

35. Rupture has a high mortality rate

For each of the following statements about chronic peptic ulcer disease (CPUD), choose whether it is TRUE or FALSE.

36. Peptic ulcers occur most commonly in the stomach

37. Peptic ulcers occur most often as solitary lesions

38. CPUD does not develop in individuals with achlorhydria

39. Genetic predisposition is demonstrated only for duodenal CPUD

40. Most patients with gastric CPUD secrete abnormally high levels of gastric acid

41. Most patients with duodenal CPUD secrete abnormally high levels of gastric acid

42. Most patients with gastric peptic ulcer also have chronic gastritis

43. Most gastric carcinomas arise in gastric peptic ulcers

44. Most duodenal carcinomas arise in duodenal peptic ulcers

For each of the following statements about diverticular disease of the colon, choose whether it is TRUE or FALSE.

45. About half of Americans older than 60 years are affected

46. Diverticula are aneurysmic outpouchings of mural smooth muscle (muscularis propria)

47. The cecum is the colonic region most frequently affected

48. The muscularis propria of the affected colonic segment is characteristically hypertrophied

49. Diverticulitis is usually initiated by diverticular perforation

50. High-fiber diets have been shown to prevent development of the disease

51. Surgical resection is required for most patients with acute inflammatory disease

For each of the following statements about carcinoma of the colon in the United States, choose whether it is TRUE or FALSE.

52. It causes more deaths than any other form of cancer

53. High incidence is related to low dietary fiber

54. The right colon is the most commonly affected site

55. The vast majority arise from adenomatous polyps

56. Stage is the most important prognostic factor

57. Carcinoembryonic antigen (CEA) is produced by most tumors

58. Tumors that produce copious mucin have a better prognosis

59. Testing for occult blood in stool is a sensitive screening modality

60. Surgical resection of early lesions is usually curative

For each of the following statements about carcinoid tumors, choose whether it is TRUE or FALSE.

61. They occur in the lung more often than in the gastrointestinal tract

62. Their degree of histologic atypia (grade) usually correlates well with their metastatic potential

63. They can be identified positively by their cytoplasmic secretory granules

64. Those arising in the appendix rarely metastasize

65. Small bowel carcinoid tumors do not produce the carcinoid syndrome in the absence of liver metastasis

66. Gastrointestinal carcinoids are associated with an increased incidence of other malignant tumors of the gastrointestinal tract

DIRECTIONS: For Questions 67 to 119, the set of lettered headings is followed by a list of numbered words or phrases. For each numbered word or phrase choose:

    A—if the item is associated with (A) only
    B—if the item is associated with (B) only
    C—if the item is associated with *both* (A) and (B)
    D—if the item is associated with *neither* (A) nor (B)

For each of the statements listed below, choose whether it describes esophageal carcinoma, gastric carcinoma, both, or neither.

    A. Esophageal carcinoma
    B. Gastric carcinoma
    C. Both
    D. Neither

67. Almost all tumors are adenocarcinomas

68. Blacks are affected more often than whites

69. Dietary factors are important in the pathogenesis

70. Cigarette smoking is a significant risk factor

71. Alcohol abuse is a significant risk factor

72. Chronic inflammation in the organ of origin is a risk factor

73. Epigastric pain typically develops as an early symptom

74. Krukenberg's tumors of the ovary occur as a complication

For each of the characteristics listed below, choose whether it describes acute gastritis, chronic gastritis, both, or neither.

    A. Acute gastritis
    B. Chronic type B environmental gastritis
    C. Both
    D. Neither

75. Associated with alcohol consumption

76. Associated with cigarette smoking

77. Causally related to autoantibodies against gastric mucosal cells

78. Causally related to gastric mucosal hypoperfusion

79. Associated with the use of aspirin

80. Productive of gastrointestinal bleeding

81. Associated with gastric peptic ulcers

82. Associated with infection by *Campylobacter pylori*

For each of the features listed below, choose whether it describes Ménétrier's disease, the Zollinger-Ellison syndrome, both, or neither.

    A. Ménétrier's disease
    B. Zollinger-Ellison syndrome
    C. Both
    D. Neither

83. Marked enlargement of gastric rugal folds is characteristic

84. Parietal and chief cell hyperplasia are common histologic features

85. Excessive protein loss is an associated complication

86. The risk of developing gastric lymphoma is increased

87. The risk of developing gastric carcinoma is increased

88. Pancreatic tumors are associated findings

89. Pheochromocytoma and medullary carcinoma of the thyroid are associated disorders

For each of the characteristics listed below, choose whether it describes hyperplastic gastric polyps, adenomatous gastric polyps, both, or neither.

    A. Hyperplastic gastric polyps
    B. Adenomatous gastric polyps
    C. Both
    D. Neither

90. Tend to be large (greater than 3 cm)

91. Usually occur in multiple numbers

92. Are commonly asymptomatic

93. Frequently undergo malignant transformation

94. Are often associated with carcinoma elsewhere in the stomach

For each of the features of inflammatory bowel disease listed below, choose whether it describes Crohn's disease, ulcerative colitis, both, or neither.

    A. Crohn's disease
    B. Ulcerative colitis

    C. Both
    D. Neither

95. Lesions occur at any level of the enteric tract

96. Organ systems other than the enteric tract are occasionally involved

97. The presence of granulomas is pathognomonic

98. Viral particles are usually found in diseased bowel

99. The disorder is associated with histocompatibility antigen HLA-B27

100. Affected bowel usually becomes thickened and narrowed

101. Toxic megacolon is an occasional complication

102. Distribution of lesions is generally discontinuous

103. Fissures and fistulas are characteristic

104. Incidence of gastrointestinal carcinoma is increased

105. Incidence of primary gastrointestinal lymphoma is increased

For each of the features listed below, choose whether it describes ischemic bowel disease producing transmural infarction, mucosal infarction, both, or neither.

    A. Transmural bowel infarction
    B. Mucosal bowel infarction
    C. Both
    D. Neither

106. Principally affects the small bowel

107. Results from venous thrombosis

108. Produced by arterial occlusion

109. Produced by atherosclerosis and hypotension

110. Produced by hypotension alone

111. Grossly appears hemorrhagic

112. Associated with a high mortality rate

For each of the characteristics listed below, choose whether it describes tropical sprue, Whipple's disease, both, or neither.

    A. Tropical sprue
    B. Whipple's disease
    C. Both
    D. Neither

113. The disease causes a malabsorption syndrome

114. History of travel to an endemic area is essential to the diagnosis

115. Small bowel biopsy frequently shows flattened villi

116. Antibiotic therapy is usually curative

117. Systemic disease is present in addition to bowel involvement

118. Macrophages laden with rod-shaped bacteria are found in the small bowel mucosa

119. The disease is associated with an increased risk of small bowel lymphoma

DIRECTIONS: Questions 120 to 151 are matching questions. For each numbered item, choose the most likely associated lettered item from those provided. Each numbered item has ONLY ONE answer. Within each group, each lettered item may be the answer to one, more than one, or none of the numbered items.

For each of the congenital gastrointestinal tract anomalies listed below, choose whether it most commonly afflicts the esophagus, stomach, small bowel, or large bowel.

    A. Esophagus
    B. Stomach
    C. Small bowel
    D. Large bowel

120. Congenital atresia

121. Congenital stenosis

122. Congenital duplication

123. Congenital diverticula

124. Congenital absence of ganglion cells

For each of the characteristics listed below, choose whether it is characteristic of the gastric cardia, corpus (body), antrum, all of these regions, or none of these.

    A. Cardia
    B. Corpus (body)
    C. Antrum
    D. All of these
    E. None of these

125. Gastrin production

126. Pepsin secretion

127. Intrinsic factor production

128. Location of endocrine (enterochromaffin) cells

129. Location of goblet cells

130. Location of Paneth's cells

For each of the features listed below, choose whether it is characteristic of the duodenum, jejunum, ileum, all of these segments of small bowel, or none of these.

    A. Duodenum
    B. Jejunum
    C. Ileum
    D. All of these
    E. None of these

131. Paneth's cells

132. Peyer's patches

133. Brunner's glands

134. Serotonin-secreting endocrine cells

135. Vitamin B_{12}-intrinsic factor absorption

136. Meckel's diverticula

137. Pancreatic rests

For each of the characteristics listed below, choose whether it describes *Salmonella* enterocolitis, *Shigella* enterocolitis, cholera, or none of these.

    A. *Salmonella* enterocolitis
    B. *Shigella* enterocolitis
    C. Cholera
    D. None of these

138. Shallow mucosal ulcers are typically produced

139. Submucosal lymphoid hyperplasia is a characteristic feature

140. Submucosal granulomas are a characteristic histologic feature

141. The causative organism does not invade the mucosal lining

142. The causative organism does not produce toxins

143. The large bowel is preferentially involved

144. The etiologic agent is a common cause of ulcero-inflammatory proctitis in homosexual males

For each of the features of colonic polyps listed below, choose whether it describes the hyperplastic polyp, tubular adenoma, villous adenoma, or hamartomatous polyp.

    A. Hyperplastic polyp
    B. Tubular adenoma
    C. Villous adenoma
    D. Hamartomatous polyp

145. Most common type of colonic polyp

146. Largest colonic polyp overall

147. Greatest likelihood of harboring cancer

148. Typically occurs in familial polyposis coli

149. Typically occurs in the Peutz-Jeghers syndrome

150. Occasionally causes a protein-losing enteropathy

151. Characterized histologically by mucin-filled cysts lined by goblet cells

The Gastrointestinal Tract

1. (A) Hiatal hernia is a disorder in which the proximal portion of the stomach herniates through the diaphragmatic hiatus into the thorax. The competence of the lower esophageal sphincter is compromised, and reflux of gastric contents into the lower esophagus occurs. Thus, acute esophagitis is commonly produced (reflux esophagitis), causing symptoms of retrosternal burning pain. In a small percentage of these patients, persistent reflux esophagitis leads to adenomatous metaplasia of the lower esophageal epithelium, a condition known as Barrett's esophagus. In severe cases, postinflammatory esophageal scarring may result. Small esophageal lacerations (Mallory-Weiss tears) have also been reported in association with underlying hiatal hernias that appear to potentiate abnormal esophageal dilatation in instances of increased intragastric pressure. Although hiatal hernia is twice as common in patients with lower esophageal ring as in the otherwise normal population, there is no increased incidence of hiatal hernia in patients with esophageal webs *(pp. 829–833)*.

2. (E) Achalasia is an uncommon disorder of esophageal motility; its pathogenesis is still poorly understood. The disease appears to represent a complex of functional abnormalities of the esophageal musculature. Primary among these defects is the failure of relaxation of the lower esophageal sphincter in advance of the propulsive peristaltic wave. In addition, diffuse esophageal spasm with aperistalsis and increased basal tone of the lower esophageal sphincter have also been noted. Although the cause remains controversial, most studies show a loss of myenteric ganglion cells in the body of the esophagus. Muscle hypertrophy of the lower esophageal sphincter is not a feature of achalasia. The obstruction in achalasia is functional/neurologic in character rather than stenotic/physical *(p. 829)*.

3. (A) Esophagitis is a common problem among cancer patients and may result from a variety of factors. Cytotoxic chemotherapeutic drugs frequently cause esophageal damage and inflammation, as does therapeutic radiation. Furthermore, anticancer therapy produces immunologic deficiencies that predispose to viral and fungal infections of the esophagus. Although antibiotic therapy may be associated with fungal infections of the esophagus, direct toxic damage to the esophageal mucosa is rarely caused by antibiotics *(p. 832)*.

4. (D) Esophageal disorders that lead to chronic regurgitation of ingested substances are often associated with pulmonary aspiration. Esophageal diverticula may become overdistended with food, leading directly to regurgitation and pulmonary aspiration. Esophageal diverticula are also associated with other disorders of esophageal motor function, including achalasia (see Question 2), hiatal hernia (see Question 1), and esophageal ring, which may themselves be primary causes of chronic regurgitation. When scleroderma (systemic sclerosis) involves the esophagus, it produces fibrosis of the submucosa and muscular wall, producing a narrowed esophagus with markedly abnormal motor function; chronic regurgitation is a common consequence. Esophageal carcinoma may lead to pulmonary aspiration through several mechanisms. Progressive dysphagia and obstruction may occur from intraluminal growth of fungating tumors, whereas infiltrating tumors may invade nerves and muscles, producing motor dysfunction. Furthermore, invasive esophageal carcinoma may occasionally produce a tracheoesophageal fistula through which ingested material can be aspirated directly into the bronchial tree. Viral esophagitis, most commonly caused by herpes simplex virus or cytomegalovirus, produces superficial mucosal disease only (small discrete ulcerations). It does not produce obstruction or motor dysfunction of the esophagus and is not associated with aspiration pneumonia *(pp. 829–831, 832, 837)*.

5. (C) Focal acute gastric mucosal ulcerations are essentially a severe form of acute erosive gastritis and are known to occur in a number of well-defined, biologically stressful situations. Those that occur in association with conditions that raise intracranial pressure, such as brain tumors, head trauma, or intracranial surgery, are known as Cushing's ulcers, after the great neurosurgeon Harvey Cushing, who described them. Increased intracranial pressure is believed to stimulate vagal nuclei, causing hypersecretion of gastric acid, a phenomenon that has only been documented with Cushing's ulcers. In addition, neurogenic or catecholamine-induced vasoconstriction with mucosal hypoperfusion and injury contributes to their pathogenesis. Morphologically indistinguishable lesions are produced in other stressful conditions such as extensive burns (Curling's ulcers) and severe sepsis.

Although Cushing's ulcers are not a feature of Cushing's syndrome (a clinical and metabolic disorder resulting from excess production of cortisol), gastric erosions may occur in association with exogenous corticosteroid ingestion. Corticosteroids, as well as other agents including aspirin, ethanol, cigarette smoke, indomethacin, and phenylbutazone, are believed to be ulcerogenic to the gastric mucosa at least in part because they potentiate the appearance of stress lesions *(p. 848)*.

6. (E) Mucosal ulceration in the affected bowel is characteristic of a number of infectious agents, including *Entamoeba histolytica*, *Campylobacter jejuni*, and *Yersinia enterocolitica*. Radiation-induced or ischemia-induced enteritis can also produce mucosal ulceration that may mimic infectious enteritis. Only when specific causes of mucosal ulceration have been ruled out can the diagnosis of idiopathic inflammatory disease (ulcerative colitis or Crohn's disease) be made.

Rotavirus is an important cause of viral gastroenteritis in infants and children. Although severe diarrhea may result, mucosal ulceration of the bowel is usually not observed *(pp. 317, 357–358, 865–867)*.

7. (D) Hirschsprung's disease is a congenital anomaly of the colon caused by failure of development of both Meissner's and Auerbach's plexuses. Neuroblasts from the neural crest fail to complete their distal migration, leaving a portion of distal colon devoid of ganglion cells. In more than 80% of cases, only the rectum or rectosigmoid colon is involved. Involvement of the entire colon is extremely rare. Hirschsprung's disease may occur as an isolated lesion but is often associated with other congenital anomalies. It is ten times more common in patients with Down's syndrome than in the general population. The disorder can be cured by surgical excision of the affected segment, which is not usually dilated. The dilated proximal bowel is usually normal; it becomes dilated with accumulated fecal material that cannot be moved through the aganglionic, aperistaltic segment *(pp. 883–884)*.

8. (D) In Figure 8–1, the numerous granulomas within the bowel wall strongly suggest the diagnosis of gastrointestinal tuberculosis, although definitive diagnosis of this entity requires the identification of acid-fast bacilli within the lesions by histochemical stain or by microbial culture. In the United States, involvement of the gastrointestinal tract by a mycobacterial organism is most commonly a secondary consequence of primary pulmonary tuberculosis. Organisms from a primary pulmonary focus are coughed up and swallowed, thereby gaining access to the gastrointestinal tract. With the eradication of *Mycobacterium bovis* infection from contaminated cows, primary bovine tuberculosis of the gastrointestinal tract has been virtually eliminated in the United States. Thus, reactivation of a previous primary gastrointestinal infection is uncommon. Although any organ may be involved in systemic infection with *Mycobacterium tuberculosis*, blood-borne spread to the gastrointestinal tract is much less common than direct infection from swallowed contaminated mucus originating from a pulmonary focus as discussed earlier *(pp. 378, 866)*.

9. (C) Neoplasms of the small intestine, whether benign or malignant, are rare entities. All together they account for only 3 to 6% of all gastrointestinal tumors. Benign tumors are even less common than malignant tumors in the small bowel. Of the benign tumors, leiomyomas are the most common, but adenomatous polyps are the most important. As in the large bowel, large adenomatous polyps often undergo transformation to adenocarcinoma. Nevertheless, the incidence of adenocarcinoma of the small bowel is very low. It occurs less frequently than either malignant carcinoid tumor or primary lymphoma in that site; thus, reports vary as to whether adenocarcinoma or primary lymphoma is the most frequent form of malignancy in the small intestine *(pp. 858–859, 872–875)*.

10. (C) Celiac sprue (gluten-sensitive enteropathy or nontropical sprue) is an immunologically mediated reaction to the gliadin constituent of dietary gluten that causes small bowel mucosal injury and malabsorption. It is known to have a genetic predisposition and is associated with HLA-B8 and HLA-D/DR3 or HLA-D/DR7 histocompatibility antigens in most cases. The disorder responds dramatically to a gluten-free diet, and definitive diagnosis is based on this characteristic. Histologically, the disorder is characterized by flattening of the small intestinal mucosal villi, although this feature is not pathognomonic for celiac sprue. Increased numbers of IgA-bearing lymphocytes and plasma cells are also present in the lamina propria. Furthermore, in many patients, antibodies to gliadin can be demonstrated in the serum. The disease is also associated with an increased incidence of primary gastrointestinal tract lymphomas as well as carcinomas.

The pathologic changes in celiac sprue are typically more pronounced in the proximal small bowel because the highest concentrations of gliadin are present there. The predominantly proximal distribution of the injury helps to differentiate celiac sprue from tropical sprue. Although tropical sprue may produce mucosal pathology indistinguishable from celiac disease, it often affects the distal small bowel exclusively *(pp. 876–877)*.

11. (C) Endoscopic or radiologic diagnosis of benign gastric ulcers is based on distinguishing (virtually diagnostic) gross features that make it possible to differentiate them with great accuracy from ulcerating gastric cancers. Gastric peptic ulcers are characteristically small (i.e., usually less than 2 cm in diameter), round to oval, sharply demarcated ("punched-out") defects with straight walls. They are most often located on the lesser curvature at the interface between the gastric antrum and body. Although 40% of gastric cancers occur on the lesser curvature, they are often larger than benign lesions (i.e., usually greater than 4 cm in diameter) and have an irregular contour. The base of a benign tumor is composed of smooth scar tissue, cleaned of debris by peptic digestion. The base of a malignant ulcer is composed of bumpy tumor tissue. The edges of benign ulcers are slightly puffy from edema and inflammation but are not unevenly heaped up and beaded like the edges of an expanding malignancy. Finally, contraction of the scar tissue at the base of a benign ulcer tends to draw the surrounding mucosa centripetally; consequently, the folds of the tethered mucosa fan out radially from the ulcer crater. This feature is characteristically lacking in malignant ulcers *(pp. 850–853, 858)*.

12. (A) The lesion pictured in Figure 8–2 is a juvenile polyp. These tumors are hamartomatous growths i.e., proliferations of cytologically normal colonic glands and lamina propria arranged in a haphazard abnormal fashion. They are easily recognized by their relatively smooth surface and rounded contour, cystically dilated mucin-filled glands and abundant lamina propria. Most commonly, they occur as solitary sporadic lesions in the rectums of children less than 5 years of age and have no malignant potential. However, in the inherited juvenile polyposis syndrome, they are multiple, distributed throughout the gastrointestinal tract, and are associated with an increased risk of colon cancer.

Polyps that occur in long-standing inflammatory bowel disease are known as inflammatory polyps or pseudopolyps. They are not neoplasms but represent mucosal reparation and proliferation in response to chronic injury.

In the Peutz-Jeghers syndrome, hamartomatous polyps occur in association with orofacial melanotic pigmentation. However, Peutz-Jeghers polyps are histologically distinct from juvenile polyps. They are composed of tightly packed, highly arborized glands with little intervening lamina propria, and their mucosa is typically partitioned by bands of smooth muscle, a component that juvenile polyps lack altogether.

In Gardner's syndrome, large numbers of colonic polyps occur in association with multiple osteomas, epidermal cysts, and fibromatosis. The polyps of Gardner's syndrome are adenomas and have a high probability of transformation. In fact, the incidence of colon cancer in Gardner's syndrome is 100% at 30 years, the same as in familial polyposis coli (the prototypic adenomatous polyposis syndrome) *(pp. 891–897)*.

13. (A) Although the lower esophageal sphincter mainly functions to prevent reflux of gastric contents into the esophagus, it opens at the proper time to allow the passage of food and fluid from the esophagus to the stomach. Relaxation of the lower esophageal sphincter requires vagal innervation and the transmission of vagal stimuli through Auerbach's plexus to the sphincter muscle. The sphincter opens in anticipation of the peristaltic wave and closes again after the swallowing reflex.

Rather than relaxing the sphincter, gastrin acts to increase the sphincter tone, maintaining sphincter competence and preventing reflux of the ingested material that stimulated the hormone's release *(p. 828)*.

14. (B) Although they occur at different levels of the esophagus, esophageal webs (upper esophagus) and esophageal rings (lower esophagus) are morphologically identical lesions. These lesions are composed of overhanging folds of esophageal mucosa, often circumferential, that constrict the lumen and produce dysphagia. Esophageal webs are found almost exclusively in women and may be associated with hypochlorhydria (the Plummer-Vinson syndrome). Although esophageal webs must be differentiated from strictures as a cause of obstruction and dysphagia, these delicate mucosal folds contrast dramatically with the postinjury subepithelial scar formation that characterizes esophageal strictures *(pp. 829–830)*.

15. (E) The most common cause of inflammatory disorder of the esophagus is reflux esophagitis. It is a multifactorial disorder and has been shown to be related to frequent and protracted reflux of gastric juice. Thus, incompetence of the lower esophageal sphincter is an important predisposing factor. Acid and pepsin as well as bile and lysolecithin in the refluxed fluid create the injury and inflammation. In addition, disordered esophageal motility contributes by permitting prolonged contact of the esophageal mucosa with caustic refluxed material *(pp. 832–834)*.

16. (C) Barrett's esophagus, a consequence of chronic gastrointestinal reflux, is characterized by metaplastic transformation of the stratified squamous epithelium of the normal esophageal mucosa to a columnar, secretory-type epithelium. Three types of metaplastic secretory epithelia have been described: (1) intestinal type with goblet cells and absorptive cells, (2) gastric antral type with mucus-secreting epithelial surface cells, and (3) gastric fundic type with both parietal cells and chief cells. The most important consequence of these metaplastic structures is an increased risk of adenocarcinoma of the esophagus, an otherwise rare entity.

Pseudomembrane formation typically occurs as a result of the severe mucosal injury of monilial esophagitis. Nuclear inclusion bodies occur in viral esophagitis produced by herpes or cytomegalovirus. Neither pseudomembranes nor intranuclear inclusions occur with esophageal reflux *(pp. 832–834)*.

17. (E) Stimuli for the secretion of gastric acid are numerous and varied. Chemical, mechanical, neurologic, and hormonal factors are known to be involved in the secretory process. Parasympathetic (vagal) stimulation of gastric parietal cells is the final common pathway for stimuli such as the sight, smell, and taste of food (the cephalic phase of stimulation) and gastric distention (mechanical stimulation during the gastric phase). Independently of vagal input, digested proteins and amino acids chemically stimulate the release of gastrins by antral endocrine cells (G cells) during the gastric phase. Gastrins are the most potent of all stimuli to gastric acid secretion. The physiologic role of histamine is still poorly understood, but it is clear that histamine acts as a potent acid secretagogue by activating adenyl cyclase and raising cyclic AMP levels within the parietal cell. In fact, blocking histamine receptors on parietal cells with chemical antagonists (e.g., cimetidine, ranitidine) effectively inhibits gastric acid secretion and is the basis of current therapy for gastritis and peptic ulcer disease. The final phase of the secretory process occurs when digested proteins enter the proximal small intestine (the intestinal phase) and cause the release of a small intestinal polypeptide hormone, which in turn stimulates gastric acid secretion.

In a normal stomach, protection against the corrosive effects of the secreted acid depends on the integrity of the tight intercellular junctions between gastric mucosal cells (the gastric mucosal barrier). Destruction of this barrier not only leads to gastric mucosal injury from back diffusion of acid, but also causes further stimulation of gastric acid secretion. Thus, a truly vicious cycle is initiated *(pp. 838–841)*.

18. (D) Although angiodysplasia of the colon is one of the most frequent causes of lower gastrointestinal bleeding in elderly patients, it has only recently received notice. Angiodysplasia is characterized by dilated, tortuous submucosal veins and venules that may easily rupture to produce bleeding. These pathologic changes are always limited to the right colon and are most often located within the cecum. Although it has been suggested that these lesions represent a congenital defect or even a neoplastic change, their pathogenesis is now believed to be related to bowel distention and increased intraluminal pressure from fecal impaction of the capacious cecum. Because these lesions are almost entirely intramucosal, they cannot be detected by conventional diagnostic methods and require selective mesenteric angiography for clinical diagnosis. Even for pathologic diagnosis, injection of mesenteric vessels with colloidal contrast agents may be needed to accurately localize lesions in surgical resection specimens *(p. 886)*.

19. (B) Melanosis coli is an innocuous condition that is virtually always asymptomatic but has an alarming gross appearance that may startle the unsuspecting colonoscopist. It is characterized by a diffuse, brown-black pigmentation of the colonic mucosa. The condition is associated with the use of cathartics of the anthracene type. It is always limited to the colon, curiously sparing the small intestine. Despite the name melanosis coli, the brown-black pigment granules contained within lysosomes of macrophages in the mucosal lamina propria probably represent lipofuscin derived from membranes of damaged colonic epithelial cells. Melanosis coli has no association with either benign or malignant melanocytic tumors *(p. 885)*.

20. (A) Pseudomembranous colitis is an inflammatory disorder of the colon characterized by focal mucosal ulceration and the formation of fibrinomucinous exudate over denuded areas. The coagulum of fibrin and mucin containing inflammatory cells and necrotic mucosal epithelial cells forms what is known as a pseudomembrane. The disorder is associated with the administration of broad-spectrum antibiotics, particularly clindamycin and lincomycin, which allow for the overgrowth of *Clostridium difficile*, a microorganism resistant to these antibiotics. Although the organism does *not* invade the bowel mucosa, it produces a toxin that is the cause of the mucosal injury. The diagnosis can be confirmed by isolation of *C. difficile* or its toxin from the stool. The disease is cured promptly by the administration of vancomycin. Prompt positive identification of the organism or its toxin is important because the colitis caused by *C. difficile* is grossly indistinguishable from other colitides that produce pseudomembranes: for example, staphylococcal, *Shigella*, or fungal *(Candida)* infection or ischemic disease *(pp. 360–361, 889–890)*.

21. (A) Acute appendicitis occurs mainly in adolescents and young adults but may affect individuals of any age. It is characterized histologically by transmural neutrophilic infiltration and, in fulminant cases, mural necrosis. Lymphoid hyperplasia of the submucosa, however, is not an indication of acute appendicitis and may be considered a variation of the normal appendiceal morphology. Clinically, acute appendicitis is most commonly confused with acute mesenteric lymphadenitis caused by *Yersinia enterocolitica* or viral enterocolitis, which is often unrecognized before surgery. Although a false-positive diagnosis may be made in 10 to 30% of cases, the risks of appendiceal perforation (with a 2% mortality rate) necessitate prompt action on the part of the surgeon and more than justify the occasional "negative" laparotomy for suspected appendicitis. Luminal obstruction of the appendix predisposes to acute appendicitis, and fecaliths, calculi, tumors, or worms can be demonstrated in 50 to 80% of inflamed appendices *(pp. 357–358, 902–903)*.

22. (A) Reflux esophagitis is the most common cause of esophageal pathology. Although some reflux of gastric contents occurs commonly in normal individuals, it does not usually produce esophagitis. Inflammation results when multiple contributing factors are present concomitantly: for example, lower esophageal sphincter incompetence, disordered esophageal motility, and increased amounts of acid, pepsin, bile acids, and/or lysolecithin in the refluxed fluid. To confirm the diagnosis, the distinctive features of reflux esophagitis may be sought on endoscopic biopsy. Characteristically, chronic reflux esophagitis produces reactive mucosal changes such as expansion (hyperplasia) of the basal zone exceeding 20% of the epithelial thickness and elongation of papillae into the upper third of the epithelium. The most sensitive and specific marker is intraepithelial eosinophils with or without neutrophils. However, none of the changes is pathognomonic of reflux esophagitis, and clinical-pathological correlation is required for diagnosis.

Submucosal varices are not a feature of any form of esophagitis. They are seen exclusively in diseases causing elevated pressures in the esophageal venous system such as occurs in cirrhosis with portal hypertension *(pp. 832, 834)*.

23. **(A)** The gastrointestinal (GI) tract is the most common site of primary extranodal lymphoma. Nevertheless, GI lymphoma is distinctly uncommon compared with other malignancies of the GI tract. Most primary GI lymphomas arise in the stomach, and almost all are B-cell lesions. Overall, GI lymphomas have a better prognosis than either GI carcinomas or lymphomas arising in other extranodal sites, and gastric lymphoma has the best prognosis of all. Many gastric lymphomas are curable with surgical resection.

Lymphomas arising in lymph nodes in the course of their dissemination may secondarily involve the GI tract, but primary GI lymphoma, by definition, arises directly from the gut-associated lymphoid tissue (GALT) within the GI tract. Conversely, of course, primary GI lymphoma may secondarily involve lymph nodes *(pp. 858–859)*.

24. **(C)** Lactase is the most important disaccharidase associated with the apical brush border of the intestinal absorptive cell. Lactase breaks lactose into its component monosaccharides, glucose and galactose, for absorption. Acquired disaccharidase deficiency represents a loss of absorptive cell-associated lactase after intestinal mucosal injury (e.g., viral or bacterial enteritis). In this situation, the osmotic gradient created by unabsorbed lactose causes watery diarrhea and malabsorption. Individuals with acquired lactose intolerance can only be treated by dietary restriction (elimination of lactose-containing foods and substitution with imitation milk products).

Disaccharidase deficiency with lactose intolerance is not a form of food allergy and is not immunologically mediated. Thus, features of hypersensitivity-mediated injury are not present (e.g., mucosal eosinophilia with abscess formation as seen in eosinophilic gastroenteritis) *(p. 880)*.

25. **(E)** The defect pictured in Figure 8–3 is an intussusception. This defect results when a segment of small bowel, while contracted in peristalsis, becomes telescoped into the lumen of the adjacent downstream segment and causes intestinal obstruction. As the intussusceptum is pushed by peristalsis deeper inside the enveloping segment, its mesentery is pulled in after it, and the resultant vascular compromise leads to infarction. Intussusception is uncommon but occurs most often in otherwise normal bowel in infants and children. In adults, intussusception may occur when an intraluminal mass (tumor or polyp) acts as a lead point for peristaltic propulsion into the distal bowel segment. Intussusception requires prompt surgical correction or resection *(p. 881)*.

26. **(E)** The broad band of collagen beneath the interglandular surface epithelium of the architecturally normal colonic mucosa in Figure 8–4 is virtually diagnostic of collagenous colitis. This disorder of unknown cause is characterized by chronic or episodic watery diarrhea in adults. Affected individuals are almost always 30 years of age or older (mean age of 60), are usually female, often have a concurrent autoimmune disease, and frequently test positively for rheumatoid factor and antinuclear antibodies. Despite the rather dramatic microscopic changes in this disease, the colonic mucosa characteristically appears unremarkable on barium enema or colonoscopy. Thus, the diagnosis is almost always made on colonoscopic biopsy *(pp. 890–891)*.

27. (True); 28. (False); 29. (True); 30. (False); 31. (True)

(27) The esophagus is lined throughout its length by stratified squamous epithelium, which does not keratinize under normal conditions. **(28)** Its outer surface lacks a serosa and is covered instead by loose connective tissue. **(29)** The muscular wall of this hollow tube is composed of striated muscle in the upper third and smooth muscle in the lower two-thirds. **(30)** Although functional studies have shown that sphincter function exists in both the upper and lower aspects of the esophagus, no anatomic counterpart for these functional sphincters has been discerned by morphologic studies. **(31)** The esophageal lumen narrows slightly at the level of the bifurcation of the trachea and at two other levels—the cricoid cartilage and the diaphragmatic hiatus *(pp. 827–828)*.

32. (True); 33. (True); 34. (False); 35. (True);

Esophageal varices are dilated, tortuous submucosal veins that are produced when flow through the hepatic portal system is compromised, increasing portal venous pressure and diverting flow through the coronary veins of the stomach into the esophageal plexus. Portal hypertension is most commonly caused by hepatic cirrhosis, yet the incidence of this complication varies markedly among the different forms of cirrhosis. **(32)** Portal hypertension and esophageal varices are most commonly found in association with alcoholic cirrhosis and occur in nearly two-thirds of the patients with this disorder. (33) Curiously, however, they rarely occur in association with biliary cirrhosis or cardiac cirrhosis. (34) Whatever the cause, esophageal varices are asymptomatic until they rupture. Thus, epigastric pain in alcoholic patients would most likely indicate acute gastritis or reflux esophagitis rather than the presence of esophageal varices, although they may well coexist. (35) Once rupture has occurred, the consequences are dire, and death occurs with the first episode of bleeding in about half of the cases. Even if the initial episode of bleeding can be controlled with medical measures or surgical ligation, rebleeding is likely to occur. Overall, only surgical procedures that reduce the pressure in the portal venous system are capable of altering the course of this highly lethal consequence of advanced cirrhosis (*p. 834*).

36. (False); 37. (True); 38. (True); 39. (True); 40. (False); 41. (True); 42. (True); 43. (False); 44. (False)

Peptic ulcers are perhaps the most common chronic gastrointestinal disorder in industrialized nations. (36) Although they may occur at any level of the gastrointestinal tract exposed to gastric acid and pepsin, they occur most commonly in the first portion of the duodenum. The second most common site is the gastric antrum. (37) Peptic ulcers occur most commonly as solitary lesions. Occasionally, however, they may be multiple, especially in such disorders as the Zollinger-Ellison syndrome.

(38) Although the pathogenesis of chronic peptic ulcers remains largely unknown, it is clear that they are associated with gastric acid and pepsin secretion. In fact, without some level of acid-pepsin secretion, peptic ulcers do not develop and, therefore, are not encountered in individuals with achlorhydria. (39) Epidemiologic evidence suggests that genetic factors are important in the predisposition to duodenal peptic ulcer but do not appear to be important in the genesis of gastric peptic ulcer. Duodenal ulcers occur approximately three times more commonly in first-degree relatives of affected patients than in the general population, and individuals with blood group O are more prone to develop these lesions than individuals with other blood types.

(40 and 41) Although some degree of gastric acid production has been shown to be requisite to the genesis of peptic ulcers, abnormally high levels of gastric acid have been demonstrated only in patients with duodenal peptic ulcers. Even in duodenal ulcer disease, this finding is not constant, and there is considerable overlap between measurements of mean basal acid output in duodenal ulcer patients and normal controls. Patients with gastric ulcers, in general, have low to normal levels of gastric acid.

(42) In 60 to 80% of cases of gastric ulceration, chronic antral gastritis is also present and frequently persists after the ulcer heals. This implies that chronic gastritis

may be the primary condition and that ulcer development is secondary. It has been suggested that both are etiologically related to the reflux of bile acids and lysolecithin into the gastric antrum, causing damage to the gastric mucosal barrier with back diffusion of gastric acid.

(43 and 44) Malignant transformation of peptic ulcers is exceedingly rare and has only been reported in gastric ulcers. Even in those cases, it is possible that the cancers did not derive from malignant transformation of benign ulcers but rather presented unrecognized malignancies from the outset. Although peptic ulcers have a characteristic gross morphology in most cases (see Question 12), differentiating benign gastric ulcers from ulcerating gastric carcinomas can be difficult in cases with overlapping features (*pp. 848–853, 858*).

45. (True); 46. (False; 47. (False); 48. (True); 49. (True); 50. (False); 51. (False)

Diverticular disease is an idiopathic disorder characterized by the development of saccular outpouchings of the colonic mucosa, usually in the distal third of the colon, that are prone to fecal impaction. (45) In industrialized Western countries, the disease is extremely common and is currently found in approximately 50% of individuals older than 60 years. The incidence of the disease increases with age and is rare before 30 years of age.

(46) Acquired colonic diverticula are aneurysmic flask-shaped outpouchings of the colonic mucosa through "weak spots" in the muscularis propria where blood vessels penetrate the colonic wall. They are herniations of mucosa and submucosa alone. An attenuated muscularis mucosa may or may not be present, but diverticula lack a muscularis propria entirely. (47) Although they may occur in any segment, 95% of colonic diverticula are located in the sigmoid colon. (48) Wherever they are found, the wall of the affected segment is commonly hypertrophied.

(49) The delicacy of these thin-walled diverticular structures makes perforation an easily understood complication. Inflammatory changes are usually produced by perforation with leakage of the contents into the adjacent pericolonic fat. The inflammatory response may be quite extensive, with pericolonic abscesses, sinus tracts, or even peritonitis. With chronic inflammation, pericolonic scarring with stricture formation may occur. Because diverticula without superimposed inflammation may be symptomatic and, conversely, inflamed diverticula may not be associated with symptoms of inflammatory disease, it is frequently impossible to differentiate between diverticulosis and diverticulitis. In fact, about half of the cases of diverticulitis do not produce fever or systemic leukocytosis. Thus, the terms "diverticulosis" and "diverticulitis" have been replaced by the more useful clinical term "diverticular disease."

(50) The morphology of diverticula suggests that they arise as a consequence of increased intraluminal pressure and subsequent herniation of the colonic mucosa

through a muscle weakness in the colonic wall. Although clinical studies have failed to confirm that increased intraluminal pressure is essential in the pathogenesis of diverticular disease, they have shown that it correlates well with symptomatic disease. Thus, high-fiber diets that increase stool bulk and decrease peristaltic activity (hence intraluminal pressure) do not prevent the development of diverticular disease but are effective in reducing the symptoms of this condition.

(51) Fortunately, most individuals with diverticular disease are asymptomatic and never come to medical attention. When inflammation does occur, however, it most often resolves spontaneously. Only a small percentage of patients require surgical intervention for obstruction, free perforation, or inflammatory complications (*pp. 884–885*).

52. (False); 53. (True); 54. (False); 55. (True); 56. (True); 57. (True); 58. (False); 59. (False); 60. (True)

(52) Adenocarcinoma of the colon is by far the most common malignant tumor of the gastrointestinal tract, but overall it is second to lung cancer as the most common cause of cancer death in the United States. (53) Its high incidence has been shown epidemiologically to be related to dietary factors such as low fiber, high carbohydrate, and high fat content.

(54) Almost three-quarters of colonic carcinomas are located in the rectum, rectosigmoid, or sigmoid colon. The remainder occur with more or less equal frequency throughout the remainder of the colon. In the past, only about 10% occurred in the right colon. However, the relative frequency of right colon cancers appears to be increasing, and is now about 20%. (55) The vast majority of colon cancers have a similar origin and histologic appearance. Except for those that arise in inflammatory bowel disease, almost all colon cancers derive from malignant transformation of colonic adenomas (adenomatous polyps). Ninety-eight per cent of all colon cancers are adenocarcinomas, and most of these are moderately to well differentiated. (56) Although stage is by far the most important indicator of outcome in colon cancer, certain histological variations may also have prognostic significance. (58) For example, tumors of the rectosigmoid that produce copious amounts of mucin (known as mucinous or colloid carcinomas) tend to have a worse prognosis. It is believed that the elaboration of pools of extracellular mucin by the tumor aids in its ability to dissect through normal tissues and increases its potential for infiltration.

(57) Although by no means unique to colonic malignancies, most of these cancers produce the glycoprotein oncofetal antigen known as carcinoembryonic antigen (CEA). With removal of the primary tumor, the serum levels of CEA usually decline. Any subsequent rise in the serum CEA level may indicate recurrent or metastatic disease.

(59 and 60) Colon cancer is a surgical problem. Radiation therapy and chemotherapy are largely considered adjuvant treatment modalities for this disease.

Although colon cancer is deadly in advanced stages, early stage disease is curable with surgical resection. Resected tumors that are limited to the mucosa have a 5-year survival rate of virtually 100% and are almost always cured. Therefore, aside from prevention, early detection is the most important issue surrounding this disease. Many tumors are within the reach of the palpating finger (thus the importance of the rectal examination), but screening for more proximal malignancies is usually done by colorimetric tests for occult blood in the stool. These tests are both nonspecific (bleeding from any cause will yield a positive test) and insensitive (intermittent bleeding produces many false-negative tests). More accurate screening tests for this disease are being sought. Nevertheless, stool examinations for occult blood are inexpensive and can easily be repeated to increase accuracy. Furthermore, blood in the stool is always pathologic and should initiate investigation for colon cancer as the possible underlying cause (*pp. 897–902*).

61. (False); 62. (False); 63. (True); 64. (True); 65. (True); 66. (True)

(61) Although they may occur in the lung as well as the breast, thymus, liver, gallbladder, ovary, or urethra, carcinoid tumors arise most often in the gastrointestinal tract. (62) No matter what their site of origin, carcinoid tumors tend to have the same histologic appearance. They are composed of a uniform population of round cells showing little cytologic atypia. The ability of these tumors to invade and metastasize cannot be predicted from their histologic appearance.

(63) Carcinoid tumor cells can be positively identified by their cytoplasmic content of secretory granules, which have a characteristic affinity for soluble silver salts. Thus, carcinoid tumors are also known as argentaffinomas. These secretory granules may contain a variety of amine and peptide products, including adrenocorticotropic hormone, histamine, serotonin, 5-hydroxytryptophan, kallikrein, or prostaglandin. Most of these products can be identified in tissue secretions of the tumor by immunohistochemistry.

(64) Although in general the biologic behavior of carcinoid tumors is somewhat unpredictable, carcinoids arising in the appendix (the most common site of gastrointestinal carcinoid tumors) are almost always indolent and rarely metastasize. Their behavior contrasts with that of extra-appendiceal carcinoid tumors, which tend to spread to local lymph nodes as well as to the liver, lungs, and bone.

(65) The carcinoid syndrome results from the systemic effects of the secretory products of carcinoid tumors, especially serotonin and histamine. Because these substances are readily metabolized in the liver, the carcinoid syndrome is rarely produced by small intestinal carcinoid tumors in the absence of liver metastases. The secretory products of hepatic metastases enter the systemic circulation directly and bypass hepatic degradation.

(66) One of the most important and unfortunate

features of gastrointestinal carcinoid tumors is their association with an increased incidence of other malignant tumors, both intestinal and extraintestinal. Concurrent malignant neoplasms are found in about 30% of patients with carcinoid tumors of the small intestine and in about 15% of those with appendiceal carcinoids. Most of these concurrent cancers are found elsewhere in the gastrointestinal tract and are usually adenocarcinomas (*pp. 872–875*).

67. (B); 68. (C); 69. (C); 70. (A); 71. (A); 72. (C); 73. (D); 74. (B)

(67) Gastric carcinomas are adenocarcinomas that arise from the glandular epithelium of the gastric mucosa. Most malignancies of the esophagus, however, are squamous cell carcinomas. Exceptions to this are represented by esophageal adenocarcinomas that arise from the metaplastic epithelium of a Barrett's esophagus or, rarely, from esophageal mucous glands.

(68) Although the reasons are completely unknown, epidemiologic studies have shown that throughout the world the incidence of esophageal carcinoma is significantly higher among blacks than whites. Racial predisposition has also been demonstrated for gastric carcinoma, and in the United States, blacks, American Indians, and native Hawaiians are at increased risk compared with whites.

(69) Dietary factors are important in the pathogenesis of both esophageal and gastric malignancy. Diets rich in nitrites, nitrates, and nitrosamines have been causally linked to both esophageal and gastric carcinoma. Other dietary factors significant in the pathogenesis of esophageal carcinoma include certain vitamin and mineral deficiencies (e.g., vitamins A and C, some B vitamins, zinc, and molybdenum) and fungal (e.g., *Aspergillus*) food contamination. Salted and smoked foods have been implicated in the pathogenesis of gastric cancer.

(70 and 71) It has been further shown by epidemiologic studies in the United States that esophageal carcinoma occurs six to seven times more frequently among smokers of cigarettes, cigars, or pipes than among nonsmokers. Alcohol abuse is well known to represent a significant risk factor for esophageal cancer. However, neither cigarette smoking nor alcohol abuse has been demonstrated to influence the incidence of gastric carcinoma.

(72) Chronic inflammation with unremitting epithelial injury, inflammation, and repair predisposes to neoplasia in both the esophagus and the stomach. Both chronic esophagitis and the fundic/autoimmune forms of chronic gastritis (types A and AB) are associated with an increased risk of malignancy, but for unknown reasons, type B (antral) gastritis does not appear to be a significant risk factor for gastric cancer.

(73) Unfortunately, both esophageal and gastric carcinoma tend to be diseases of insidious onset and rarely produce symptoms that bring the patient to early clinical attention. Both diseases are characteristically asymptomatic until late in their course, when pain may develop as a symptom.

(74) Bilateral metastatic adenocarcinomas in the ova-

ries are known as Krukenberg's tumors. Although the primary tumor may originate from any abdominal viscus, it is most frequently poorly differentiated (signet ring) gastric adenocarcinomas that give rise to this metastatic pattern. Squamous carcinoma of the esophagus, by definition, never gives rise to Krukenberg's tumors. Even adenocarcinoma of the esophagus, however, rarely produces this metastatic pattern (*pp. 835–838, 854–858*).

75. (C); 76. (A); 77. (D); 78. (A); 79. (A); 80. (A); 81. (B); 82. (B)

Acute gastritis is an acute mucosal inflammatory process that may be accompanied by hemorrhage and/or erosion. It is usually symptomatic (sometimes dramatically so) but transient. Acute gastritis commonly resolves completely after reversal of the causative condition or removal of the causative agent. Chronic gastritis, however, is defined histologically. It refers to a group of conditions that produce a continuum of increasing mucosal inflammation (characteristically lymphoplasmacytic) and atrophy of the gastric mucosa, often accompanied by metaplastic and/or dysplastic changes. Chronic gastritis is associated with an extended clinical course, but it commonly has ill-defined symptoms or may even be asymptomatic. Two types are defined: (1) Type A is an autoimmune-mediated fundal gastritis, and (2) type B (the most common form) is a nonimmune antral gastritis. Chronic gastritis of either type has a limited potential for reversibility and is associated with an increased incidence of gastric carcinoma, particularly when intestinal metaplasia or dysplasia is present.

(75, 76, 79) Acute gastritis may be produced by excessive alcohol consumption or heavy smoking. Alcohol, cigarette smoke, and aspirin, the three most common causes of acute gastritis, all are agents known to damage the gastric mucosal barrier. They disrupt the tight junctions between mucosal cells and allow back diffusion of gastric acids. Consequently, mucosal edema and inflammation and erosion of the gastric mucosal cells are produced. Although chronic type B gastritis has also been linked to alcohol abuse, cigarette smoking has not been defined as a causative factor in this disorder.

(77) The production of autoantibodies directed against gastric mucosal cells is a feature associated exclusively with chronic type A fundal gastritis. In particular, patients with chronic fundal gastritis and pernicious anemia typically produce antibodies directed against gastric parietal cells and intrinsic factor. Patients with chronic antral gastritis do not have these circulating autoantibodies. Whether these antibodies represent a secondary response to exposed antigens on damaged gastric mucosal cells or whether they are the causative agents in type A gastritis is still unclear.

(78) Primary among the factors necessary for maintenance of the gastric mucosal barrier is adequate blood flow. Shock and consequent hypoperfusion of the gastric mucosa are major contributory factors leading to mucosal

injury in acute gastritis, but ischemia is not known to have a causative role in chronic gastritis.

(80) Only the acute form of gastritis, with its gastric epithelial cell damage, mucosal denudation, and exposure of delicate submucosal vessels, is associated with gastrointestinal bleeding. In chronic forms of gastritis, mucosal atrophy is the rule, but the mucosa characteristically remains intact.

(81 and 82) Only the antral form of chronic gastritis is commonly associated with concurrent gastric peptic ulcers or with infection by *Campylobacter pylori (pp. 842–845).*

83. (C); 84. (B); 85. (A); 86. (D); 87. (A); 88. (B); (D)

Both Ménétrier's disease and the Zollinger-Ellison syndrome are considered forms of so-called hypertrophic gastritis, even though neither is inflammatory in origin. (83) Although they represent opposite ends of the histologic spectrum of disorders producing hyperplasia of the gastric epithelium, both Ménétrier's disease and the Zollinger-Ellison syndrome are characterized grossly by striking cerebriform enlargement of rugal folds.

(84 and 88) The Zollinger-Ellison syndrome is caused by gastrin-producing endocrine tumors, usually of pancreatic origin. With continued excessive gastrin stimulation, hyperplasia of gastric glands occurs with increased numbers of both parietal and chief cells. Hypersecretion of gastric acid by parietal cells is induced, leading to the production of numerous intractable peptic ulcers, the hallmark of the syndrome. (86) In Ménétrier's disease, the hypertrophic rugal folds are composed predominantly of hyperplastic surface mucous cells. These cells secrete excessive amounts of mucus, and in some patients, the loss of mucoprotein is severe enough to produce hypoproteinemia. Thus, Ménétrier's disease sometimes constitutes a form of protein-losing gastroenteropathy.

(86) Although the heaped-up mucosal folds of Ménétrier's disease and the Zollinger-Ellison syndrome may bear a superficial morphologic resemblance to the mucosal thickening seen in gastric lymphoma, neither disorder is actually associated with lymphoma. (87) Ménétrier's disease, however, does impose a slightly increased risk of gastric carcinoma.

(89) The gastrin-producing pancreatic endocrine tumors of the Zollinger-Ellison syndrome may be part of a multiple endocrine neoplasia (MEN) syndrome. MEN syndromes can be divided into two major categories: those composed primarily of tumors of neural crest origin and those arising in endocrine organs that are not derived from the neural crest. The pancreatic adenomas of the Zollinger-Ellison syndrome belong to the latter group. They are associated with adenomas of the pituitary gland, the parathyroid, and the adrenal cortex. In contrast to this group of neoplasms, pheochromocytoma and medullary carcinoma of the thyroid are examples of tumors of neural crest origin and do not occur in association with pancreatic adenomas. Ménétrier's disease has no association with MEN syndromes *(pp. 847, 1007–1008).*

90. (B); 91. (A); 92. (C); 93. (B); 94. (A)

Although gastric polyps are in fact rare, they are among the most common benign neoplasms of the stomach. Histologically, gastric polyps are classified as either hyperplastic or adenomatous; the hyperplastic variety account for 80 to 90% of all gastric polyps. (90) Adenomatous polyps, which are true neoplasms, tend to be large and may grow as large as 3 to 4 cm in diameter. Hyperplastic polyps are seldom larger than 1 cm in diameter. (91) Hyperplastic polyps are usually multiple, whereas adenomatous polyps tend to occur singly. However, multiple adenomatous polyps may be present as part of an inherited polyposis syndrome such as familial polyposis coli. (92) All gastric polyps tend to be asymptomatic and are usually discovered incidentally. (93) The major significance of adenomatous gastric polyps is their tendency to undergo malignant transformation. Hyperplastic polyps represent regenerative non-neoplastic lesions and rarely, if ever, undergo malignant transformation. (94) Curiously, however, hyperplastic polyps are associated with coexistent gastric carcinoma elsewhere in the stomach, constituting perhaps the most significant feature of this otherwise innocuous lesion *(pp. 853–854).*

95. (A); 96. (C); 97. (D); 98. (D); 99. (D); 100. (A); 101. (B); 102. (A); 103. (A); 104. (C); 105. (C)

Both Crohn's disease and ulcerative colitis are idiopathic disorders with systemic manifestations that produce inflammatory disease of the bowel as their primary consequence. Although they have many overlapping features, leading to the hypothesis that the two diseases may actually represent opposite ends of the spectrum of host response to the same disease entity, in their classic forms the two processes can be distinguished on a number of bases.

(95) The distribution of the two diseases is usually quite distinctive. On the one hand, Crohn's disease involves the terminal ileum in most cases (65 to 75%) and frequently affects the colon concurrently. The colon alone is involved in 20 to 30% of cases, but the lesions of Crohn's disease may be found at any level of the gastrointestinal tract, including the stomach. On the other hand, ulcerative colitis is a process largely limited to the large intestine, although the terminal ileum is involved in 10% of cases.

(96) Extraintestinal involvement may occur in both conditions. The systemic complications are similar in both diseases and include migratory polyarthritis, sacroiliiitis, ankylosing spondylitis, uveitis, hepatic involvement, and skin lesions.

(97) One of the primary pathologic features that distinguishes Crohn's disease from ulcerative colitis is the presence of granulomas. These appear in affected bowel segments in approximately 60% of the cases. However, the presence of granulomas is by no means pathognomonic. When granulomas are observed, specific causes of granulomatous enterocolitis such as tuberculosis must be considered, and special stains for organisms should be performed. In Crohn's disease,

special stains for bacteria, fungi, parasites, or acid-fast bacilli fail to reveal microorganisms.

(98) The search for a specific etiologic microorganism in ulcerative colitis and Crohn's disease has proved unfruitful. Although various viruses have been suspected to be causative agents, the evidence for a viral cause of inflammatory bowel disease is inconclusive. Although viruses have been cultured from diseased portions of bowel in a small number of cases, electron and immunohistochemical microscopic studies have failed in most cases to confirm the presence of viral particles in diseased tissue. Moreover, the issue is further clouded by the possibility that viral particles, when present, represent only secondary infection of diseased bowel.

(99) Crohn's disease and ulcerative colitis share many epidemiologic similarities, including age, race, and sex distribution, but no specific HLA profiles have been identified in association with these diseases. Although previous reports linked HLA-B27 to Crohn's disease with ankylosing spondylitis, it is now clear that the antigen is associated only with the latter disorder with or without Crohn's disease.

(100) In general, the gross appearance of the affected bowel in the two diseases differs in several specific aspects. In Crohn's disease, the inflammation is characteristically transmural and leads to marked fibrosis (scarring) of the submucosa and muscularis propria. The wall of the affected bowel becomes rigid, thickened, and narrowed. (101) In ulcerative colitis, the inflammatory process is usually limited to the mucosa, and the bowel wall is not significantly thickened. Occasionally, however, a severe acute attack of fulminant ulcerative colitis may produce sudden cessation of bowel function, dilatation of the colon, and acute transmural inflammation with fraying and thinning of the muscularis propria (toxic megacolon). The danger of perforation in this situation is great, and the consequences may be lethal. Curiously, this drastic complication of ulcerative colitis is virtually never seen in Crohn's disease.

(102) The distribution of lesions in the involved bowel is another major distinguishing feature between ulcerative colitis and Crohn's disease. The lesions of Crohn's disease are typically discontinuous; affected areas are interrupted by uninvolved patches of bowel (known as skip lesions). This pattern contrasts with that of ulcerative colitis, in which the lesions are usually continuous. The ulceration characteristically begins in the rectum and progressively involves the proximal mucosa in a confluent manner. (103) The transmural nature of the inflammatory process in Crohn's disease leads to the formation of deep mural fissures and fistulous tracts, which are among the most important complications of this disease. Ulcerative colitis does not produce these deeply penetrating lesions; it is characterized instead by shallow superficial mucosal ulcerations.

(104) One of the most important yet most unfortunate similarities between ulcerative colitis and Crohn's disease is the increased frequency of colonic carcinoma with which they both are associated. The overall risk of gastrointestinal carcinoma is much smaller in Crohn's disease than in ulcerative colitis, but in both disorders the risk increases with increasing duration of the disease. (105) In addition, both Crohn's disease and ulcerative colitis impose an increased risk of primary gastrointestinal lymphoma (*pp. 867–872, 886–889*).

106. (A); 107. (A); 108. (A); 109. (C); 110. (B); 111. (C); 112. (A)

"Ischemic bowel disease" is a broad term used to describe hypoxic injury to the gastrointestinal tract caused by any disorder that leads to enteric hypoperfusion. In general, the extent of the injury produced in the bowel is directly related to the severity of the reduction in blood flow. On the one hand, transmural infarction represents maximal injury to the bowel, producing ischemic necrosis of all layers of the bowel wall. Mural infarction, on the other hand, is the result of minimal ischemic damage, involving only that layer of the wall that is most remote in the end-arterial system. Thus in mucosal infarction, ischemic injury and necrosis are limited to the mucosa and submucosa and spare the muscularis and the serosa.

(106) Mucosal infarction may occur at any level of the bowel from stomach to anus without particular predilection for any specific region. Transmural infarction, however, most commonly affects the small bowel. Unlike the colon, which throughout most of its length receives collateral circulation from the posterior abdominal wall to which it is attached, the small bowel depends entirely on the mesenteric vascular supply.

(107 and 108) Although transmural infarction is most often produced by arterial occlusion with total or almost total reduction in blood flow, it occurs as a result of venous thrombosis in a minority of cases. In contrast to total arterial or venous occlusion, which completely halt the flow of blood, conditions that reduce but do not arrest the flow of blood may produce mucosal injury but rarely lead to transmural infarction. (109) The combination of atherosclerosis and hypotension may, according to the severity of these elements, produce any degree of ischemic injury, from mucosal to transmural infarction. (110) In the absence of significant atherosclerosis, hypotension alone virtually never produces transmural infarction. Conversely, low-flow states (shock) with reflex splanchnic vasoconstriction are the major causes of mucosal infarction.

(111) Ischemic bowel disease, no matter what the level of injury, commonly appears hemorrhagic. In mucosal infarction, the hemorrhage is limited to the superficial layers of the gut, but in transmural infarction hemorrhage may be seen throughout the deeper levels as well. (112) Because the hemorrhagic necrosis of mucosal infarction is limited and superficial, it rarely has grave consequences. Transmural infarction, in contrast, is a highly lethal disorder that is associated with a mortality of 50 to 75%. It requires prompt diagnosis and surgical intervention (*pp. 863–865*).

113. (C); 114. (A); 115. (A); 116. (C); 117. (B); 118. (B); 119. (D)

(113) Tropical sprue and Whipple's disease are two uncommon causes of malabsorption that are suspected to be of infectious cause, but a microbiologic pathogen has not yet been identified for either disease. (114) Only tropical sprue is associated with travel to an endemic area (the Caribbean, for example). Because the pathologic changes in the small bowel are not pathognomonic, a history of travel to an endemic area is essential to its diagnosis. (115) Small bowel biopsy in tropical sprue usually shows flattening of villi as in celiac sprue, whereas villi in Whipple's disease are usually distended with macrophages, giving the mucosa a shaggy appearance.

(116) Despite the fact that no etiologic microorganism has been identified for either disease, both tropical sprue and Whipple's disease can be cured by antibiotic therapy. The dramatic response of these diseases to antibiotics strongly suggests that they are indeed of bacterial origin. (117) Although Whipple's disease was once thought to be a process limited to the small bowel, it is now clear that the disorder is systemic in distribution. The skin, central nervous system, joints, heart, blood vessels, kidney, lungs, serosal membranes, lymph nodes, spleen, and liver all may be involved. Tropical sprue, in contrast, produces disease only in the small intestine. (118) One of the primary pathologic features of Whipple's disease is the presence of periodic acid-Schiff (PAS)-positive glycoprotein-laden macrophages in the small bowel mucosa that contain unidentified, rod-shaped bacilli. Although it is suspected that these rod-shaped bacteria are the causative agents, this remains to be confirmed. (119) Neither disease is associated with an increased risk of gastrointestinal lymphoma or carcinoma *(pp. 877–880)*.

120. (C); 121. (B); 122. (C); 123. (C); 124. (D)

Congenital anomalies may occur at any level of the gastrointestinal tract and lead to bowel obstruction and other serious gastrointestinal problems in the neonate. Because many of these developmental defects are life threatening and must be recognized early, knowledge of the most prevalent lesions and their most common sites of occurrence is critical. (120) Congenital atresia (failure of a bowel segment to develop, leaving behind a solid cord-like remnant) occurs most often in the small intestine.

(121) Intestinal stenosis refers to luminal narrowing due to any cause. The most frequent developmental abnormality producing intestinal stenosis is hypertrophy of the gastric pylorus. Hypertrophic pyloric stenosis is unique among the congenital stenoses, because most of the others are caused by hypoplastic, rather than hyperplastic, segments of bowel wall or luminal strictures.

(122) Congenital duplication occurs as a consequence of a defect in transformation from the solid to the hollow luminal phase of bowel development early in gestation. Although rare, this anomaly occurs most frequently in the small intestine.

(123) Congenital diverticula, which represent herniations or outpouchings of the intestinal wall, are uncommon lesions and are often asymptomatic. The most common congenital diverticulum, known as Meckel's diverticulum, is located in the small intestine and represents a remnant of the vitelline duct. Other congenital diverticula represent primary defects in the bowel wall and are unrelated to antecedent embryologic structures.

(124) Ganglion cells, which are critical to the transmission of the parasympathetic stimulus to peristalsis, migrate into the gut from the neural crest. Most commonly, they fail to reach the most distal bowel segment, the rectosigmoid region of the large bowel. The aganglionic segment cannot propagate a peristaltic wave and acts as a functional bowel obstruction (see Question 7) *(pp. 861–862, 883)*.

125. (C); 126. (B); 127. (B); 128. (D); 129. (E); 130. (E)

(125) Gastrin, a peptide hormone that stimulates hydrochloric acid production by gastric parietal cells, is primarily produced in the gastric antrum, which itself is devoid of parietal cells. (126) Pepsin is produced by the zymogenic chief cells of the gastric glands in the body and fundus of the stomach. (127) The gastric parietal cells are also located in the gastric glands of the body and fundus of the stomach. In addition to the production of hydrochloric acid, parietal cells elaborate intrinsic factor—a glycoprotein that plays an essential part in the absorption of vitamin B_{12}. (128) Gastric endocrine cells (enterochromaffin cells) are scattered throughout the glands of all the gastric regions and indeed throughout the entire gut, making the gastrointestinal tract the largest endocrine organ in the body. (129) The goblet cell, however, is a cell type characteristically found in the small and large intestine but not in the normal stomach. Mucus-secreting surface cells and neck cells of the gastric glands contain finely dispersed mucigen granules rather than a single large mucin-containing apical vacuole that characterizes the intestinal goblet cell. (130) Similarly, in the normal gastrointestinal tract, Paneth's cells are found only in the small intestine. Therefore, the appearance of Paneth's cells or goblet cells in the gastric mucosa indicates a pathologic metaplastic change and usually occurs in association with chronic gastritis *(pp. 838–839, 845)*.

131. (D); 132. (C); 133. (A); 134. (D); 135. (C); 136. (C); 137. (D)

(131) Two microscopic features that are unique to the normal small intestine allow for its ready histologic identification. On a cytologic level, the easily recognizable, intensely eosinophilic Paneth's cells, which occur almost exclusively in the small bowel, can be identified in the mucosal crypts of all small bowel segments. The second singular feature of the small bowel is the unique architectural arrangement of the surface mucosal epithelium into projections known as villi. (132) Peyer's patches are prominent lymphoid nodules (germinal centers) that characterize the ileal segment of small bowel,

whereas (133) Brunner's glands, elaborately branched submucosal mucus glands, are found only in the duodenal segment.

(134) Endocrine cells (argentaffin or enterochromaffin cells), many of which secrete serotonin, are found in the mucosal crypts throughout the length of the small intestine. Although histologically identical, endocrine cells represent a family of unique cell types, each capable of elaborating a particular gut hormone. Besides serotonin, these cells are known to produce gastrin, somatostatin, substance P, vasoactive intestinal peptides, bombesin, and other hormones. However, serotonin-producing endocrine cells do not appear to be anatomically segregated from endocrine cells producing any of these other intestinal hormones and are found scattered among other argentaffin cells in all small bowel segments.

(135) Like the intestinal endocrine cells, mucosal absorption cells in the small bowel are histologically identical but, at least in some aspects, functionally unique. The best-studied example of such functional uniqueness is that of vitamin B_{12}–intrinsic factor absorption by the surface absorptive cells of the ileum. These cells produce a specific receptor protein for intrinsic factor–vitamin B_{12} complex, which they display on the luminal surface of their cell membrane. The receptor protein is not produced by absorptive cells elsewhere in the small intestine; thus, vitamin B_{12} deficiency is a common consequence of ileal resection.

(136) Meckel's diverticulum is a remnant of the omphalomesenteric duct, an embryologic structure that connects the primitive gut with the yolk sac. Although it may vary slightly in position, it is always located in the ileal segment of small bowel, usually within 12 inches of the ileocecal valve. (137) Pancreatic rests, on the other hand, may occur anywhere in the small bowel. They occur as small foci of ectopic, yet normal, pancreatic tissue that are considered to be congenital anomalies but, unlike Meckel's diverticula, have no normal embryologic counterpart. Their occurrence may have clinical significance, however, as they may give rise to acute pancreatitis or even pancreatic adenocarcinoma (*pp. 860–861, 862*).

138. (B); 139. (A); 140. (D); 141. (C); 142. (D); 143. (B); 144. (D)

The pathologic characteristics of bacterial enterocolitides vary according to three basic properties of the infecting agent: (1) invasive potential, (2) toxin production, and (3) antigenic potential (ability to elicit immune responses in the host). The infective enterocolitides produced by *Salmonella*, *Shigella*, and *Vibrio cholerae* organisms are major causes of infectious gastrointestinal disease that represent classic examples of these three pathogenetic features. (138) The *Shigella* bacillus is the cause of the clinical syndrome known as bacillary dysentery. This organism directly penetrates the bowel mucosa through the epithelial cells and replicates within the lamina propria. Here the organism liberates an endotoxin that is cytodestructive and leads to shallow

mucosal ulcerations, the characteristic feature of *Shigella* enterocolitis. (139) Although *Salmonella* organisms are capable of mucosal penetration and liberation of endotoxins, mucosal ulceration is not a prominent feature. Instead, *Salmonella* enterocolitis is characterized by an intense immune response producing massive hypertrophy of submucosal lymphoid follicles. In the prototypic *Salmonella* gastroenteritis, typhoid fever, *Salmonella typhi* organisms tend to localize within the Peyer's patches of the ileum, which become greatly hypertrophied and are seen grossly as plaque-like mucosal elevations often 6 to 8 cm in diameter. The mucosa overlying these hypertrophied follicles undergoes secondary necrosis, presumably as a result of pressure-induced ischemia but not as a direct consequence of bacterial toxicity.

(140) Granulomatous inflammation is not produced by any of these three organisms. The presence of granulomas would suggest infection with mycobacteria (tuberculosis), fungi, or, rarely, strains of bacteria, such as *Brucella*, that induce granulomatous inflammation.

(141) Enterocolitis produced by *Vibrio cholerae* causes few anatomic changes in the affected bowel. Because the organism does not invade the bowel mucosa, no mucosal ulcerations are produced. The profuse watery diarrhea that is the hallmark of this infection is caused by an enterotoxin elaborated by the bacillus. The enterotoxin activates membrane-bound adenyl cyclase, causing increased intracellular levels of cAMP. Thus, salt and water absorption are inhibited, and active secretion of water, chloride, and bicarbonate by mucosal crypt cells is stimulated.

(142) As indicated above, all three of these organisms are capable of toxin production. In *Shigella* enterocolitis and cholera, toxin production by the causative organism is the principal pathogenetic factor.

(143) Among these three forms of enterocolitis, only shigellosis preferentially involves the large bowel. The tissue damage in *Shigella* enterocolitis is almost entirely limited to the mucosa of the colon, although the ileum is sometimes involved. *Salmonella* enterocolitis classically involves both the small and large intestine, whereas cholera is primarily a disease of the small bowel.

(144) Although ulceroinflammatory proctitis of infectious origin may be encountered among homosexual males, it is not particularly associated with any of the previously described forms of bacterial enterocolitis. The most common causative agents are *Treponema pallidum*, *Neisseria gonorrhoeae* (gonococci), *Chlamydia*, and herpes simplex virus (*pp. 865–867*).

145. (A); 146. (C); 147. (C); 148. (B); 149. (D); 150. (C); 151 (D)

Any benign proliferation of colonic mucosal elements that has an exophytic growth pattern and protrudes above the level of the surrounding mucosa is called a colonic polyp. The term, however, refers only to the gross morphology of the lesion. Microscopically, colonic polyps can be divided into two basic categories: hyperplastic lesions and true neoplasms (adenomas). Among the adenomas, several different morphologic types may be distinguished, corresponding to differing tendencies to undergo neoplastic transformation.

(145) The hyperplastic polyp is the most common type of colonic polyp, accounting for 90% of all colonic epithelial polyps at autopsy. Clinically, they are usually only discovered incidentally, because they are virtually always asymptomatic. Hyperplastic polyps are not considered to be true neoplasms but rather reactive proliferations of mature, well-differentiated, non-neoplastic epithelial cells separated by connective tissue resembling the lamina propria.

(146) Although the definitive identification of any colonic polyp depends on its histologic appearance, the gross size and configuration of the polyp often provide clues to the recognition of specific types. Overall, villous adenomas are the largest. They are slow-growing velvety lesions that, unlike other types of adenomatous polyps, are rarely pedunculated. In general, hyperplastic polyps are the smallest lesions. Tubular adenomas and hamartomatous polyps tend to be intermediate in size between hyperplastic polyps and villous adenomas.

(147) In true adenomatous polyps (tubular adenomas, villous adenomas, and tubulovillous adenomas, a histologic composite of these two types), there is a positive correlation between the size of the lesion and the probability of neoplastic transformation. Thus, villous adenomas, the largest of the adenomatous polyps, have the highest likelihood of containing carcinoma. Non-adenomatous polyps (hyperplastic polyps and hamartomatous polyps) virtually never undergo neoplastic transformation.

(148) Familial polyposis is a hereditary autosomal dominant disorder characterized by the formation of extremely large numbers of adenomatous polyps in the colon and occasionally the small bowel and stomach as well. Typically, the entire colonic mucosa is covered by closely packed polyps, giving the surface a shaggy appearance. The vast majority of the polyps are small tubular adenomas, although an occasional villous adenoma may occur. Eventual malignant transformation of one or more of these polyps is virtually inevitable in this disease; therefore, it is commonly treated with total colectomy at an early age.

(149) The Peutz-Jeghers syndrome is also an autosomal dominant disorder characterized by diffuse intestinal polyposis. In contrast to familial polyposis coli, however, the polyps of Peutz-Jeghers syndrome occur mainly in the small intestine and are of the hamartomatous variety.

(150) Villous adenomas in general tend to be symptomatic more often than other adenomatous polyps and often cause rectal bleeding. Villous adenomas may occasionally be associated with copious mucin production, causing a protein-losing enteropathy, a complication not usually associated with other types of colonic polyps.

(151) Although the hamartomatous polyps of the Peutz-Jeghers syndrome resemble tubular adenomas grossly, they are easily differentiated from the latter by histologic examination. Instead of the closely aggregated neoplastic glands of tubular adenomas, hamartomatous polyps are composed of tightly packed, highly arborized glands that are lined primarily by normal-appearing goblet cells. The glands are often separated by strands of smooth muscle. As the name implies, hamartomatous polyps are composed of proliferations of the three normal elements of the colonic mucosa: mucosal epithelial cells, loose connective tissue (lamina propria), and smooth muscle (muscularis mucosae) *(pp. 891–897).*

The Liver, Biliary Tree, and Pancreas

9

DIRECTIONS: For Questions 1 to 12, choose the ONE BEST answer to each question.

1. All of the following predispose to cholesterol gallstone formation EXCEPT:

A. Exogenous estrogen exposure
B. Crohn's disease
C. Clofibrate therapy
D. Obesity
E. Ulcerative colitis

2. All of the following characteristically cause fatty change in the liver EXCEPT:

A. Reye's syndrome
B. Diabetes mellitus
C. Total parenteral nutrition
D. Tetracycline toxicity
E. Acute B viral hepatitis

3. Which of the following histologic features of hepatocellular injury is prognostically LEAST favorable?

A. Councilman body formation
B. Bile infarct formation
C. Collagen formation
D. Ballooning of hepatocytes
E. Lobular inflammatory cell infiltrates

4. The hepatorenal syndrome refers to which of the following?

A. Functional failure of a morphologically normal kidney associated with severe liver disease
B. Simultaneous toxic damage to the liver and kidneys with functional failure of both
C. Immune complex glomerulopathy from chronic antigenemia associated with chronic viral hepatitis

D. Acute tubular necrosis due to hypotension after a gastrointestinal bleed in a cirrhotic patient
E. All of these

5. Which one of the following statements about central hemorrhagic necrosis of the liver is true?

A. Pressure necrosis from distended central veins and sinusoids is the major causal factor
B. Congestive heart failure is the most common cause
C. Its gross appearance is identical to that of nutmeg toxicity (nutmeg liver)
D. In chronic cases, micronodular cirrhosis frequently develops
E. Severe involvement with bridging necrosis is known as an infarct of Zahn

6. All of the following statements about fulminant viral hepatitis are true EXCEPT:

A. It is more common than fulminant hepatitis caused by drugs
B. Its severity is proportional to the immune response to the virus
C. Death usually occurs within 24 hours of the onset of symptoms
D. Histologically, it is commonly indistinguishable from drug-induced fulminant hepatitis
E. Survivors usually have lifelong immunity to recurrent infection

7. The liver condition pictured in Figure 9–1 predisposes to all of the following disorders EXCEPT:

A. Hemorrhoids
B. Cholesterol gallstones

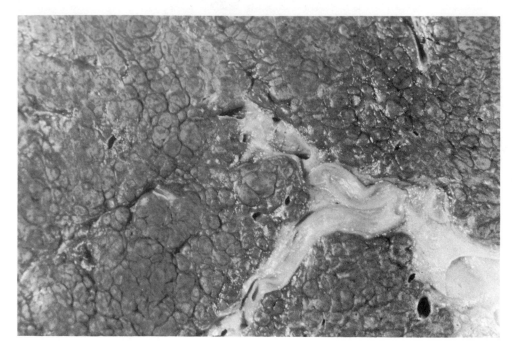

Figure 9–1

C. Hyperaldosteronism
D. Splenomegaly
E. Hepatocellular carcinoma

8. Causes of cirrhosis in infancy include all of the following EXCEPT:

A. Wilson's disease
B. Alpha$_1$-antitrypsin deficiency
C. Total parenteral nutrition
D. Extrahepatic biliary atresia
E. Galactosemia

9. All of the following statements about Wilson's disease are true EXCEPT:

A. It is caused by increased copper absorption
B. Kayser-Fleischer rings in the eyes are diagnostic

C. Excess copper in the liver is rarely visible on liver biopsy
D. Cirrhosis eventually develops in virtually all patients
E. Serum ceruloplasmin levels are characteristically low

10. All of the following features are associated with hepatocellular carcinoma EXCEPT:

A. Bile production
B. Alpha-fetoprotein production
C. Mucin production
D. Tumor embolization to the lung
E. Intraperitoneal hemorrhage

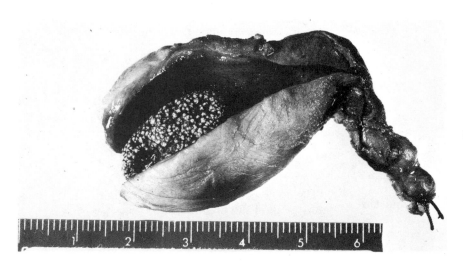

Figure 9–2

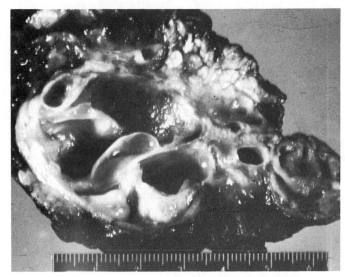

Figure 9–3

11. All of the following predispose to the disorder pictured in Figure 9–2 EXCEPT:

A. Obesity
B. Crohn's ileitis
C. Diabetes mellitus
D. Clofibrate therapy
E. Chronic hemolytic anemia

12. The lesion pictured in Figure 9–3 was removed from the head of the pancreas and was lined by epithelium forming papillary projections. This lesion is associated with:

A. Angiomas of the retina and cerebellum
B. Pancreatitis
C. Mucin-producing adenocarcinoma
D. Cystic fibrosis
E. Cysts in the liver and kidney

DIRECTIONS: For Questions 13 to 22, ONE or MORE of the completions given correctly finishes the incomplete statement. Choose:

A—if only *1, 2, and 3* are correct
B—if only *1 and 3* are correct
C—if only *2 and 4* are correct
D—if only *4* is correct
E—if all are correct

13. In which of the following conditions is the unconjugated (indirect) fraction of bilirubin increased more than the conjugated (direct) fraction?

1. Primary biliary cirrhosis
2. Recurrent jaundice of pregnancy
3. Rotor syndrome
4. Thalassemia

A. 1,2,3   B. 1,3   C. 2,4   D. 4 Only   E. All

14. Metabolic effects of alcohol that contribute to fatty change in the liver include:

1. Increased lipid absorption from the small bowel
2. Increased lipid mobilization from adipose tissue
3. Decreased triglyceride formation in hepatocytes
4. Decreased fatty acid oxidation

A. 1,2,3   B. 1,3   C. 2,4   D. 4 Only   E. All

15. In which of the following conditions is Mallory's hyaline found within hepatocytes?

1. Carbon tetrachloride toxicity
2. Wilson's disease
3. Viral hepatitis
4. Alcoholic liver disease

A. 1,2,3   B. 1,3   C. 2,4   D. 4 Only   E. All

16. Hepatic encephalopathy is a metabolic disorder that:

1. Characteristically causes asterixis
2. Frequently responds to antibiotic treatment
3. Is frequently associated with generalized cerebral edema
4. Does not occur when serum ammonia levels are normal

A. 1,2,3   B. 1,3   C. 2,4   D. 4 Only   E. All

17. Hepatic disorders that are incompatible with survival to adulthood include:

    1. Crigler-Najjar syndrome type 1
    2. Gilbert's disease
    3. Extrahepatic biliary atresia
    4. Wilson's disease

    A. 1,2,3   B. 1,3   C. 2,4   D. 4 Only   E. All

18. Hepatitis A virus infection is a disease that:

    1. Does not produce a viral carrier state
    2. Does not produce chronic hepatitis
    3. Is usually acquired by ingestion of contaminated food or water
    4. Sometimes produces fatal fulminant hepatitis

    A. 1,2,3   B. 1,3   C. 2,4   D. 4 Only   E. All

19. Causes of chronic active hepatitis include:

    1. Wilson's disease
    2. Methyldopa
    3. Alpha$_1$-antitrypsin deficiency
    4. Alcohol

    A. 1,2,3   B. 1,3   C. 2,4   D. 4 Only   E. All

20. Acetaminophen hepatotoxicity is related to:

    1. Dose of the drug
    2. Glutathione content of the liver cell
    3. Previous alcohol ingestion
    4. T-cell sensitization to the drug

    A. 1,2,3   B. 1,3   C. 2,4   D. 4 Only   E. All

21. Primary idiopathic hemochromatosis is a hereditary disorder that:

    1. Produces cirrhosis
    2. Is associated with HLA-A3
    3. Predisposes to hepatocellular carcinoma
    4. Commonly occurs in diabetic patients

    A. 1,2,3   B. 1,3   C. 2,4   D. 4 Only   E. All

22. Carcinoma of the pancreas is correctly described as:

    1. Arising from pancreatic acinar cells
    2. Decreasing in incidence in the United States
    3. Occurring most often in the tail of the pancreas
    4. Associated with spontaneous venous thrombosis

    A. 1,2,3   B. 1,3   C. 2,4   D. 4 Only   E. All

DIRECTIONS: For Questions 23 to 41, you are to decide whether EACH choice is TRUE or FALSE.

For each of the following statements about hepatitis B virus (HBV) infection, choose whether it is TRUE or FALSE.

23. The virus causes cytotoxic damage to the liver cells

24. Antibody production to the HBV surface antigen is defective in HBV carriers

25. Antibody production to the HBV core antigen confers lifelong immunity

26. The presence of HBV e antigen in serum indicates infectivity

27. HBV is the only hepatotropic virus associated with an asymptomatic carrier state

28. The histologic finding of ground-glass cytoplasm in liver cells is diagnostic of hepatitis B

29. HBV is the most common cause of virally induced chronic active hepatitis

30. Infection with delta virus occurs only in HBV-infected individuals

31. Co-infection with delta virus protects against chronic complications of HBV disease

For each of the following statements about extrahepatic biliary obstruction, choose whether it is TRUE or FALSE.

32. The increased serum levels of alkaline phosphatase help to differentiate it from primary biliary cirrhosis

33. The increased serum levels of conjugated bilirubin cause pruritus

34. The associated bleeding diathesis is a result of platelet dysfunction

35. The associated darkening of the urine differentiates it from hemolytic causes of jaundice

36. It is most frequently produced by impaction of a gallstone in the cystic duct

For each of the following statements about acute cholecystitis, choose whether it is TRUE or FALSE.

37. Virtually all patients with gallstones eventually develop acute cholecystitis

38. Bacterial infection is the initiating factor in acute cholecystitis in most cases

39. Chronic cholecystitis is usually preceded by repeat episodes of acute cholecystitis

40. Right upper quadrant pain is the most common presentation of acute cholecystitis

41. Surgical removal of the gallbladder is the treatment of choice

DIRECTIONS: For Questions 42 to 67, the set of lettered headings is followed by a list of numbered words or phrases. For each numbered word or phrase choose:

A—if the item is associated with (A) only
B—if the item is associated with (B) only
C—if the item is associated with *both* (A) and (B)
D—if the item is associated with *neither* (A) nor (B)

For each of the following characteristics, choose whether it describes hepatic vein thrombosis, portal vein thrombosis, both, or neither.

A. Hepatic vein thrombosis
B. Portal vein thrombosis
C. Both
D. Neither

42. The mortality rate is high

43. The disorder is known as the Budd-Chiari syndrome

44. An enlarged and tender liver is characteristic

45. Intra-abdominal tumor is a risk factor

46. Pregnancy is a risk factor

47. Peritoneal sepsis is a risk factor

48. Cirrhosis is a predisposing factor

For each of the statements listed below, choose whether it describes cholangitis, pericholangitis, both, or neither.

A. Cholangitis
B. Pericholangitis
C. Both
D. Neither

49. Characterized by a neutrophilic inflammatory infiltrate

50. Associated with cholelithiasis (gallstones)

51. Associated with inflammatory bowel disease

52. Produces an elevated serum alkaline phosphatase

53. Usually accompanied by bile stasis

54. Responds to antibiotic therapy

55. Predisposes to cholangiocarcinoma

For each of the characteristics listed below, choose whether it describes primary biliary cirrhosis, sarcoidosis, both, or neither.

A. Primary biliary cirrhosis
B. Sarcoidosis
C. Both
D. Neither

56. Productive of granulomas in the liver

57. Associated with Sjögren's syndrome

58. Associated with a hyperglobulinemia

59. Associated with cutaneous anergy

60. Associated with antimitochondrial antibody

For each of the characteristics listed below, choose whether it describes acute cholecystitis, acute pancreatitis, both, or neither.

A. Acute cholecystitis
B. Acute pancreatitis
C. Both
D. Neither

61. Strongly resembles perforated peptic ulcer on clinical presentation

62. Associated with gallstones

63. Associated with hyperlipidemia

64. Associated with hypercalcemia

65. Associated with alcoholism

66. Causes markedly elevated serum amylase levels

67. Causes adult respiratory distress syndrome

DIRECTIONS: Questions 68 to 81 are matching questions. For each numbered item, choose the most likely associated lettered item from those provided. Each numbered item has ONLY ONE answer. Within each group, each lettered item may be the answer to one, more than one, or none of the numbered items.

For each of the characteristics listed below, choose whether it describes liver cell adenoma, hepatocellular carcinoma, hepatic cholangiocarcinoma, gallbladder carcinoma, or none of these.

    A. Liver cell adenoma
    B. Hepatocellular carcinoma
    C. Hepatic cholangiocarcinoma
    D. Gallbladder carcinoma
    E. None of these

68. Associated with cirrhosis

69. Associated with cholelithiasis

70. Usually produces elevated serum levels of alpha-fetoprotein

71. Associated with Thorotrast exposure

72. Associated with oral contraceptive use

73. Occasionally causes the Budd-Chiari syndrome

74. Usually produces elevated serum levels of human chorionic gonadotropin

For each of the following causes of hepatic injury, choose the histologic feature with which it is commonly associated:

    A. Fatty change
    B. Cholestasis
    C. Councilman bodies
    D. Granulomas
    E. None of these

75. Hepatic duct obstruction

76. Hypersensitivity response to sulfa drugs

77. Toxicity from anovulatory steroids ("the pill")

78. High-dose corticosteroid toxicity

79. Yellow fever

80. Acute viral hepatitis

81. Cardiogenic shock

The Liver, Biliary Tree, and Pancreas

ANSWERS

1. **(E)** Most gallstones (approximately 85%) are composed largely of cholesterol. Cholesterol is a water-insoluble substance. Its solubility in bile depends on combination with bile salts and phospholipids, hydrophilic molecules that coat the cholesterol to form water-soluble micelles. In normal bile, the ratio of concentration of bile salts and phospholipids to cholesterol usually exceeds 13:1. When this equilibrium is disturbed by either an increase in the concentration of cholesterol or a decrease in bile salts or lecithin, cholesterol may precipitate out and form stones. Estrogens inhibit bile acid synthesis and increase cholesterol secretion as well. Thus, women are twice as often affected by gallstones as men, and exogenous estrogen administration increases the risk of gallstone formation in either sex. Clofibrate is a drug used to lower serum cholesterol levels in the treatment of hyperlipidemia and atherosclerosis; however, it increases cholesterol secretion by the liver and predisposes to gallstone formation. Obesity and high-calorie diets are related but independently variable risk factors for gallstones; both cause increased hepatic cholesterol secretion. Crohn's disease predisposes to gallstone formation through the depletion of bile salts. The ulceroinflammatory process of Crohn's disease mainly involves the terminal ileum—the site of bile salt resorption—leading to loss of bile salts from the enterohepatic circulation. Ulcerative colitis, on the other hand, produces disease largely limited to the colon and does not interfere with the enterohepatic circulation of bile salts *(pp. 967–969)*.

2. **(E)** The accumulation of fat within liver cells is one of the most common patterns of hepatic injury. Although the pathogenesis is not fully understood in some cases such as Reye's syndrome, most conditions that cause fatty liver are believed to involve one or more of the following metabolic/biochemical abnormalities in hepatocyte lipid metabolism: (1) excessive entry of free fatty acids into the liver; (2) interference with conversion of fatty acids to phospholipids; (3) increased esterification of fatty acids to triglycerides; (4) decreased apoprotein synthesis; (5) impaired coupling of lipid with apoproteins; and (6) impaired lipoprotein secretion from the liver.

Among systemic diseases causing hepatocellular fatty change, diabetes mellitus is one of the most common. Diabetes causes excessive breakdown of fat stores and an increased presentation of fatty acids to the liver. Total parenteral nutrition is associated with fatty change because the lipid content of the solutions presents an increased free fatty acid load to the liver. Many drugs cause fatty change in the liver, and tetracycline is thought to do so by reducing apoprotein synthesis.

Fatty change is not an unusual feature in acute viral hepatitis, however. Hepatotropic viruses cause lymphocyte-mediated immune attack on infected liver cells, producing diffuse liver cell injury and patchy necrosis. Although non-A, non-B hepatitis may cause mild fatty change in the affected liver, hepatitis with significant lipid accumulation usually suggests an alcoholic or drug-related cause *(pp. 20–21, 944–945, 963–964)*.

3. **(C)** The liver is an organ with impressive regenerative capacity and may recover fully from disorders that cause liver cell death. However, the severity, duration, and type of injury are counterbalancing factors in the recovery process. Chronic or profound injuries frequently lead to scar (collagen) formation in the damaged liver. Although fibrosis is reversible to a variable extent during the early stages of chronic injury if the source of the injury is removed, removal of the injurious agent is frequently difficult (alcoholism) or impossible (chronic active viral hepatitis or primary biliary cirrhosis). Thus, collagen formation often heralds the development of

cirrhosis and is prognostically the least favorable histologic feature of hepatic injury.

Councilman body formation and ballooning degeneration of hepatocytes are the histologic manifestations of coagulative necrosis or intracellular edema, respectively. A bile "infarct" refers to confluent necrosis of groups of hepatocytes from chemical (bile) injury. The liver, through regeneration, may recover fully from any of these events.

Lobular inflammatory infiltrates may be the cause or the result of hepatocyte necrosis and are a variable feature of hepatocyte injury. They may resolve completely or contribute to the formation of fibrosis. Thus, their prognostic significance is more variable than fibrosis itself *(pp. 16–17, 29, 917–918, 945)*.

4. (A) The hepatorenal syndrome is defined as functional renal failure in the absence of morphologically overt renal damage occurring in patients with severe liver disease (most often advanced cirrhosis) or undergoing surgery for biliary tract obstruction. Although the pathogenesis of the hepatorenal syndrome has not been fully elucidated, there is evidence that it may be related to generalized renal vasoconstriction, which is more marked in the cortex than in the medulla. The cause of the vasoconstriction may be multifactorial: increased production of vasoconstrictive thromboxane A_2 and decreased synthesis of vasodilator PGE_2; decreased circulating blood volume due to ascites causing elevated renin and aldosterone levels; and/or vasoconstriction mediated by endotoxin that is produced by intestinal organisms and that has escaped hepatic clearance. Although hepatic and renal failure may occur simultaneously in toxic or immune complex disorders, these specific cases are defined by their underlying cause and are not included in the concept of the hepatorenal syndrome. Likewise, acute tubular necrosis due to hypotension following a gastrointestinal bleed in a patient with cirrhosis would be excluded according to the above definition *(p. 918)*.

5. (B) Central hemorrhagic necrosis of the liver is a severe form of chronic passive centrilobular congestion and is most commonly caused by congestive heart failure. Necrosis of hepatocytes in the centrilobular zone is primarily the result of hypoxia secondary to arteriolar hypoperfusion, although pressure necrosis may have a secondary role. Grossly, the cut surface of the liver has a mottled pattern of deep red, blood-filled centrilobular zones rimmed by pale tan zones of necrotic hepatocytes in a background of normal red-brown parenchyma. Oddly, the resultant pattern resembles the cut surface of a nutmeg and thus has become known as nutmeg liver. (Eggnog drinkers note: Nutmeg is not a hepatotoxin.) In cases of chronic hypoperfusion and passive congestion, delicate centrilobular scarring may result, but true cirrhosis rarely develops. Infarcts of Zahn are sharply demarcated areas of red-blue discoloration of the hepatic parenchyma caused by occlusion of an intrahepatic branch of the portal vein. They are not related to central hemorrhagic necrosis. In fact, they are not associated with necrosis at all and, therefore, are not even true infarcts *(p. 921)*.

6. (C) Fulminant hepatitis is an uncommon but often lethal form of hepatocellular disease characterized by submassive to massive necrosis of liver cells and precipitous hepatic failure. Most cases (about 50 to 65%) are caused by viral hepatitis, but 25 to 30% of cases are related to drugs and chemicals. In contrast to the drug-induced form of fulminant hepatitis, in which the damage may be caused either by a hypersensitivity reaction to the drug or by direct toxic damage from a metabolite of the offending compound, fulminant viral hepatitis is most often an immunologically mediated phenomenon. Except for delta virus, none of the hepatotropic viruses are cytotoxic. Liver injury in viral hepatitis is produced by the immune response to the virally infected, antigenically altered hepatocytes, and the severity of the injury is proportional to the strength of the immune response.

Histologically, all forms of fulminant hepatitis tend to look alike. Massive "dropout" necrosis (liquefactive necrosis) of the liver cells occurs, leaving only a collapsed reticulin framework and intact portal structures. The severity and distribution of the necrosis tend to be variable. Although the mortality rate in fulminant viral hepatitis is high, those who do survive almost never become carriers but acquire lifelong immunity to recurrent infection.

Fulminant hepatitis causes rapidly progressive hepatic insufficiency, resulting in death 2 to 3 weeks after the onset of symptoms. Although rapidly fatal, fulminant liver failure does not produce sudden death (within 24 hours after onset) *(pp. 932–933, 937–939)*.

7. (B) Micronodular cirrhosis, the form of cirrhosis most commonly caused by alcohol abuse, is illustrated in Figure 9–1. The fibrous scarring and regenerative nodules of the sclerotic liver greatly increase resistance to flow through the portal venous system, and the hydrostatic pressure in the portal vein increases. With the rising portal pressure, flow is diverted into the systemic venous system through common portosystemic collateral channels. The principal sites of these portosystemic shunts are the veins around the rectum (hemorrhoids), gastroesophageal junction (esophageal varices), retroperitoneum, and the falciform ligament of the liver (periumbilical or abdominal wall varices). Blood flow is also preferentially diverted into the splenic vein, which is a major tributary of the portal vein, and congestive splenomegaly results. Secondary hyperaldosteronism and sodium retention also occur in association with cirrhosis. It is thought to be due to sequestration of blood within the splanchnic bed, decreasing the circulating blood volume. Renal perfusion is decreased, and renin is released from the juxtaglomerular cells, causing increased aldosterone secretion. In addition, impaired hepatic metabolism and excretion of the hormone contribute to the hyperaldosteronism.

Cirrhosis predisposes to the development of hepatocellular carcinoma. In the United States, about 80 to 90% of liver cell carcinomas arise in cirrhotic livers. The risk of developing hepatocellular carcinoma varies with different etiologic types of cirrhosis, but all forms impose some risk. Worldwide, cirrhosis following chronic active hepatitis from hepatitis B virus infection imposes the greatest risk of subsequent development of hepatocellular carcinoma. In the United States, where persistent hepatitis B virus infection is relatively infrequent, other forms of cirrhosis such as pigment cirrhosis (hemochromatosis) are relatively more frequently associated with hepatocellular carcinoma.

Cholesterol gallstones may be associated with cirrhosis because they can cause the condition, but cirrhosis is not a risk factor for their formation. Although secondary biliary cirrhosis is caused by chronic impaction of gallstones and large duct obstruction, this situation is now unusual because surgical therapy for cholelithiasis is widely available. Cholesterol gallstones result from hepatic production of bile with abnormal proportions of cholesterol and bile salts, a problem not typically associated with cirrhosis. For obscure reasons, alcoholic cirrhosis predisposes to the formation of pigment (bilirubin) gallstones, but this complication is infrequent and usually clinically inconsequential (*pp. 941–942, 968*).

8. (A) A wide variety of hereditary metabolic defects, congenital anomalies, and iatrogenic disorders can produce severe liver injury early in life and cirrhosis in infancy or early childhood. Although the hepatic manifestations of alpha$_1$-antitrypsin deficiency are extremely varied, neonatal hepatitis and childhood cirrhosis are produced in severe cases. Prolonged total parenteral nutrition administered in infancy is now known to produce significant hepatocellular damage, and cases of cirrhosis have been reported. Extrahepatic biliary atresia is a congenital condition characterized by defective development of the extrahepatic biliary tree, which may be incomplete and/or lack luminal patency. This rare and catastrophic condition is incompatible with life unless surgically corrected before the inevitable production of secondary biliary cirrhosis. Galactosemia and tyrosinemia are two of the more common errors of metabolism that produce cirrhosis in infancy if survival is sustained long enough.

Wilson's disease, in contrast, is an autosomal recessive disorder of copper metabolism that rarely becomes symptomatic before 5 to 10 years of age and in half of the patients remains asymptomatic until adolescence. Although copper accumulates in many tissues, the liver, brain, and eyes are principally affected (see Question 9). Ultimately, cirrhosis is produced, and Wilson's disease is among the most common causes of cirrhosis in older children. However, the disease is usually compatible with survival into adulthood. With early diagnosis and chelating drug (e.g., penicillamine) therapy, the buildup of copper in the liver, brain, and other organs is prevented and life expectancy is normal (*pp. 955–957, 964–966*).

9. (A) Wilson's disease (hepatolenticular degeneration) is a hereditary defect of copper metabolism with impaired excretion of copper by the liver. Copper accumulates in the parenchyma of various organs, most importantly the liver and brain. Deposition of copper granules in Descemet's membrane close to the limbus of the cornea produces one of the most characteristic and diagnostic features of Wilson's disease, Kayser-Fleischer rings. Although toxic accumulations of copper in the liver may first produce active hepatitis, the disease inevitably produces cirrhosis. Ironically, however, copper may be difficult to identify on liver biopsy in Wilson's disease. Copper is rarely visible in routine histologic preparations and may or may not be demonstrable with special histochemical techniques. A more easily identified abnormality consistently present in all patients with Wilson's disease is a reduction of the serum ceruloplasmin level. Absorbed copper is bound to ceruloplasmin, an alpha$_2$-globulin produced by the liver, before release into the circulation. Ceruloplasmin accounts for 90% to 95% of the total plasma copper. Normally, the ceruloplasmin-bound copper is then recycled to the liver for excretion through the bile. In Wilson's disease, copper is absorbed normally but biliary excretion of copper is defective. Copper accumulates in hepatocytes, causing injury and suppression of ceruloplasmin production. Thus, serum ceruloplasmin levels are consistently reduced. Nevertheless, total serum copper remains relatively normal because free copper loosely bound to albumin is proportionately increased. Free copper is the toxic culprit that causes all the extrahepatic tissue damage in Wilson's disease and is the target of chelating drug therapy (*pp. 956–957*).

10. (C) Hepatocellular carcinoma (hepatoma) often displays some of the distinctive features reminiscent of its cell of origin, the liver cell. Among normal cells, bile production is a feature unique to hepatocytes. Likewise, bile production by malignant cells identifies them as hepatocellular in origin. The production of alpha-fetoprotein by hepatocellular carcinoma is also highly characteristic but not diagnostic because other tumor types, such as germ cell tumors, may also manufacture this protein. The production of alpha-fetoprotein by hepatocellular carcinoma recapitulates the characteristic production of this protein by the embryonic liver.

Another distinctive feature of hepatocellular carcinoma is its striking propensity for venous invasion. It commonly invades the hepatic vein and may extend into the inferior vena cava. Fragments of intravascular tumor may then break off and embolize to the lung, a phenomenon associated with only a few other tumors, including renal cell carcinoma, choriocarcinoma, and gastric or breast carcinoma metastatic to the liver. Another common pattern of growth that hepatocellular carcinomas exhibit is direct extension through the liver capsule with penetration of surrounding structures. Capsular penetration may give rise to severe intraperitoneal bleeding, which is occasionally the presenting feature of the disease.

It is important to recognize, however, that hepatocellular carcinoma is not a mucin-secreting adenocarcinoma. Primary hepatic mucin-secreting adenocarcinomas originate from the bile duct epithelium and are known as cholangiocarcinomas. Rarely, hepatocellular carcinoma and cholangiocarcinoma may exist simultaneously in a so-called mixed pattern, but the two elements may be differentiated on the basis of bile production and mucin production, respectively. A bigger problem in differential diagnosis is distinguishing cholangiocarcinoma from the far more common metastatic adenocarcinomas of the liver. There are usually no distinctive features for either one, and they cannot be differentiated from each other on histopathologic grounds alone *(pp. 959–962).*

11. (E) The gallbladder pictured in Figure 9–2 contains a large crystalline, yellow-flecked, cholesterol gallstone. Cholesterol stones are by far the most common type of gallstone and account for about 85% of biliary calculi. Many contain varying amounts of bile salts, bilirubin, protein, or inorganic salts and are called mixed cholesterol stones. Nevertheless, their primary constituent is cholesterol, a water-insoluble molecule, which crystallizes out of a supersaturated bile. Thus, conditions that affect lipid metabolism and increase the cholesterol content of the bile, such as obesity, diabetes mellitus, and clofibrate therapy, predispose to the formation of cholesterol-containing stones (see Question 1).

In normal bile, cholesterol is kept in solution by bile salts and lecithin. These polar molecules form a hydrophilic shell around cholesterol, and the resultant water-soluble complex is known as a micelle. Conditions that lead to loss of bile salts from the enterohepatic circulation and reduce their availability for micelle formation also predispose to cholesterol calculus formation.

Therefore, diseases such as Crohn's disease that primarily affect the ileum, the principal site of bile salt resorption, increase the risk of stone formation.

Chronic hemolytic anemia is an example of a disorder that increases only the bilirubin content of the bile and predisposes to the formation of pigment (calcium bilirubinate) stones but not cholesterol-based calculi. Pigment stones are small, occur multiply, and are jet black *(pp. 967–970).*

12. (C) The lesion shown in Figure 9–3 is a multiloculated neoplastic pancreatic cyst known as a cystadenoma. These lesions are uncommon but are important to recognize because of their premalignant potential. The typical papillary epithelial lining of these tumors may be either serous or mucinous, the mucinous variety having the greatest premalignant potential. Extensive histologic examination of these tumors is required to rule out the presence of a mucin-producing adenocarcinoma in some portion of the wall. These lesions must be differentiated clinically from pseudocysts, by far the most common cystic lesion of the pancreas, and from congenital cysts or retention cysts. Only pseudocysts are invariably associated with pancreatitis. They are caused by severe inflammation, with focal necrosis and

fluid accumulation that is subsequently walled off by fibrosis. A cystic lesion without a true epithelial lining develops (therefore, a pseudocyst rather than a true cyst). Congenital cysts of the pancreas are believed to develop from anomalous pancreatic ducts. They may occur singly or multiply and are frequently associated with cysts in the liver and kidney as well. Rarely, they occur as part of an entity called von Hippel-Lindau disease. In this syndrome, angiomas are found in the retina and cerebellum or brain stem in association with cysts of the pancreas as well as cysts of the liver and kidney. Retention cysts are dilated pancreatic ducts that develop from ductal obstruction, such as occurs in cystic fibrosis from inspissated secretions. They are lined by ductal epithelium. Pseudocysts, congenital cysts, and retention cysts all tend to be unilocular lesions. The presence of a multilocular cyst, such as the one pictured in the figure, suggests a neoplastic lesion, a cystadenoma, or a cystadenocarcinoma *(pp. 989–990).*

13. (D) Bilirubin is a catabolic product of heme metabolism. It is delivered to the liver bound to albumin, taken up by the hepatocytes, conjugated with glucuronide, and excreted in bile. Disorders that cause defects in the excretion of bile from the hepatocyte or block its flow through the biliary tree cause an increase in serum levels of conjugated bilirubin (direct fraction). Unconjugated bilirubin (indirect fraction) is elevated in disorders that increase the amount of bilirubin delivered to the liver, impair hepatic uptake of unconjugated bilirubin, or impair the conjugation process within the liver cells. In thalassemia, for example, bilirubin production is greatly increased as a result of hemolysis, the conjugation capacity of the liver is overwhelmed, and the indirect fraction of bilirubin in the serum rises.

Primary biliary cirrhosis, recurrent jaundice of pregnancy, and Rotor's syndrome all cause increases in the direct fraction of bilirubin. They are examples of underexcretion rather than overproduction of bilirubin. The capacity of the liver cells to conjugate bilirubin is unimpaired in these conditions. In primary biliary cirrhosis, intrahepatic bile ducts are injured and flow through the injured duct is consequently impaired. In Rotor's syndrome and recurrent jaundice of pregnancy, secretion of bile into the bile canaliculus is impaired. Consequently, bilirubin conjugated in the hepatocytes cannot be eliminated and backs up into the serum. The secretory defect of the liver cells is hereditary in Rotor's syndrome and in recurrent jaundice of pregnancy is believed to be induced by an exaggerated response to estrogens *(pp. 913–915, 916–917, 921).*

14. (C) Alcohol consumption is the most common cause of fatty change in the liver. The abnormal accumulation of neutral fat in the hepatocytes is the result of a combination of pathogenetic mechanisms. Alcohol causes increased mobilization of lipid from adipose tissue stores, leading to excessive entry of free fatty acids into the liver. Concomitantly, alcohol increases the esterification of fatty acids to triglycerides while reducing fatty acid oxidation. In addition, the formation of lipoproteins and their release from the hepatic cells are also impaired by alcohol. Alcohol has no known effect on lipid absorption from the small bowel, however *(pp. 20–21)*.

15. (C) Mallory's hyalin is a finely granular eosinophilic material that is found in the liver cell cytoplasm in certain forms of hepatocellular injury. It is considered to be highly characteristic of alcoholic injury but also occurs in less common disorders such as Wilson's disease, primary biliary cirrhosis, chronic cholestatic syndromes, Indian childhood cirrhosis, focal nodular hyperplasia, and hepatocellular carcinoma. Mallory's hyalin is composed primarily of aggregates of prekeratin intermediate filaments. These aggregates result from alcohol-induced depolymerization of tubulin and defective assembly of microtubules required for intracytoplasmic transport of proteins. This pattern of injury occurs in relatively few hepatocellular disorders, however, and is not seen in carbon tetrachloride toxicity or viral hepatitis *(pp. 29, 945)*.

16. (A) Hepatic encephalopathy, a complication of liver failure, is a metabolic disorder of the central nervous system characterized by alteration in consciousness, neurologic signs, and electroencephalographic changes. It characteristically produces a flapping tremor of the upper extremities known as asterixis. Although the pathogenesis of these manifestations is uncertain, it is believed to be related to the production of a toxin in the intestine derived from protein metabolism by intestinal bacteria. With cirrhosis and portal hypertension, toxic substances absorbed from the bowel would be shunted into the inferior vena cava from the portal system through intra- or extrahepatic anastomoses, bypassing liver cells and escaping detoxification. Support for this concept is derived from the observations that high protein intake exacerbates the encephalopathy, whereas low protein intake and/or antibiotics administered to reduce the intestinal flora are effective in its treatment. Although ammonia has been implicated as the toxic agent, hepatic encephalopathy may occur in the absence of hyperammonemia. Pathologic findings in the brain are inconsistent in hepatic encephalopathy but usually include generalized cerebral edema as well as alterations in neurons and laminar necrosis. The changes are reversible if hepatic function is restored *(pp. 918–919)*.

17. (B) The Crigler-Najjar syndrome type 1 is characterized by the near complete impairment of glucuronyl transferase. Death inevitably occurs in infancy as a result of extensive brain damage caused by severe unconjugated hyperbilirubinemia. Extrahepatic biliary atresia inevitably leads to secondary biliary cirrhosis in infancy and causes death from hepatic failure unless surgical correction is possible. Gilbert's disease, in contrast, is a benign hereditary disorder producing mild defects in hepatocyte uptake of unconjugated bilirubin, mild deficiencies in glucuronyl transferase, and in 50% of the cases a mildly increased hemolysis. There are no patho-

logic alterations in the liver, and the disease is usually asymptomatic, at most producing a mild jaundice. Wilson's disease, although a much more serious condition, usually remains asymptomatic until adolescence. Wilson's disease is caused by an impairment in hepatic excretion of copper, leading to the accumulation of toxic levels of this metal in the liver, brain, and other organs. However, the process of accumulation is usually slow and is compatible with prolonged survival. Although the liver damage (hepatitis or cirrhosis) usually becomes manifest during childhood or adolescence, the degenerative changes in the brain generally develop during adulthood (see Question 9) *(pp. 919–920, 956–957)*.

18. (E) In the vast majority of cases, hepatitis A virus infection is a benign, transient disease from which lifelong immunity is acquired. The hepatitis A virus produces neither a carrier state nor a chronic disease process. In about 25% of cases, the infection is contracted by the fecal-oral route from infected humans, the natural reservoir of the virus, during the stage of fecal viral shedding. More often, the infection is contracted from contaminated food, water, milk, or shellfish. Only rarely does infection with hepatitis A virus produce fulminant hepatitis; thus, the mortality rate for this disease is less than 0.1%. Overall, hepatitis A virus is responsible for about 2 to 4% of fulminant hepatitis of viral origin and less than 1% of all fulminant hepatitis *(p. 925)*.

19. (E) Chronic active hepatitis is a serious disorder of varied etiology that is characterized by chronic destructive inflammation and fibrosis in the liver. It is a progressive disorder that often ends in cirrhosis and death. Although known to occur in about 3% of cases of acute hepatitis B and about 50% of all non-A, non-B hepatitis, chronic active hepatitis may also occur in association with Wilson's disease, drug toxicity or hypersensitivity, alpha$_1$-antitrypsin deficiency, autoimmune (lupoid) hepatitis, and alcoholic liver disease. The most common drugs known to cause chronic active hepatitis are methyldopa, oxyphenacetin, isoniazid, and acetaminophen *(pp. 935–937, 962–963)*.

20. (A) Acetaminophen hepatotoxicity is an example of liver injury produced by the bile transformation of the drug by the liver into a toxic product. This pattern of drug injury is called direct hepatotoxicity to distinguish it from indirect drug-related hepatotoxicity, in which the drug acts as a hapten to convert an intracellular protein into an immunogenic molecule. T-cell sensitization to the immunogen in turn effects an immune attack on the hapless liver cell.

In acetaminophen hepatotoxicity, the extent of hepatic injury is related to (1) the dose of the drug, (2) the glutathione content of the hepatocyte, and (3) previous ingestion of substances such as alcohol that induce the P-450 enzymes of the mixed-function oxidase system. Glutathione, a molecular constituent of the hepatocyte cytoplasm, is the keystone of one of the major drug detoxification systems in the liver. Conjugation of drug metabolites to glutathione renders them nontoxic, water soluble, and amenable to excretion in the urine. When the glutathione content of liver cells is exhausted, toxic drug metabolites accumulate in the cytoplasm. Because most drugs are metabolized by the mixed-function oxidase system of the hepatocyte, induction of this enzymatic system by one drug (e.g., alcohol or barbiturate) will accelerate metabolic transformation of other drugs by the same activated enzymes. In the case of acetaminophen, the greater the rate of metabolic biochemical transformation, the greater the production of the toxic metabolite. T-cell sensitization to acetaminophen with indirect hepatocellular injury is not believed to contribute to the hepatotoxicity of this drug *(p. 963)*.

21. (A) Primary idiopathic hemochromatosis is a hereditary disorder of iron metabolism transmitted as an autosomal recessive trait and closely linked with the histocompatibility gene HLA-A3. Severe systemic iron overload is produced, but the precise metabolic defect is still undefined. Profound parenchymal damage due to iron toxicity occurs in the liver, pancreas, myocardium, pituitary, adrenal, thyroid and parathyroid, joints, and skin. Micronodular "pigment" cirrhosis results from damage to the liver, characteristically the most severely affected organ. Pigment cirrhosis poses a considerable risk to the subsequent development of hepatocellular carcinoma, which is one of the leading causes of death due to hemochromatosis. Treatment (phlebotomy) reduces but does not eliminate the risk of hepatoma when cirrhosis is already present.

In the pancreas, iron is deposited in both the exocrine and the endocrine cells. The pancreas undergoes atrophy and fibrosis. Loss of pancreatic islets produces a secondary type of diabetes late in the course of the disease. Primary idiopathic diabetes mellitus, however, is unrelated to primary hemochromatosis. In short, diabetes commonly occurs in primary hemochromatosis, but hemochromatosis does not commonly occur in diabetic patients *(pp. 950–953)*.

22. (D) Carcinoma of the pancreas entails neoplastic transformation of the pancreatic ductal elements. Pancreatic acini may give rise to malignant tumors but do so rarely and make up less than 1% of all pancreatic malignancies. Pancreatic endocrine (islet cell) tumors are separately categorized neoplasms that are pathogenetically distinctive, not always malignant, and not generally designated as pancreatic carcinoma. The pathogenesis of pancreatic carcinoma is still obscure, but the threefold rise in incidence of this malignancy during the past 40 years is thought to be related to smoking, diet, and chemical carcinogen exposure. Most tumors (60 to 70%) arise in the head of the pancreas and may cause early obstructive symptoms. Although only 5 to 10% arise in the tail, these tumors are particularly insidious. They often grow silently for long periods and are usually metastatic by the time a patient comes to clinical attention.

One of the most characteristic paraneoplastic syndromes associated with pancreatic carcinoma is sponta-

neous venous thrombosis, also referred to as migratory thrombophlebitis and known clinically as Trousseau's sign. The pathogenesis of this condition is thought to be related to a tissue thromboplastic factor produced by the malignancy, leading to a hypercoagulable state *(pp. 990–992)*.

23. (False);   **24. (True);**   **25. (False);**   **26. (True);**
27. (False);   **28. (True);**   **29. (False);**   **30. (True);**
31. (False)

(23) Hepatitis B virus (HBV) is one of a small group of hepatotropic viruses that themselves are not cytotoxic for liver cells. Damage to the liver is produced by the host immune responses mounted against the virally infected liver cells. **(24)** Individuals who fail to respond immunologically to HBV harbor the virus indefinitely but fail to sustain liver disease. Such individuals are known as "healthy" carriers. **(25)** Antibody to the HBV core antigen is usually produced early in the course of the disease in normally responding individuals, but it serves only as a marker of current or recent infection. It does not confer immunity to the virus. Only antibody to the hepatitis B surface antigen is capable of eradicating the HBV infection and conferring lifelong immunity. **(26)** HBV e antigen is associated with the DNA-containing viral core but is immunologically distinct from both HBV core antigen and surface antigen. The e antigen is detectable in the serum early in the course of acute infection, when the disease is most transmissible, and disappears before the onset of recovery. Thus, it is a marker of infectivity.

(27) Although HBV is associated with an asymptomatic carrier state as outlined earlier, it is not the only hepatotropic virus to produce such a condition. The less well defined non-A, non-B viruses have been shown by epidemiologic evidence to occasionally produce a chronic carrier state. There is, however, no known chronic carrier state for hepatitis A virus.

(28) Overall, the histologic findings in acute viral hepatitis are similar whether produced by hepatitis A virus, HBV, or non-A, non-B. Because the histologic findings are so nonspecific in these three disease states, the best way to distinguish them is through serologic studies. Occasionally, however, hepatocytes infected with HBV may show an amorphous eosinophilic area within their cytoplasm known as ground-glass cytoplasm. This finding represents focal collections of virions and is pathognomonic of HBV infection. Unfortunately, it is usually seen only in chronic carrier states and is only infrequently present in acute hepatitis B.

(29) Chronic active hepatitis, a progressive fibrosing inflammatory disorder, follows about 3% of cases of acute hepatitis B, but about 50% of non-A, non-B hepatitis evolves to chronic active disease. Hepatitis A has not been known to produce chronic active hepatitis.

(30 and 31) Delta virus is a very small, defective RNA virus that can only replicate or cause infection when it is encapsulated by hepatitis B surface antigen. Thus, it can only infect HBV carriers or those with HBV hepatitis. It exacerbates any form of HBV infection: Healthy HBV carriers develop acute hepatitis, mild hepatitis progresses to fulminant disease, and the incidence of chronic progressive hepatitis and subsequent cirrhosis increases *(pp. 924–931).*

32. (False); 33. (False); 34. (False); 35. (True); 36. (False)

Extrahepatic biliary obstruction causes hepatic cholestasis, secondary hepatocellular dysfunction, and malabsorption as a result of the absence of bile acids in the gut. It is characterized by hyperlipidemia with increased plasma levels of cholesterol and phospholipids. (32) Increased serum levels of alkaline phosphatase originating from damaged ductal epithelial cells occur in extrahepatic duct obstruction but do not help to differentiate this disorder from other causes of cholestasis. Indeed, in primary biliary cirrhosis, significant elevations of alkaline phosphatase result from the widespread destruction of bile ducts, the hallmark of this disease. (33) One of the most characteristic clinical features of extrahepatic cholestasis is the development of pruritus, believed to be caused by the accumulation of bile acids in the serum. The elevated serum levels of conjugated bilirubin occurring in extrahepatic cholestasis cause jaundice, not pruritus.

(34) The absence of bile salts from the intestine seriously affects the absorption of fat and fat-soluble vitamins, including vitamin K. The synthesis of prothrombin and other vitamin K-dependent coagulation factors may become seriously impaired in extrahepatic cholestasis and may cause a bleeding diathesis. Platelet function is not known to be altered, however.

(35) In hemolytic causes of jaundice, excessive production of bilirubin results in an unconjugated hyperbilirubinemia. Unconjugated bilirubin is water insoluble and is bound to albumin in the serum; thus it is not filtered across the glomerulus into the urine. In extrahepatic biliary obstruction, however, jaundice is produced by conjugated hyperbilirubinemia. Because conjugated bilirubin is water soluble, it appears in the glomerular filtrate and produces a characteristically dark-colored urine (choluric jaundice).

(36) By far the most common cause of obstruction of the extrahepatic biliary tree is gallstones. In order to cause cholestasis in the liver, however, the stone must lodge in either the hepatic duct or the common bile duct. If lodged in the cystic duct, it may give rise to acute cholecystitis, but because hepatic biliary drainage is unimpaired, extrahepatic cholestasis does not occur *(pp. 916–918, 970).*

37. (False); 38. (False); 39. (False); 40. (True); 41. (True)

(37) Although the great majority (about 90%) of cases of acute cholecystitis are associated with gallstones, the converse is not true. In fact, most cases of cholelithiasis (perhaps 80%) are asymptomatic.

(38) Bacterial infection may be a contributing factor to the pathogenesis of acute cholecystitis in 5 to 10% of cases; however, the major causative factor in most cases is direct chemical irritation of the gallbladder wall by concentrated bile.

(39) Although repeat attacks of acute cholecystitis may result in chronic changes with fibrosis of the gallbladder wall, this rarely occurs. Chronic cholecystitis is classically an insidious disorder producing vague complaints and is not associated with acute bouts of severe inflammation.

(40) In contrast to the intolerance to fatty foods, belching, and epigastric distress that characterize chronic cholecystitis, acute cholecystitis usually manifests itself as an acute abdominal emergency. It commonly produces right upper quadrant pain, often referred to the right shoulder.

(41) The treatment of choice in acute cholecystitis is surgical removal of the gallbladder to prevent catastrophic complications such as perforation of the gallbladder with pericholecystic abscess formation, generalized peritonitis, ascending cholangitis, liver abscess formation, subdiaphragmatic abscesses, or septicemia *(pp. 970–972).*

42. (A); 43. (A); 44. (A); 45. (C); 46. (A); 47. (B); 48. (B)

(42, 43, 44) The Budd-Chiari syndrome is a rare but catastrophic event caused by thrombosis of the hepatic veins. Because the liver has a dual blood supply from the hepatic artery and from the portal vein but has a single venous outflow, occlusion of the hepatic veins has more serious consequences than any other major form of hepatic vascular occlusion. It is associated with a high mortality, many patients dying within days of its onset, most dying within months. The liver is enlarged and tender, and intractable ascites is produced. In contrast, portal vein thrombosis is much better tolerated. The liver is neither enlarged nor tender, and the outlook for survival is good when the problem is corrected surgically with a splenorenal shunt.

(45) One of the most common causes of thrombosis of either the portal or hepatic vein is vascular invasion by tumor. Hepatic vein thrombosis is frequently caused by tumors with a propensity for invasion of the vena cava, such as hepatocellular, renal cell, or adrenal carcinoma, whereas portal vein thrombosis is caused most often by tumors arising within the abdominal cavity.

(46) About half the cases of hepatic vein thrombosis are linked to conditions that are associated with thrombotic tendencies such as polycythemia vera, pregnancy and the postpartum state, oral contraceptive use, paroxysmal nocturnal hemoglobinuria, and intra-abdominal malignancies (in order of frequency). Vascular invasion from intra-abdominal malignancy is also a common cause of portal vein thrombosis, but it is the only major risk factor shared with hepatic vein thrombosis.

(47) Intrahepatic rather than peritoneal infections are common causes of hepatic vein thrombosis. Portal vein thrombosis, in contrast, is associated with intraperitoneal sepsis and secondary portal phlebitis. Furthermore, because the portal vein is anatomically continuous with the splenic vein, disorders that initiate thrombosis in the splenic vein, such as pancreatitis or pancreatic carcinoma, may produce portal vein thrombosis through retrograde propagation of the thrombus. Pancreatitis,

however, does not cause thrombosis of the hepatic veins. (48) Cirrhosis is the most common intrahepatic cause of portal vein thrombosis, but it does not predispose to hepatic vein thrombosis *(pp. 922–923).*

49. (A); 50. (A); 51. (B); 52. (C); 53. (A); 54. (A); 55. (D)

(49) Cholangitis is a suppurative inflammation of the intrahepatic or extrahepatic bile ducts and is characterized histologically by neutrophilic inflammatory infiltrates within the walls or lumina of affected ducts. (50) Cholangitis is almost always produced by extrahepatic duct obstruction, which is most commonly caused by impaction of a gallstone in the common bile duct.

(51) Pericholangitis, as the name implies, refers to inflammatory infiltrates in portal triads around, but not involving, bile ducts. In contrast to cholangitis, the inflammatory infiltrates in pericholangitis consist predominantly of lymphocytes and macrophages. Although pericholangitis is a rather common and nonspecific histologic finding, its strongest association is with inflammatory bowel disease.

(52) Both cholangitis and pericholangitis produce elevated serum alkaline phosphatase levels. Compared with cholangitis, however, the degree of alkaline phosphatase elevation occurring with pericholangitis is usually modest.

(53) Because cholangitis is almost always caused by extrahepatic duct obstruction, it is almost invariably accompanied by bile stasis. In pericholangitis, bile stasis may occur but is a much less predictable feature.

(54) Antibiotic therapy is usually effective in cholangitis, a process caused by direct bacterial infection of the bile duct. In contrast, pericholangitis is believed to be caused by drainage of bacterial products or other toxic substances through the portal system or peribiliary lymphatics and does not commonly respond to antibiotic therapy. (55) Neither cholangitis nor pericholangitis is associated with subsequent neoplastic transformation of bile ducts *(pp. 939–940, 970).*

56. (C); 57. (A); 58. (C); 59. (C); 60. (A)

(56) Both primary biliary cirrhosis and sarcoidosis are idiopathic diseases that are associated with abnormal immunologic findings and may produce granulomas in the liver. (57) Primary biliary cirrhosis is thought to be an autoimmune disease whose primary target is the intrahepatic biliary tree. The disease is associated with other autoimmune diseases such as rheumatoid arthritis, Hashimoto's thyroiditis, and Sjögren's syndrome. Sarcoidosis is characterized by hyperreactive cellular and humoral immunity but is not believed to be autoimmune in character. (58) Both diseases are associated with hyperglobulinemia. In sarcoidosis, abnormally high levels of antibodies to commonly encountered antigens typically occur. In primary biliary cirrhosis, the hyperglobulinemia is usually of the IgM class. (59) Abnormal cellular immunity is also observed in both diseases, and impaired T-cell reactivity with cutaneous anergy is characteristic. (60) Primary biliary cirrhosis can usually be distinguished, however, on the basis of the histologic

picture of a nonsuppurative injury to bile ducts and by the presence of an antimitochondrial antibody in the serum of 95% of patients with this disorder *(pp. 427–429, 953–954).*

61. (C); 62. (C); 63. (C); 64. (B); 65. (B); 66. (B); 67. (B)

(61) Acute cholecystitis and acute pancreatitis are diseases that may closely resemble one another at presentation, because the onset of both diseases is usually marked by the sudden development of acute abdominal pain, a situation known as an "acute abdomen." Thus, they must be differentiated not only from one another but from other common causes of acute abdomen such as perforated peptic ulcer or bowel infarction. (62) The two diseases share some etiologic factors as well. Gallstones are implicated in the pathogenesis of almost all (90%) cholecystitis, and in the United States are second only to alcohol consumption as the most common cause of acute pancreatitis. However, only a small percentage of patients with gallstones develop either of these conditions. Direct damage to the organ caused by bile salts and lecithin is believed to be the underlying causative factor in both disorders.

(63) Both acute cholecystitis and pancreatitis are also more common among individuals with hyperlipidemia. Type IV hyperlipidemia predisposes to biliary calculus formation, which, as mentioned, is strongly related to the pathogenesis of acute cholecystitis. Types I and V hyperlipidemia are more closely associated with acute pancreatitis. In contrast to acute cholecystitis, acute pancreatitis associated with hyperlipidemia is believed to develop from activation of pancreatic lipase, with local production of free fatty acids that are toxic to acinar cells and blood vessels. (64) Similarly, direct activation by calcium of another pancreatic enzyme, trypsinogen, is believed to be the underlying cause of acute pancreatitis associated with hypercalcemia. Trypsin, in turn, is able to activate most proenzymes in the pancreas, such as proelastase and prophospholipase, initiating a catastrophic process of autodigestion in the pancreas. Very rarely, calcium may be the major constituent of gallstones (calcium carbonate gallstones), conceivably causing duct obstruction and acute cholecystitis. However, the formation of these calculi is poorly understood and does not appear to be related to hypercalcemia.

(65) One of the conditions most strongly associated with acute pancreatitis is chronic alcoholism. Although the exact role of alcohol in the pathogenesis of this disorder is unclear, alcohol is known to be a potent stimulator of pancreatic secretion and has been postulated to have direct toxic effects on acinar cells. At the same time, alcohol may increase pancreatic sphincteric tone, leading to partial pancreatic ductal obstruction. Alcoholism does not appear to be related to the pathogenesis of acute cholecystitis, however.

(66) Amylase is one of many pancreatic enzymes released into the serum during an attack of acute pancreatitis. Elevation of serum amylase usually occurs within the first 24 hours of an acute attack and serves as an early marker for the disease. Although amylase is

somewhat less specific for pancreatic disease than other pancreatic enzymes, assay methods for amylase are simple and widely used. Serum amylase remains elevated during the active phase of the disease and declines to basal levels 2 to 5 days after the acute attack. Amylase is not an enzyme produced by the gallbladder or associated with cholecystitis.

(67) The adult respiratory distress syndrome (diffuse alveolar damage in the lungs) is an ominous complication of acute pancreatitis. The pathogenesis is thought to be related to enzymatic destruction of pulmonary surfactants by circulating pancreatic phospholipase released into the serum during an acute attack of pancreatitis (*pp. 970–972, 983–987*).

68. (B); 69. (D); 70. (B); 71. (C); 72. (A); 73. (B); 74. (E)

(68) Chronic infection with hepatitis B virus is the most common condition associated with hepatocellular carcinoma on a worldwide basis. However, in countries such as the United States, where the hepatitis B virus is not endemic, cirrhosis is the most common predisposing condition and is present in 85 to 90% of cases of hepatoma. The risk of developing hepatocellular carcinoma varies among the specific forms of cirrhosis. Hepatoma occurs with high frequency in pigment cirrhosis and postnecrotic cirrhosis. Although alcoholic cirrhosis is the most common form of cirrhosis in the United States, hepatocellular carcinoma is relatively rare in this disease, perhaps because the natural course of the disease is usually relatively short.

(69) Gallstones are present in most cases (75 to 90%) of carcinoma of the gallbladder. It is postulated that chronic inflammation of the gallbladder associated with gallstones may be an important factor in the pathogenesis of gallbladder carcinoma. Furthermore, metabolic derivatives of cholic acid, a bile component, are known to be potent carcinogens and may also contribute to the origin of this malignancy.

(70) High serum levels of alpha-fetoprotein are present in as many as 75% of patients with hepatocellular carcinoma. Although mildly elevated serum levels of alpha-fetoprotein may occur in nonmalignant liver disease, very high levels (greater than 1000 ng/ml) strongly suggest the presence of either of the two malignant tumors known to produce large quantities of this protein: hepatocellular carcinoma and yolk sac tumors of germ cell origin.

(71) Hepatic cholangiocarcinoma (carcinoma of the intrahepatic bile ducts) occurs with increased frequency in individuals exposed to Thorotrast, a contrast agent formerly used in radiography of the biliary tree. Thorotrast exposure is also associated with angiosarcoma of the liver which is otherwise rare, but does not increase the risk of any other hepatobiliary malignancies.

(72) Liver cell adenoma used to be a very rare tumor. Although still uncommon, it now appears more frequently in women who are between 20 and 40 years of age and who have used oral contraceptives.

(73) Hepatocellular carcinoma has a propensity for hepatic vein invasion and may even extend into the inferior vena cava and right side of the heart. With extensive hepatic vein invasion, venous outflow from the liver is blocked and the Budd-Chiari syndrome is produced.

(74) With rare exceptions, the only malignancies that produce elevated levels of human chorionic gonadotropin are those that originate from germ cells and have trophoblastic differentiation. The primary hepatic and biliary neoplasms discussed do not produce this hormone (*pp. 958–962, 974–977*).

75. (B); 76. (D); 77. (B); 78. (A); 79. (C); 80. (C); 81. (E)

(75) Very few histologic patterns of liver injury are pathognomonic for a given disease process. However, many causes of liver injury do predictably produce patterns that suggest the diagnosis. Hepatic duct obstruction, for example, characteristically produces cholestasis in the liver. Cholestasis is first seen in centrilobular zones and, if the obstruction persists, progressively involves the peripheral zones of the lobule and portal bile ducts. Although cholestasis may occur in other forms of liver disease, extrahepatic bile duct obstruction occasionally produces an additional unique feature called bile lakes or bile infarcts. These are produced by leakage of bile from small portal bile ducts with necrosis of surrounding liver cells. Bile infarcts are diagnostic of extrahepatic duct obstruction but occur in only 20% of cases.

(76) Drug-induced hepatic injuries fall into two basic categories: toxic injury and hypersensitivity reactions. In general, toxic injuries produce predictable pathologic changes. Hypersensitivity reactions are much less consistent in the pattern of injury they produce. They may result in cholestasis, nonspecific eosinophilic inflammation, granuloma formation, or injury resembling viral hepatitis ranging in severity from focal to massive hepatocellular necrosis. A few drugs tend to be more predictably associated with a specific type of hypersensitivity response than others. Reactions to sulfonamides, for example, most frequently produce a granulomatous hepatitis.

(77 and 78) Anovulatory steroids and high-dose corticosteroids are examples of agents that produce toxic liver injury. They commonly produce cholestasis and fatty change, respectively.

(79) Yellow fever is an acute viral disease that classically causes focal coagulative necrosis of liver cells. The dead hepatocytes become small, rounded, eosinophilic masses called Councilman bodies, after the renowned pathologist who first described them. This feature is not specific for yellow fever, however. It occurs in numerous other types of liver disease as well. (80) Acute viral hepatitis caused by any of the hepatotropic viruses, for example, produces focal random necrosis of liver cells with Councilman body formation. (81) Cardiogenic shock typically produces marked centrilobular congestion in the liver and may result in centrilobular zonal necrosis. However, it is not characteristically associated with fatty change, cholestasis, Councilman body formation, or granulomas (*pp. 916–917, 921, 933, 963*).

The Kidneys and Urinary Tract

DIRECTIONS: For Questions 1 to 8, choose the ONE BEST answer to each question.

1. All of the following substances are components of the glomerular basement membrane EXCEPT:

    A. Fibronectin
    B. Heparan sulfate
    C. Laminin
    D. Type IV collagen
    E. Fibrin

2. Most forms of chronic renal failure produce increased serum levels of all of the following substances EXCEPT:

    A. Calcium
    B. Aldosterone
    C. Phosphate
    D. Parathormone
    E. Renin

3. Uremia is associated with all of the following abnormalities EXCEPT:

    A. Peripheral neuropathy
    B. Gastritis
    C. Polycythemia
    D. Pericarditis
    E. Diffuse alveolar damage

4. Glomerular injury caused by circulating complexes occurs with all of the following disorders EXCEPT:

    A. Syphilis
    B. Goodpasture's syndrome
    C. Hepatitis B
    D. Systemic lupus erythematosus
    E. Lung cancer

5. Diabetes mellitus is associated with all of the following renal disorders EXCEPT:

    A. Diffuse glomerulosclerosis
    B. Nodular glomerulosclerosis
    C. Benign nephrosclerosis
    D. Urate nephropathy
    E. Acute pyelonephritis

6. Clinical manifestations associated with the kidney tumor pictured in Figure 10–1 include all of the following EXCEPT:

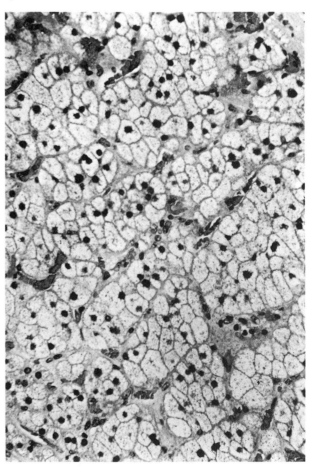

Figure 10–1

A. Hyperlipidemia
B. Cushing's syndrome
C. Polycythemia
D. Hypercalcemia
E. Femininization

7. All of the following conditions predispose to urolithiasis EXCEPT:

A. Sickle cell nephropathy
B. Hyperparathyroidism
C. Gout
D. Proteus pyelonephritis
E. Enteric hyperoxaluria

8. Of the conditions listed below, the one *least* likely to cause acute pyelonephritis is:

A. Pregnancy
B. Nephrolithiasis
C. Catheterization of the bladder
D. Prostatic hypertrophy
E. Septicemia

DIRECTIONS: For Questions 9 to 21, ONE or MORE of the completions given correctly finishes the incomplete statement. Choose:

Λ—if only *1, 2, and 3* are correct
B—if only *1 and 3* are correct
C—if only *2 and 4* are correct
D—if only *4* is correct
E—if all are correct

9. Mesangial cells are known to:

1. Ingest macromolecules
2. Connect with lacis cells
3. Be contractile
4. Make renin

   A. 1,2,3 B. 1,3 C. 2,4 D.4 Only E. All

10. In immunologically mediated glomerulonephritis, which of the following factors contribute to glomerular injury?

1. Substances secreted by macrophages
2. Substances released by platelets
3. Neutrophilic enzymes
4. Substances released by mesangial cells

   A. 1,2,3 B. 1,3 C. 2,4 D. 4 Only E. All

11. Systemic lupus erythematosus gives rise to glomerular lesions that are histologically identical to which of the following primary glomerular diseases?

1. Focal sclerosis
2. Membranous glomerulonephritis
3. Lipoid nephrosis
4. Membranoproliferative glomerulonephritis

   A. 1,2,3 B. 1,3 C. 2,4 D. 4 Only E. All

12. Renal papillar necrosis usually occurs in the *absence* of infection in:

1. Urinary tract obstruction
2. Analgesic abuse nephropathy
3. Diabetes mellitus
4. Sickle cell anemia

   A. 1,2,3 B. 1,3 C. 2,4 D. 4 Only E. All

13. Chronic pyelonephritis is a kidney inflammation that:

1. Causes symmetrically scarred kidneys
2. Is associated with vesicoureteral reflux in most cases
3. Characteristically spares the calyces and pelvis
4. Typically produces thyroidization of tubules

   A. 1,2,3 B. 1,3 C. 2,4 D. 4 Only E. All

14. Analgesic nephritis:

1. Is associated with ingestion of about a kilogram of analgesic per year
2. Is caused most commonly by phenacetin alone
3. Produces sterile pyuria
4. Predisposes to the development of renal cell carcinoma

   A. 1,2,3 B. 1,3 C. 2,4 D. 4 Only E. All

15. Substances that are produced by the kidney and that raise blood pressure include:

1. Platelet-activating factor
2. Kininogen
3. Prostaglandins
4. Renin

   A. 1,2,3 B. 1,3 C. 2,4 D. 4 Only E. All

16. Factors predisposing to essential hypertension include:

1. Positive family history
2. Chronic renal disease
3. High dietary sodium intake
4. Pheochromocytoma

   A. 1,2,3 B. 1,3 C. 2,4 D. 4 Only E. All

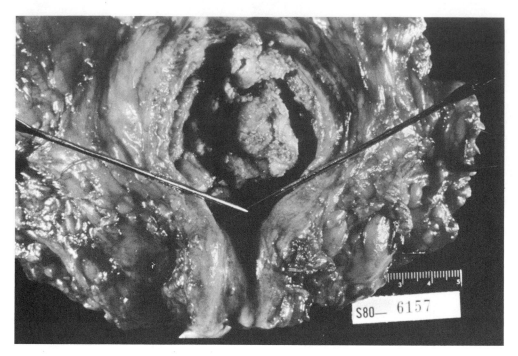

Figure 10–2

17. Histologic features of malignant nephrosclerosis include:

    1. Fibrinoid necrosis of arterioles
    2. Intimal thickening of arterioles
    3. Necrotizing glomerulitis
    4. Fibromuscular dysplasia of the renal artery

    A. 1,2,3 B. 1,3 C. 2,4 D. 4 Only E. All

18. Renal artery stenosis is correctly described as:

    1. The most common curable form of hypertension
    2. Usually caused by atherosclerotic plaque
    3. Producing high renin levels in the venous blood of the ischemic kidney
    4. Treated by surgical removal of the ischemic kidney

    A. 1,2,3 B. 1,3 C. 2,4 D. 4 Only E. All

19. Obstetric complications carry an increased risk of developing:

    1. Diffuse cortical necrosis

    2. Adult hemolytic uremic syndrome
    3. Acute tubular necrosis
    4. Hydronephrosis

    A. 1,2,3 B. 1,3 C. 2,4 D. 4 Only E. All

20. Hematuria is a characteristic clinical feature of:

    1. Glomerulonephritis
    2. Nephrolithiasis
    3. Renal cell carcinoma
    4. Bladder papilloma

    A. 1,2,3 B. 1,3 C. 2,4 D. 4 Only E. All

21. The tumor pictured in Figure 10–2 is associated with:

    1. Exposure to azo dyes
    2. *Schistosoma haematobium* infection
    3. Cigarette smoking
    4. Von Hippel-Lindau disease

    A. 1,2,3 B. 1,3 C. 2,4 D. 4 Only E. All

DIRECTIONS: For Questions 22 to 26, you are to decide whether EACH choice is TRUE or FALSE.

For each of the following statements about acute tubular necrosis (ATN), choose whether it is TRUE or FALSE.

22. Ischemic ATN commonly complicates massive hemorrhage

23. Nephrotoxic ATN is associated with thiazide diuretics

24. In toxic ATN, distal tubules are most severely damaged

25. Oliguria is the sine qua non of diagnosis of ATN

26. Recovery depends on compensatory hypertrophy of uninjured tubules

DIRECTIONS: For Questions 27 to 33, the set of lettered headings is followed by a list of numbered words or phrases. For each numbered word or phrase choose:
A—if the item is associated with (A) only
B—if the item is associated with (B) only
C—if the item is associated with *both* (A) and (B)
D—if the item is associated with *neither* (A) nor (B)

For each of the conditions associated with kidney disease listed below, choose whether it is a cause of rapidly progressive glomerulonephritis, the nephrotic syndrome, both, or neither.

A. Rapidly progressive glomerulonephritis
B. Nephrotic syndrome
C. Both
D. Neither

27. Streptococcal infection

28. Henoch-Schönlein purpura

29. Penicillamine therapy

30. Synthetic penicillin (e.g., methicillin) therapy

31. Wegener's granulomatosis

32. Goodpasture's syndrome

33. Systemic lupus erythematosus

DIRECTIONS: Questions 34 to 50 are matching questions. For each numbered item, choose the most likely associated lettered item from those provided. Each numbered item has ONLY ONE answer. Within each group, each lettered item may be the answer to one, more than one, or none of the numbered items.

For each of the following statements about cystic disease of the kidney, choose whether it describes childhood polycystic disease, adult polycystic disease, medullary sponge kidney, all of these, or none of these.

A. Childhood polycystic disease
B. Adult polycystic disease
C. Medullary sponge kidney
D. All of these
E. None of these

34. The disease is inherited as an autosomal dominant trait

35. Renal function is usually normal

36. Berry aneurysms are associated anomalies

37. Cysts arising from collecting ducts are present in the medulla

38. Cysts arising from proximal tubules are present in the cortex

For each of the characteristics of primary glomerular disease listed below, choose whether it describes lipoid nephrosis, membranous glomerulonephritis, membranoproliferative glomerulonephritis, IgA nephropathy, or none of these.

A. Lipoid nephrosis
B. Membranous glomerulonephritis
C. Membranoproliferative glomerulonephritis
D. IgA nephropathy
E. None of these

39. The most common cause of the nephrotic syndrome in children

40. The most common cause of the nephrotic syndrome in adults

41. Normal-appearing glomeruli by light microscopy

42. Basement membrane splitting in glomeruli by light microscopy

43. Cellular crescents in glomeruli by light microscopy

44. Subendothelial electron-dense deposits in glomeruli

45. Mesangial electron-dense deposits in glomeruli

46. Association with malignant epithelial tumors

47. Association with prophylactic immunizations

48. Association with thyroiditis

49. Association with primary activation of the alternate complement pathway

50. Very good long-range prognosis

The Kidneys and Urinary Tract

ANSWERS

1. (E) The glomerular basement membrane is the structure that is primarily responsible for the molecular size-dependent permeability barrier in the glomerulus. Its normal biochemical components include fibronectin, heparan sulfate (the most important of the polyanionic proteoglycans responsible for the charge-dependent glomerular filtration barrier), laminin, and type IV collagen, which gives structural support to the capillary wall. Fibrin is not a normal component of the glomerular basement membrane; its presence would indicate a pathologic alteration of glomerular permeability with leakage of fibrinogen such as occurs in glomerulonephritis (GN). Fibrinogen is a high-molecular-weight protein that is normally excluded from filtration across the glomerulus. With glomerular injury, fibrinogen may leak into Bowman's space, where it may itself serve as a mediator of further glomerular damage. Fibrinogen and fibrin stimulate cell proliferation in the glomerulus, and in some experimental models of GN, pretreatment with anticoagulants prevents proliferative glomerular lesions. The rationale for using anticoagulant therapy in the treatment of human GN is based on this observation *(pp. 1012, 1028)*.

2. (A) Chronic renal disease due to any cause manifests the same major physiologic consequences and clinical abnormalities. Hyperaldosteronism is produced as a consequence of increased renin production and compounds the problem of salt and water retention that results from impaired glomerular filtration. Phosphate begins to be retained as soon as the glomerular filtration rate drops below 25% of normal and overt uremia develops. Increased serum phosphate leads to increased entry of calcium into bone and a decrease in serum calcium levels. The failing kidney further contributes to hypocalcemia by its inability to synthesize 1,25-dihydroxyvitamin D_3, the active metabolite of vitamin D, which increases calcium absorption from the gut (see Chapter 3, Question 4). Hypocalcemia, in turn, stimulates the production of parathormone by the parathyroid glands, producing secondary hyperparathyroidism and renal osteodystrophy *(pp. 1016–1017)*.

3. (C) Uremia is a *clinical* syndrome resulting from chronic renal failure. It encompasses a host of metabolic and endocrine abnormalities that complicate the biochemical derangements of end-stage chronic renal disease. The severity of the clinical manifestations of uremia correlates only roughly with the degree of azotemia (elevation of blood urea nitrogen levels).

Uremia produces clinical abnormalities in almost every major organ system as well as systemic derangements of fluid, electrolyte, and acid-base balance. Neurologic abnormalities include peripheral neuropathy, myopathy, and encephalopathy. In the gastrointestinal tract, gastritis, esophagitis, and colitis are the major abnormalities. Cardiopulmonary abnormalities commonly include uremic pericarditis and less commonly diffuse alveolar damage with hyaline membrane formation (uremic pneumonitis).

On the one hand, uremia is associated with an *increase* in one of the two major endocrine functions of the kidney—that is, renin production. On the other hand, erythropoietin production, the second major endocrine function, is diminished. Therefore, anemia (not polycythemia) is the major hematologic manifestation of uremia *(pp. 1016–1017)*.

4. (B) Nephritis initiated by circulating antigen-antibody complexes is known to occur as a secondary consequence of various diseases. In nephritis of this type, the antibodies have no immunologic specificity for glomerular constituents. The complexes are simply trapped in the glomerulus because of their physicochemical properties and glomerular hemodynamic forces. Once the immune complexes have localized in the glomerulus, injury is mediated by various mechanisms including complement activation, neutrophil and monocyte infiltration, platelet activation, and fibrin deposition (see Question 10).

The underlying immune response in circulating immune complex nephritis may be directed against either exogenous or endogenous antigens. Diseases in which the inciting antigen is microbial in origin include syphilis, hepatitis B, malaria, and certain streptococcal infections, to name a few. Immune complex nephritis-associated diseases characterized by the production of antibodies against endogenous antigens include systemic lupus erythematosus and cancer, the antibody targets being native DNA and tumor-specific or tumor-associated antigen, respectively.

The glomerular injury in Goodpasture's syndrome is not the result of circulating immune complexes. On the contrary, autoantibodies against intrinsic components of the glomerular basement membrane (GBM) form immune complexes in situ as they are filtered through the glomerulus. It is the archetypal example of anti-GBM nephritis (*pp. 1024–1025, 1027–1028*).

5. (D) Diabetes mellitus is the systemic disease that produces the widest variety of renal lesions. The spectrum of diabetic nephropathy includes glomerular, vascular, and tubulointerstitial disease. Diabetic glomerulosclerosis may be either diffuse or nodular, the latter known as the Kimmelstiel-Wilson syndrome. The microangiopathy associated with diabetes is often more pronounced in the kidney than in other organs, producing arteriolosclerosis and benign nephrosclerosis. Acute pyelonephritis also occurs more frequently in diabetic than nondiabetic persons and may be associated with necrotizing papillitis (see Question 12), a consequence of the coincidence of acute bacterial infection and impaired papillary circulation.

Urate nephropathy is caused by precipitation of uric acid crystals in the kidneys of individuals with hyperuricemia. Urate crystals may precipitate in the tubules causing obstruction of nephrons, may deposit in the medullary interstitium, or may form stones in the collecting system. Hyperuricemia and urate nephropathy are principally associated with primary or secondary gout (e.g., chemotherapeutic treatment of leukemias and lymphomas with cell destruction and the elaboration of uric acid) (see Chapter 15, Questions 26 through 32). Urate nephropathy is not associated with diabetes mellitus (*pp. 1044–1047, 1055, 1059–1060*).

6. (A) The photomicrograph in Figure 10–1 illustrates the typical clear cell appearance of renal cell carcinoma. This tumor, which arises from tubular epithelium, is the most common renal cancer in adults. It is also one of the great mimics in medicine, because it is capable of manufacturing a wide variety of hormones that produce a number of diverse systemic syndromes. For example, Cushing's syndrome may result from the secretion of glucocorticoids by the tumor. Polycythemia may result from the production of erythropoietin. Secretion of a parathyroid-like hormone leads to hypercal-

cemia. Femininization or masculinization may occur if gonadotropins are elaborated by the tumor. Although renal cell carcinomas are known to contain a large amount of lipid and glycogen, giving them a clear cell appearance on histologic section, they do not secrete lipid and are not associated with hyperlipidemia (*pp. 1075–1076*).

7. (A) Although stones may be formed at any level in the urinary tract, most originate in the kidney. The majority of urinary stones (75 to 85%) are composed of calcium salts and occur in association with conditions producing hypercalcemia and/or hypercalciuria such as hyperparathyroidism. Five percent of calcium-containing stones are associated with hyperoxaluria, either primary (hereditary) or acquired by increased intestinal absorption of oxalates (enteric hyperoxaluria).

Primary or secondary gout increase serum urate levels and predispose to the formation of urate stones. Infections by urea-splitting bacteria, such as *Proteus mirabilis*, which convert urea to ammonia and create an alkaline urine, predispose to precipitation of magnesium ammonium phosphate salts in the urine. The result is the formation of very large urinary stones, frequently staghorn calculi.

Sickle cell nephropathy causes a spectrum of renal changes including hematuria, decreased concentrating ability, proteinuria, and even papillary necrosis but, unlike the above disorders, does not predispose to stone formation (*pp. 1070, 1073–1074*).

8. (E) Acute pyelonephritis is suppurative inflammation of the renal pelvis, tubules, and interstitium caused by bacterial infection. Ascending infection from the lower urinary tract is by far the most common cause. Infection is frequently associated with specific predisposing conditions, especially those that cause urinary tract obstruction such as pregnancy, stones, prostatic hypertrophy (see Chapter 11, Question 7), or tumors. Instrumentation of the urinary tract, most commonly catheterization of the bladder, also predisposes to acute pyelonephritis in the absence of obstruction or preexisting renal lesions.

Hematogenous infection of the kidney is much less common and usually occurs only in debilitated patients or in the presence of an underlying renal abnormality such as ureteral obstruction or previous renal injury. Septicemia alone rarely causes acute pyelonephritis because the kidney is remarkably resistant to blood-borne organisms (*pp. 1051–1055*).

9. (A) In addition to forming a branching cellular framework that supports the glomerular capillary tufts, mesangial cells have other important functions. They ingest macromolecules that have leaked across the glomerulus. They are also contractile and may thereby serve to regulate intraglomerular blood flow. They are connected with the lacis cells of the juxtaglomerular apparatus, the organelle that senses changes in afferent arteriolar pressure and is the principal source of renin production. Mesangial cells themselves, however, do not elaborate renin (*p. 1014*).

10. (E) Most glomerulonephritis is caused by antibody-mediated mechanisms of damage. Once immune complexes, either circulating and passively trapped (see Question 4) or formed in situ, are localized in the glomerulus, glomerular injury is produced by a combination of secondary mechanisms. Activation of complement produces neutrophil chemotactic agents. Neutrophils, in turn, release proteases and other enzymes that cause cellular and basement membrane damage. Macrophages and monocytes also infiltrate the glomerulus and release a large number of biologically active molecules, which contribute to glomerular damage. Platelets that aggregate in the glomerulus during immune-mediated injury release arachidonic acid metabolites and growth factors believed to act as mediators of glomerular injury. Even resident mesangial cells are believed to have a role. Mesangial cells can be stimulated to produce inflammatory mediators such as oxygen free radicals, interleukin-1, arachidonic acid metabolites, and growth factors that are capable of mediating glomerular inflammation and injury *(p. 1028)*.

11. (C) Systemic lupus erythematosus (SLE) gives rise to a number of forms of glomerular injury, including renal lesions that are indistinguishable from idiopathic membranous glomerulonephritis (membranous GN of SLE) or membranoproliferative glomerulonephritis (diffuse proliferative GN of SLE). Other patterns include typical crescentic GN (see Question 27), focal proliferative GN, and mesangial lupus GN, but lesions morphologically identical to focal sclerosis or lipoid nephrosis are not produced by SLE *(pp. 198, 1031, 1034, 1042, 1043)*.

12. (C) Renal papillary necrosis (necrotizing papillitis) is a distinctive, dramatic form of tubulointerstitial disease resulting in necrosis and sloughing of renal papillae. It occurs only in well-defined sets of circumstances. Most notably, it occurs in the absence of infection in analgesic abuse nephropathy and sickle cell anemia. In these conditions, the necrosis is a direct result of toxic or anoxic damage, respectively. Although papillary necrosis may occur with urinary tract obstruction or diabetes mellitus, it is rarely produced in the absence of superimposed infection in these conditions *(pp. 1004, 1055, 1057, 1070)*.

13. (C) Chronic pyelonephritis (CPN) refers to chronic tubulointerstitial inflammation associated with vesicoureteral reflux (VUR) or urinary obstruction, usually involving chronic bacterial infection. By far the more common underlying disorder in CPN is VUR. Irreversible parenchymal injury and scarring involving the calyces and pelvis are the characteristic result in both types of CPN. Pelvocalyceal involvement is an especially distinctive feature among the tubulointerstitial renal diseases, as it is encountered only in CPN and analgesic nephropathy.

CPN typically causes asymmetric, irregular renal scarring in contrast to the symmetrically scarred kidneys of chronic glomerular disease. An important cause of end-stage kidney disease, CPN accounts for about 11 to 20% of cases of renal failure. Most renal failure (about 50%) is caused by chronic glomerulonephritis.

Although the diagnosis is best made from gross examination of the kidneys, typical microscopic changes include patchy tubular atrophy and dilatation with interstitial inflammation and fibrosis. Dilated tubules may be filled with colloid casts and resemble thyroid follicles; thus, the pattern is referred to as tubular thyroidization *(pp. 1055–1057)*.

14. (B) Analgesic nephritis (analgesic abuse nephropathy) is a form of chronic tubulointerstitial nephritis with renal papillary necrosis caused by excessive intake of analgesic mixtures that include phenacetin. Intriguingly, the disease is almost always caused by drug mixtures and is rarely produced by single drugs alone. The offending mixtures commonly contain aspirin, acetaminophen (a phenacetin metabolite), or codeine in addition to phenacetin. The minimum requirements for the development of renal damage range between 2 and 3 kg of a phenacetin-containing analgesics over a period of 3 years. Pyuria is an early clinical manifestation and occurs in virtually every patient. Although the pyuria is often sterile, bacterial infection complicates about 50% of cases. If the drug abuse is continued, renal failure often ensues. If drug use is discontinued and infectious complications are properly treated, renal function will stabilize or even improve. Unfortunately, even with discontinued drug use, neoplastic complications may develop. Specifically, transitional papillary carcinoma of the renal pelvis has been found to occur with increased frequency in long-term survivors of this disorder. Increased risk of development of renal cell carcinoma, however, has not been noted *(pp. 1058–1059)*.

15. (D) In addition to their central role in the regulation of fluids and electrolytes that maintain extracellular fluid and blood volume, the kidneys further participate in the control of blood pressure by secretion of substances that have pressor effects as well as substances that lower blood pressure.

Renin secretion in response to decreased pressure in afferent arterioles, decreased sodium or chloride load delivered to the macula densa, or adrenergic stimulation is the major renal mechanism for increasing blood pressure. Renin raises blood pressure in two ways: (1) It catalyzes the first step in the enzymatic conversion of angiotensinogen to angiotensin II, a potent vasoconstrictor and the major effector molecule of the renin-angiotensin system; and (2) it stimulates aldosterone secretion by the adrenal cortex, thereby producing sodium retention.

Vasodepressor (antihypertensive) substances secreted by the kidneys include platelet-activating factor, kininogen (the basis of the urinary kallikrein-kinin system), prostaglandins, and some neutral renomedullary lipids. The vasodepressor substances are believed to counterbalance the vasopressor effects of angiotensin II *(pp. 1063–1064)*.

16. (B) Essential (primary) hypertension, by definition, occurs in the absence of any renal, endocrine, vascular, or neurogenic conditions known to produce increased systemic blood pressure. Thus, hypertension associated with endocrine causes such as pheochromocytoma or renal causes such as chronic renal disease is defined as secondary. It seems clear, however, that essential hypertension has both genetic and environmental contributory factors. In persons with a genetic predisposition, a high sodium intake contributes to the generation of hypertension *(pp. 1064–1066)*.

17. (A) Malignant nephrosclerosis refers to renal disease associated with malignant or accelerated hypertension. It may develop in previously normotensive individuals but is more commonly superimposed on preexisting essential hypertension or chronic renal disease. Characteristic histologic alterations produced include fibrinoid necrosis of arterioles (necrotizing arteriolitis), intimal proliferation and thickening in larger interlobular arteries (hyperplastic arteriolitis, also known as "onionskinning"), and glomerular thrombosis and necrosis (necrotizing glomerulitis).

Fibromuscular dysplasia of the renal artery is a cause of nephrogenic hypertension rather than an effect of accelerated systemic hypertension. It refers to a heterogeneous group of lesions of unknown cause characterized by fibrous or fibromuscular thickening of the renal artery leading to stenosis (see Question 18) *(pp. 1066–1068)*.

18. (A) Although its occurrence is relatively uncommon, renal artery stenosis is the most common curable form of hypertension. It is most frequently caused by an atheromatous plaque at the origin of the renal artery. The resultant reduction in blood flow to the kidney stimulates the renin-angiotensin system, which in turn elevates blood pressure. Elevated renin levels in the plasma or in renal vein blood from the stenotic side are typical, and a fall in blood pressure in response to administration of angiotensin antagonists can be demonstrated in almost all patients. About 60 to 75% of patients with atherosclerotic renal artery stenosis are cured after removal of the kidney on the nonstenotic side and surgical correction of the stenosis. The kidney on the stenotic side is protected from the arteriosclerotic effects of hypertension, which takes its toll on the contralateral kidney. When the stenosis is the result of fibromuscular hyperplasia, the postoperative cure rate is about 90% *(pp. 1068–1069)*.

19. (E) A number of renal disorders occur as obstetric complications. Delivery-associated disorders include diffuse cortical necrosis, acute tubular necrosis, and the adult hemolytic uremic syndrome, all basically ischemic in character. Diffuse cortical necrosis is a complication of disseminated intravascular coagulation (DIC; see Chapter 7, Question 5) and vasoconstriction. As an obstetric complication, DIC may be initiated by either release of tissue factor and activation of the extrinsic coagulation pathway (e.g., retained dead fetus or placenta) or by widespread injury to endothelial cells and activation of the intrinsic pathway (e.g., septic abortion, amniotic fluid embolism, toxemia). Diffuse cortical necrosis is a more severe form of injury in which DIC is associated is combined with vasoconstriction. It occurs most frequently after obstetric emergencies such as abruption placentae (premature placental separation from the uterine wall), septic shock, or extensive surgery. When bilateral, it is fatal.

The adult hemolytic uremic syndrome is a disorder characterized by widespread thrombosis in larger renal vessels such as interlobular arteries as well as afferent arterioles and glomeruli, together with necrosis and thickening of vessel walls and a microangiopathic hemolytic anemia. As in DIC, the intravascular coagulation is initiated by such problems as placental hemorrhage or retained placental fragments.

Hydronephrosis (dilatation of the renal pelvis and calyces due to obstruction to the outflow of urine) is a complication not of delivery but of normal pregnancy *(pp. 699, 1048, 1069, 1070–1072)*.

20. (E) Hematuria is an important but nonspecific indicator of renal disease. It occurs in a large number of renal disorders, including glomerulonephritis, nephrolithiasis, or tumors (benign or malignant) of the kidney or lower urinary tract, to name only a few. Although red blood cells in the urine may originate from anywhere in the urinary tract, red blood cell casts formed in the renal tubules are indicative of intrarenal (either glomerular or tubular) disease and are useful in the differential diagnosis of hematuria *(pp. 1023, 1074, 1076, 1094)*.

21. (B) The fungating bladder tumor pictured in Figure 10–2 is a transitional cell carcinoma of the bladder, by far the most common type of bladder neoplasm. Almost all (95%) bladder tumors are epithelial in origin (i.e., carcinomas). Transitional cell carcinoma constitutes about 90% of bladder carcinomas; 5% are squamous cell carcinomas, and 5% are mixed. Transitional cell carcinoma of the bladder has been shown to be related to a number of environmental carcinogenic agents. It has been clearly established that azo dyes contain a number of chemical compounds that dramatically increase the incidence of bladder cancer in exposed individuals. Azo dyes are used in textile, plastics, rubber, printing, and cable industries. Tobacco smoking has also been identified as a risk factor for bladder cancer, the incidence of bladder tumors being two to four times greater in smokers than in nonsmokers.

Schistosoma haematobium infection has long been known to increase the risk of bladder cancer. However, the vast majority of schistosoma-induced cancers are squamous cell carcinomas rather than transitional cell carcinomas. Von Hippel-Lindau disease is associated with dramatically increased risk of developing renal cell carcinoma, often bilaterally, but is not associated with an increased risk of bladder cancer *(pp. 1076, 1090–1091)*.

22. (False); **23.** (False); **24.** (False); **25.** (False); **26.** (False)

Acute tubular necrosis (ATN) is a syndrome of renal tubular damage (destruction of tubular epithelial cells) on a toxic or ischemic basis producing acute renal failure. It is particularly important not only because it is a *major* form of acute renal failure but also because it is a *reversible* form of renal failure.

(22) Ischemic ATN occurs most commonly after an episode of shock produced by severe bacterial infection, large cutaneous burns, massive crush injuries, or any acute event complicated by peripheral circulatory collapse (shock). It is of note, however, that ATN rarely occurs when the shock is due to massive hemorrhage alone. Therefore, it seldom complicates arterial rupture or laceration.

(23) Nephrotoxic ATN is caused by a wide variety of agents, including heavy metals, organic solvents, antibiotics, anesthetics, chemotherapeutic agents, radiographic contrast media, insecticides, and herbicides. Thiazide diuretics are not included in the list of drugs known to cause ATN. They are, however, associated with acute drug-induced (hypersensitivity) interstitial nephritis.

(24) Histologically, toxic ATN can be differentiated from the ischemic pattern by its characteristically targeted injury to the proximal tubules, generally sparing the distal tubular segments of the nephron. Ischemic ATN, in contrast, is characterized by focal tubular necrosis at multiple points along the entire nephron. Because shock and ischemia frequently complicate toxic ATN, ischemic damage to the distal nephron may be superimposed.

(25) Although acute suppression of renal function (renal "failure") is often accompanied by oliguria or rarely by anuria, up to 50% of patients with ATN actually have an increased urine output. Nonoliguric ATN is particularly common in nephrotoxic ATN and generally tends to have a milder clinical course.

(26) Recovery from ATN occurs with regeneration of injured tubules, because tubular cells have the capacity to divide. Tubular regeneration is compatible with full recovery from this disorder. Of course, the underlying cause must be reversed, and the patient supported with dialysis during the oliguric phase of the injury *(pp. 1048–1051, 1057–1058)*.

27. (A); **28.** (C); **29.** (B); **30.** (D); **31.** (A); **32.** (A); **33.** (C)

Rapidly progressive glomerulonephritis (RPGN) is a syndrome of glomerular damage characterized clinically by hematuria with a rapid and progressive decline in renal function and pathologically by a marked accumulation of cells in Bowman's space, forming crescents. The nephrotic syndrome is characterized clinically by massive proteinuria, hypoalbuminemia, edema, and hyperlipidemia, but the glomerular pathology is variable.

(27) Immunologically mediated glomerular damage occurring in association with nephritogenic streptococcal infection typically takes the form of an acute nephritis rather than the nephrotic syndrome. In a small propor-

tion of patients with poststreptococcal glomerulonephritis, however, rapid renal failure develops, and the classic clinical and pathologic features of RPGN are seen.

(28 and 33) Henoch-Schönlein purpura and systemic lupus erythematosus are two noteworthy examples of systemic diseases that may produce either a nephritic or nephrotic syndrome and are well-known causes of rapidly progressive glomerulonephritis. Henoch-Schönlein purpura is a syndrome of immune complex-induced necrotizing vasculitis principally involving the skin, the gastrointestinal tract, the joints, and the kidneys. The renal disease is quite variable, ranging from mesangial proliferation with the nephrotic syndrome to typical crescentic glomerulonephritis. Systemic lupus erythematosus is even more variable in its renal manifestations, which range from normal renal function with minimal proteinuria and hematuria to an overt nephrotic syndrome or RPGN with corresponding differences in the associated histologic lesions.

(29) Penicillamine is one of several drugs including gold and "street heroin" that are known to cause glomerular damage productive of the nephrotic syndrome. **(30)** Synthetic penicillin (e.g., methicillin), on the other hand, is one of a long list of drugs that are more apt to cause tubular damage or interstitial inflammation. Methicillin is a well-known cause of both nephrotoxic acute tubular necrosis and acute drug-induced hypersensitivity interstitial nephritis but is not associated with glomerular disease.

(31 and 32) Both Wegener's granulomatosis, a syndrome of necrotizing vasculitis, and Goodpasture's syndrome, a disease produced by autoantibodies directed against basement membranes, typically involve both the lung and kidney as their primary targets of injury. They are both well-known causes of crescentic glomerulonephritis (RPGN), which can be differentiated only on the basis of their immunofluorescent and electron microscopic characteristics. The antiglomerular basement membrane antibodies of Goodpasture's syndrome produce a diagnostic pattern of linear immunofluorescence and uniform basement membrane thickening not seen in Wegener's granulomatosis *(pp. 198–199, 1029–1034, 1043–1044, 1057)*.

34. (B); **35.** (C); **36.** (B); **37.** (D); **38.** (B)

Diseases that produce cystic changes in the kidneys vary widely in their etiologies and clinical consequences. **(34, 36, 37, 38)** Adult polycystic disease is an inherited autosomal dominant disorder in which cysts arise from any portion of the nephron. Thus, in contrast to childhood polycystic disease and medullary sponge kidney in which cysts develop only from collecting tubules, adult polycystic disease produces proximal and distal tubular cysts in addition to those of collecting tubule origin. The cysts typically involve only portions of the nephrons so that renal function is maintained until the fourth or fifth decade of life and affected individuals remain entirely asymptomatic until renal insufficiency commences. Although a third of the patients with this disease die with chronic renal failure, as many as 10%

succumb to the rupture of a berry aneurysm, an associated congenital anomaly present in 10 to 30% of patients.

(35) In contrast to the adult and childhood polycystic diseases, which produce profound abnormalities in renal function and ultimately lead to renal failure, medullary sponge kidney rarely causes any abnormality in renal function and is usually discovered incidentally or in relation to secondary complications such as infection or stone formation (*pp. 1018–1022*).

39. (A); 40. (B); 41. (A); 42. (C); 43. (E); 44. (C); 45. (D); 46. (B); 47. (A); 48. (B); 49. (C); 50. (A)

Most of the primary forms of glomerular disease produce the nephrotic syndrome and are differentiated on the basis of their clinical manifestations and morphologic patterns of injury. **(39, 41, 47, 50)** Lipoid nephrosis (minimal change disease) is the most common cause of the nephrotic syndrome in children. Clinically, it is associated with prophylactic immunizations and respiratory tract infections and with therapeutic response to corticosteroids and immunosuppressive agents, suggesting an immunologic basis for the disease. However, affected glomeruli do not contain immunoglobulins or complement and appear normal by light microscopy. The only morphologic lesion is the fusion of glomerular epithelial cell foot processes, a nonspecific change also present in other proteinuric disorders. In contrast to the other forms of idiopathic glomerular diseases, which frequently evolve to chronic glomerulonephritis and renal failure, lipoid nephrosis usually responds rapidly to therapy and has an excellent long-term prognosis.

(40, 46, 48) Membranous glomerulonephritis (GN) is the most common cause (40% of cases) of the nephrotic syndrome in adults. It is associated with certain malignant epithelial tumors (particularly carcinoma of the lung and colon and melanoma) and autoimmune disorders such as thyroiditis and lupus. Immune complexes formed from tumor-, DNA-, or thyroid-derived antigens respectively localize in the glomerulus in the form of subepithelial electron-dense deposits, a characteristic ultrastructural feature of membranous GN.

(42, 44, 49) Membranoproliferative glomerulonephritis accounts for 5 to 10% of cases of idiopathic nephrotic syndrome in children and adults. It is characterized morphologically by basement membrane "splitting," the result of protrusion of mesangial cell processes into the basement membrane of the capillary loops (mesangial interposition). In two-thirds of cases, subendothelial electron-dense deposits are seen by electron microscopy (type I MPGN). A second variant of MPGN is characterized by the deposition of electron-dense material in the lamina densa of the glomerular basement (type II MPGN or dense-deposit disease). Most patients with type II MPGN have abnormalities that suggest primary activation of the alternate complement pathway; neither C1q nor C4 is present in the glomeruli.

(45) IgA nephropathy, or Berger's disease, a recently recognized cause of proteinuria and the nephrotic syndrome, is characterized by the presence of prominent IgA deposits in the mesangial regions of affected glomeruli.

(43) Although a rare patient with IgA nephropathy may present with rapidly progressive glomerulonephritis (RPGN) with crescents, none of these forms of glomerulonephritis typically produces crescentic RPGN (*pp. 1033–1041*).

The Reproductive System

DIRECTIONS: For Questions 1 to 7, choose the ONE BEST answer to each question.

1. All of the following problems occur as complications of pelvic inflammatory disease EXCEPT:

A. Infertility
B. Intestinal obstruction
C. Appendicitis
D. Peritonitis
E. Endocarditis

2. Which of the following lesions of the female genital tract is considered precancerous?

A. Senile cystic endometrial atrophy
B. Endocervical polyp
C. Microglandular endocervical hyperplasia
D. Endometrial polyp
E. Adenomatous endometrial hyperplasia

3. Leiomyomas are benign tumors that:

A. Usually occur singly
B. Are well encapsulated
C. Require progesterone for growth
D. Usually grow rapidly during pregnancy
E. Give rise to most leiomyosarcomas of the uterus

4. Endometrial carcinoma is associated with all of the following EXCEPT:

A. Diabetes mellitus
B. Infertility
C. Oral contraceptive steroid use

D. Hypertension
E. Obesity

5. Factors that predispose to the development of ectopic pregnancy include all of the following EXCEPT:

A. Previous appendicitis
B. Endometriosis
C. Previous pelvic surgery
D. Gonorrheal salpingitis
E. Fetal chromosomal abnormalities

6. Seminoma and dysgerminoma share all of the following features EXCEPT:

A. Origin from primordial germ cells
B. Peak incidence in the fourth decade
C. Lack of endocrine function
D. Lymphocytic infiltration of the tumor stroma
E. High degree of radiosensitivity

7. Which of the following statements about benign prostatic hypertrophy is INCORRECT?

A. It originates in the periurethral portion of the prostate
B. Hyperplasia of both glands and stroma is seen histologically
C. It occurs in about 90% of males over 70 years of age
D. Less than 10% of those affected require surgical treatment
E. It is a risk factor for prostatic adenocarcinoma

DIRECTIONS: For Questions 8 to 13, ONE or MORE of the completions given correctly finishes the incomplete statement. Choose:

A—if only *1,2, and 3* are correct
B—if only *1 and 3* are correct
C—if only *2 and 4* are correct
D—if only *4* is correct
E—if all are correct

8. Risk factors for cervical carcinoma include:

1. Early age at first intercourse
2. Use of oral contraceptive steroids
3. Multiple sexual partners
4. Postmenopausal estrogen use

A. 1,2,3 B. 1,3 C. 2,4 D. 4 Only E. All

9. Invasive cervical carcinoma may be correctly described as:

1. Increasing in incidence
2. On the decline as a cause of cancer death
3. Originating from cervical dysplasia in most cases
4. The end result of most cervical dysplasias

A. 1,2,3 B. 1,3 C. 2,4 D. 4 Only E. All

10. Causes of dysfunctional uterine bleeding include:

1. Inadequate luteal phase
2. Adenomyosis
3. Anovulatory cycle
4. Endometrial hyperplasia

A. 1,2,3 B. 1,3 C. 2,4 D. 4 Only E. All

11. Factors that contribute to the etiology of hypertension in toxemia of pregnancy include:

1. Release of placental tissue thromboplastin
2. Decreased placental prostaglandin production
3. Increased maternal catecholamine production
4. Increased placental renin production

A. 1,2,3 B. 1,3 C. 2,4 D. 4 Only E. All

12. Which of the following diseases of the male genitalia are associated with human papillomavirus?

1. Bowenoid papulosis
2. Giant condyloma
3. Penile carcinoma
4. Balanoposthitis

A. 1,2,3 B. 1,3 C. 2,4 D. 4 Only E. All

13. Which of the following conditions are associated with an increased risk of testicular cancer?

1. Testicular irradiation
2. Testicular dysgenesis
3. Semen outflow obstruction
4. Cryptorchidism

A. 1,2,3 B. 1,3 C. 2,4 D. 4 Only E. All

DIRECTIONS: For Questions 14 to 34, you are to decide whether EACH choice is TRUE or FALSE.

For each of the following statements about the normal menstrual cycle, decide whether it is TRUE or FALSE.

14. The basal third of the endometrium does not respond to ovarian steroids

15. The endometrium in the lower uterine segment does not respond to ovarian steroids

16. After ovulation, endometrial glands contain numerous mitotic figures

17. After ovulation, estrogen levels rise to their highest peak

18. The length of the postovulatory phase of the menstrual cycle is the same in all women

For each of the following statements about herpes simplex virus type II (HSVII) infection, choose whether it is TRUE or FALSE.

19. It is the most common cause of sexually transmitted disease in the United States

20. After exposure, lesions usually appear after a symptom-free interval of about a month

21. Relapsing infection often leads to infertility

22. Relapse of latent infection is usually prevented by acyclovir

23. Herpetic cervicitis is causally related to cervical carcinoma

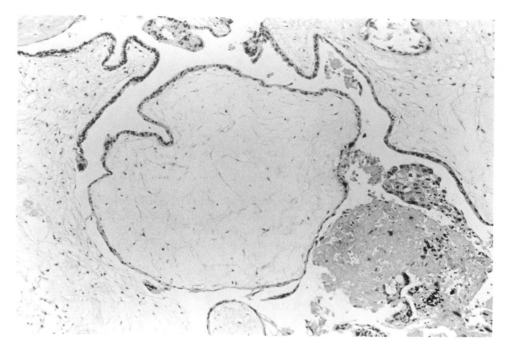

Figure 11–1

For each of the following statements about the lesion pictured in Figure 11–1, choose whether it is TRUE or FALSE.

24. It is a rare complication of gestation

25. It is usually accompanied by a developing fetus

26. It typically has a normal female karyotype

27. Its entire chromosome complement usually comes from the sperm

28. It is the most common precursor of choriocarcinoma

29. It is usually associated with higher serum gonadotropin levels than choriocarcinoma

For each of the following statements about prostate cancer, choose whether it is TRUE or FALSE.

30. About 30% of men older than 50 years have a stage A prostate cancer

31. Prognosis correlates well with the histologic grade of the tumor

32. Most tumors originate from the periurethral region of the gland

33. Serum chemistry for acid phosphatase is a useful screening tool for localized disease

34. Osteoblastic bone lesions in men with prostatic cancer are virtually diagnostic of metastatic disease

DIRECTIONS: For Questions 35 to 52, the set of lettered headings is followed by a list of numbered words or phrases. For each numbered word or phrase choose:

A—if the item is associated with (A) only
B—if the item is associated with (B) only
C—if the item is associated with *both* (A) and (B)
D—if the item is associated with *neither* (A) nor (B)

For each of the features listed below, choose whether it describes adenomyosis, endometriosis, both, or neither.

A. Adenomyosis
B. Endometriosis
C. Both
D. Neither

35. Characterized by endometrial tissue in an abnormal location

36. Almost never occurs in women over 50 years of age

37. Often produces dysmenorrhea

38. Often results in infertility

39. Caused by increased estrogen exposure

For each of the characteristics listed below, choose whether it describes serous ovarian tumors, mucinous ovarian tumors, both, or neither.

    A. Serous tumors of the ovary
    B. Mucinous tumors of the ovary
    C. Both
    D. Neither

40. Oral contraceptive steroid use is a predisposing factor

41. Most tumors exhibit cystic growth

42. Most tumors are malignant

43. Most tumors are bilateral

44. "Borderline" variants of low malignant potential are recognized

45. Simultaneous endometrial carcinoma is an associated complication

46. Malignant variants tend to spread by direct seeding throughout the peritoneal cavity

47. Psammoma bodies are a common histologic feature

48. Serum alpha-fetoprotein levels provide a useful clinical tumor marker

For each of the characteristics of ovarian stromal tumors listed below, choose whether it describes granulosa cell tumors, hilus cell tumors, both, or neither.

    A. Granulosa cell tumors
    B. Hilus cell tumors
    C. Both
    D. Neither

49. Usually cause virilization

50. Greatly predispose to endometrial carcinoma

51. Are characterized histologically by cytoplasmic crystalloids of Reinke

52. Seldom exhibit malignant biologic behavior

DIRECTIONS: Questions 53 to 62 are matching questions. For each numbered item, choose the most likely associated lettered item from those provided. Each numbered item has ONLY ONE answer. Within each group, each lettered item may be the answer to one, more than one, or none of the numbered items.

For each of the descriptions below, decide whether it refers to a Gartner's duct cyst, a nabothian cyst, a Bartholin's cyst, a hydatid cyst of Morgagni, or none of these.

    A. Gartner's duct cyst
    B. Nabothian cyst
    C. Bartholin's cyst
    D. Hydatid cyst of Morgagni
    E. None of these

53. Inflamed vulvovaginal gland with blocked duct

54. Mesonephric duct remnant of the vagina

55. Inflamed endocervical gland with a blocked duct

56. Endometriosis of the ovary

57. Wolffian duct remnant of the fallopian tube

For each of the characteristics of germ cell tumors listed below, choose whether it describes teratoma, choriocarcinoma, embryonal carcinoma, yolk sac tumor, or none of these.

    A. Teratoma
    B. Choriocarcinoma
    C. Embryonal carcinoma
    D. Yolk sac tumor
    E. None of these

58. Most common malignant germ cell tumor in men

59. Most common benign germ cell tumor in women

60. Struma ovarii is a specialized variant

61. Produces only alpha-fetoprotein

62. Produces only human chorionic gonadotropin

The Reproductive System

1. (C) Pelvic inflammatory disease (PID), a severe ascending infection of the female genital tract, may be transmitted sexually or occur as a septic complication of abortion or delivery. The severity of the disease depends somewhat on the causal organism and the route of infection, postabortion and postpartum infections typically being difficult to control. The consequences of uncontrolled PID, especially that caused by pyogenic, destructive organisms, can be severe. Local complications include peritonitis, bowel obstruction (due to adhesions between the inflamed pelvic organs and the adjacent intestinal loops), and infertility (due to pelvic adhesions and scarring of the genital organs). With septicemia, systemic complications such as infective endocarditis, meningitis, or suppurative arthritis may ensue.

The pelvic pain caused by PID may sometimes be severe enough to present as an acute abdomen and may mimic acute appendicitis. However, PID is not a *cause* of appendicitis (*pp. 1132–1133*).

2. (E) Endometrial hyperplasia refers to a spectrum of excessive proliferative changes in the endometrial glands and stroma. It is caused by elevated and prolonged levels of estrogenic stimulation, with diminished or absent progesterone production. It often occurs around the time of menopause and produces abnormal uterine bleeding. It may also occur as a result of an adrenal or ovarian disorder (see Question 50) or as a consequence of iatrogenic administration of estrogenic substances.

Beyond its production of abnormal uterine bleeding, endometrial hyperplasia is especially important because of the association of the more complex and atypical forms with endometrial carcinoma. In its mildest form, known as simple endometrial hyperpla-

sia, the proliferated glands lack atypia, and the disorder rarely progresses to endometrial carcinoma. In its more severe form, known as complex or adenomatous hyperplasia, the proliferated glands are more crowded and tortuous. When, in addition, the glandular epithelium is cytologically atypical (atypical hyperplasia or adenomatous/complex hyperplasia with atypia), the disorder is considered precancerous. Although endometrial carcinoma develops in only 2% of cases of untreated adenomatous hyperplasia without atypia, 23% of atypical hyperplasias progress to malignancy. In general, the greater the degree of atypia, the greater the risk appears to be.

Senile cystic endometrial atrophy is a postmenopausal change in the endometrial glands that can be confused with simple endometrial hyperplasia because the glands are cystically dilated in both conditions. However, in contrast to simple hyperplasia, the epithelium in senile cystic atrophy is flattened (versus tall and multilayered in hyperplasia), and the stroma is atrophic. Senile cystic atrophy is not believed to have malignant potential.

Endocervical polyps are completely benign lesions consisting of hypertrophied endocervical glands in a loose fibromyomatous stroma. They may cause irregular vaginal bleeding but are cured by simple curettage.

Microglandular endocervical hyperplasia is a benign cervical lesion occurring in women taking progesterone-containing oral contraceptive agents and sometimes occurring in women without this exposure. Clinically, it resembles a cervical polyp. Histologically, however, its tightly packed glands or tubules (sometimes showing cytologic atypia) can be confused with endocervical adenocarcinoma, to which it is unrelated. It has no known malignant potential.

Endometrial polyps are benign lesions consisting of hyperplastic endometrium, mostly of the mild, cystic variety. Although malignant change in an initially benign endometrial polyp may occur, it is extremely rare. Thus, endometrial polyps are not generally considered precancerous lesions *(pp. 1141, 1149–1152)*.

3. (D) Leiomyomas are the most common tumors in females, occurring in about 25% of premenopausal women. These benign smooth muscle tumors are well circumscribed but not encapsulated. In the great majority of cases, multiple leiomyomas are present. Leiomyomas are known to be hormone-dependent tumors that require estrogen for growth and are thought to be caused by excessive estrogen stimulation. Thus, during pregnancy they tend to increase rapidly in size and tend to atrophy after menopause or castration. Malignant transformation of leiomyomas is extremely rare. The malignant counterpart of this tumor, the leiomyosarcoma, almost always arises directly from the myometrium *(pp. 1152–1153, 1155)*.

4. (C) Endometrial carcinoma is rising in incidence and now accounts for almost 10% of all cancer in women. It is the most common invasive tumor of the female genital tract. A number of important risk factors for this disease have been defined: diabetes mellitus, infertility, hypertension, and obesity. Overt diabetes mellitus is present in about 10% of patients with endometrial carcinoma, and abnormal glucose tolerance in more than 60%. Infertility and a clinical history of menstrual irregularities consistent with anovulatory cycles tend to be common among those who develop this disease. Fifty percent of patients with endometrial carcinoma have hypertension, and 50% weigh more than 180 pounds.

There is substantial evidence that endometrial carcinoma is related to prolonged estrogen stimulation in some patients. In the past, an increased risk of endometrial carcinoma was reported with sequential contraceptive regimens consisting of potent estrogens in high dose, but these have since been withdrawn from prescription use. Present formulations of oral contraceptive steroids do not increase the risk for development of endometrial carcinoma *(pp. 1153–1155)*.

5. (E) Ectopic pregnancy refers to implantation of the fetus in any site other than the normal uterine location. It occurs most commonly in the fallopian tubes, usually the consequence of an acquired postinflammatory tubal abnormality. The most important predisposing condition is pelvic inflammatory disease (PID; see Question 1). As many as 50% of patients have PID-related chronic salpingitis, often of gonococcal origin. Less commonly, previous appendicitis, surgery, or endometriosis produces peritubal fibrous adhesions that interfere with tubal function. Whether intrauterine contraceptive devices also predispose to ectopic pregnancy is controversial.

In contrast to these maternal abnormalities, fetal abnormalities do not contribute appreciably to the development of ectopic pregnancy. They are, however, responsible for most spontaneous abortions *(p. 1171)*.

6. (B) Seminoma and dysgerminoma are the most common types of malignant germ cell tumors in men and women, respectively. Despite their different names, these tumors are identical in biologic type and are believed to arise from primordial germ cells. They are composed of sheets of uniform, undifferentiated germ cells that are divided into poorly demarcated lobules by lymphocyte-laden, fibrous tissue septa. The tumor cells themselves lack endocrine function. Occasionally, however, syncytiotrophoblastic cells, which produce human chorionic gonadotropin, may occur within the tumor.

In addition to their histologic similarities, seminomas and dysgerminomas share biologic traits as well. They have an excellent prognosis when excised while still localized within the gonad. Furthermore, because they both are highly radiosensitive, neoplasms that extend beyond the gonad can be well controlled or even eradicated by radiation therapy in most cases.

The greatest biologic difference between these tumors is the age-group in which they are most likely to occur. Although 75% of dysgerminomas occur in the second and third decades, seminomas peak in the fourth decade, distinctly later than the peak occurrence of dysgerminoma and somewhat later than the collective peak for other testicular germ cell tumors *(pp. 1109, 1167)*.

7. (E) Benign prostatic hypertrophy (BPH) refers to a process of stromal and glandular hyperplasia that originates from and is most severe within the periurethral portion of the prostate. It is an extremely common disorder in men over the age of 50 years and increases in frequency with increasing age. Thus, about 90% of men older than 70 years have BPH. However, the condition is clinically insignificant in the great majority of cases. Only about 5 to 10% of men with BPH require surgical treatment for relief of urinary tract obstruction. Although it was once held that BPH was a precursor to prostatic carcinoma, it is no longer believed that the two conditions are causally related. The coexistence of the two lesions is believed to be a reflection of the ubiquitous occurrence of BPH in older men *(pp. 1118–1121)*.

8. (B) Cervical carcinoma is now strongly suspected to be a sexually transmitted disease, related to infection by human papillomavirus. Thus, among the important risk factors for this neoplasm are early age of onset of sexual relations, multiple sexual partners, and high-risk sexual partners (i.e., males who are promiscuous, who have a former sexual partner with cervical carcinoma, or who have a history of penile condylomata).

The use of oral contraceptive steroids or estrogenic supplements after menopause is not associated with increased risk of cervical carcinoma. However, postmenopausal estrogen use may increase the risk of endometrial carcinoma through its induction of endometrial hyperplasia, a premalignant lesion (see Question 2) *(pp. 1142, 1150)*.

9. (A) The realization that epithelial malignancies could arise from precursor lesions of increasingly disordered epithelial growth and differentiation (dysplasia) came from studies of cervical carcinoma. It is now recognized that cervical carcinoma is the end stage of a continuum of progressive cervical dysplasia in the vast majority of cases. Thus, early diagnosis and treatment of premalignant lesions and in situ neoplasms have greatly improved the cure rate for cervical cancer and resulted in a dramatic decline in the death rate from this disease despite its increasing frequency.

Although most cervical dysplasias progress to higher-grade lesions with time, it appears that progression is not necessarily inevitable or may be extremely slow. Some cervical dysplasias followed over time remain static, without progression. Mild lesions and flat condylomata may even regress. However, the likelihood of developing invasive carcinoma with severe dysplasia/carcinoma in situ (cervical intraepithelial neoplasia grade 3, or CIN 3) is high. About 70% of women with untreated CIN 3 followed for a minimum of 12 years have been reported to develop invasive cervical carcinoma *(pp. 1141–1145)*.

10. (A) Dysfunctional uterine bleeding encompasses a group of disorders that produce abnormal uterine bleeding in the absence of an organic lesion. Among these disorders are various abnormalities of ovarian function, including anovulatory cycles, inadequate progesterone production by the corpus luteum (inadequate luteal phase), and irregular perimenopausal endometrial shedding.

In contrast to dysfunctional uterine bleeding, bleeding due to endometrial hyperplasia is accompanied by an organic lesion of the endometrium, namely a variety of disordered glandular and stromal growth patterns. Other organic lesions that cause abnormal uterine bleeding include adenomyosis, leiomyomas, endometrial polyps, and endometrial carcinoma *(pp. 1148–1149)*.

11. (C) Toxemia of pregnancy (preeclampsia) refers to a syndrome of hypertension, proteinuria, and edema that occurs in about 6% of pregnant women. A subset of these patients become seriously ill, developing coma or convulsions, a situation known as eclampsia. Many but not all patients with eclampsia develop disseminated intravascular coagulation (DIC).

The pathogenesis of toxemic hypertension appears to involve abnormalities in the physiologic adaptations of the renin-angiotensin system, which usually occur during pregnancy. The normal pregnant woman develops a resistance to the vasoconstrictive and hypertensive effects of angiotensin through the protective effect of prostaglandins of the E series produced in the uteroplacental vascular bed. In toxemia of pregnancy, placental prostaglandin production is decreased and placental renin production increased compared to normal pregnancy, and hypertension is the result. Catecholamines are not known to contribute to the pathogenesis of toxemia.

DIC is a consequence rather than a cause of toxemia of pregnancy. It occurs as a result of placental ischemia leading to increased output of thromboplastic substances *(p. 1172)*.

12. (A) As in the female uterine cervix, a spectrum of diseases of the penis, from inflammatory to precancerous to malignant, are believed to be causally related to human papillomavirus (HPV) infection. Among them are condyloma acuminatum, giant condyloma (Buschke-Lowenstein tumor), bowenoid papulosis, and squamous cell carcinoma of the penis.

Bowenoid papulosis is a penile lesion that appears clinically as multiple pigmented papules and histologically as a squamous cell carcinoma in situ. They are premalignant lesions associated with HPV type 16 infection. HPV type 16 DNA sequences can be detected in greater than 80% of lesions, although viral antigens are infrequently detected, suggesting that the level of virus production is low.

Like condylomata acuminata (venereal warts), giant condylomata are believed to be causally related to HPV types 6 and 11. In contrast to condylomata acuminata, giant condylomata are locally invasive tumors that may cover and destroy much of the penis. However, unlike invasive squamous cell carcinomas of the penis, giant condylomata do not metastasize. Thus, they are lesions intermediate between benign warts and true malignancy.

In addition to the demonstrated associations of HPV types 6 and 11 with precancerous penile lesions, there is also evidence linking HPV types 16 and 18 with penile malignancy. It has been hypothesized that the protective effect of circumcision in preventing penile carcinoma may be related to improved penile hygiene and reduced likelihood of infection by HPV.

Balanoposthitis is *bacterial* infection of the glans penis and/or prepuce. It is not related to HPV *(pp. 1100–1103)*.

13. (C) Testicular germ cell tumors occur with greatly increased frequency in pathologic conditions associated with gonadal maldevelopment. Testicular dysgenesis and cryptorchidism are the two most important. Testicular dysgenesis is a rare condition associated with endocrine abnormalities in which the seminiferous tubules fail to develop. Germ cell tumors arise in about 25% of dysgenetic testes. Cryptorchidism (undescended testis) represents failure of descent of the intra-abdominal testis into the scrotal sac. It occurs in as much as 0.8% of the male population and is unilateral in 75% of cases. Cryptorchidism greatly increases the risk of developing testicular carcinoma, and as many as 10% of all testicular tumors are associated with this disorder. The risk of carcinogenesis is 10- to 40-fold greater in the undescended testis than in the descended gonad. In general, the higher the location, the greater the risk. However, the contralateral, normally positioned testis is also at increased risk compared to normal testes, suggesting an underlying intrinsic defect in testicular development and cellular differentiation unrelated to anatomic position. Surgical correction does not reduce these risks but is recommended to attempt to preserve fertility and for ease of tumor surveillance.

Testicular irradiation and obstruction to the outflow of semen are examples of conditions that, like cryptorchidism, cause testicular atrophy but are not associated with an increased risk of testicular carcinoma *(pp. 1103–1104, 1108–1109)*.

14. (True); 15. (True); 16. (False); 17. (False); 18. (True)

The cyclic rise and fall of ovarian hormones normally produce a regular sequence of histologic changes in the endometrium. **(14)** Because the basal third of the endometrium does not respond to ovarian steroids, it remains behind after the menstrual flow and gives rise to the regenerated surface epithelium during the next cycle. **(15)** Not all regions of the uterus participate in this phenomenon, however. The endometrium in the lower uterine segment, an ill-defined zone located just above the endocervix, is not responsive to ovarian hormones and does not participate in the cyclic changes of the functional endometrium.

(16) During the preovulatory, proliferative phase of the cycle, the regenerating endometrial glands contain numerous mitotic figures. **(17)** Endometrial growth is stimulated by the estrogen production of the enlarging ovarian follicle. Estrogen rises progressively, reaches a peak just before ovulation, and then declines. After ovulation, estrogen levels again rise briefly at the end of the first postovulatory week, but the level is never as high as the preovulatory peak.

(18) Although the preovulatory phase of the menstrual cycle varies in length from woman to woman or even in the same woman during different cycles, postovulatory events occur according to a fixed physiologic schedule 14 days in length. Thus, glandular secretions, stromal predecidualization, and menstruation all normally occur in a highly predictable temporal sequence after ovulation *(pp. 1128–1130)*.

19. (False); 20. (False); 21. (False); 22. (False); 23. (False)

(19) The leading cause of sexually transmitted disease in the United States is gonorrhea. In fact, gonorrhea is the most common reportable communicable disease in the United States. Genital viral diseases have been rising dramatically in incidence over the past two decades, however. Herpes simplex virus type II (HSV II) infection, in particular, has become common among younger individuals and those with multiple sexual partners.

(20) Lesions consisting of painful red papules usually appear within 3 to 7 days after exposure. The papules progress to vesicles and coalesce to form ulcers. During the latter two stages, the lesions contain numerous viral particles, and a high transmission rate is the rule. **(21)** Unlike gonorrhea, which may produce infertility as one of its most feared complications, HSV II infection is usually limited to the vulva, vagina, and cervix and does not compromise reproductive function.

(22) Unfortunately, there is no known cure or prevention for HSV II infection. Although initial lesions heal spontaneously within 1 to 3 weeks, latent infection persists, and relapses occur in most cases. Topical or intravenous treatment with the antiviral agent acyclovir shortens the duration of viral shedding and accelerates healing of lesions but does not prevent relapse of latent infection.

(23) Although HSV II infection was once suspected to be causally related to cervical cancer and dysplasia, human papillomavirus (HPV) is now believed to be the important transmissible factor in cervical oncogenesis. HPV DNA is detectable by hybridization techniques in 75 to 100% of cervical condylomata, precancerous dysplasia, and invasive carcinomas of the cervix *(pp. 319–320, 1132, 1142)*.

24. (False); 25. (False); 26. (True); 27. (True); 28. (True); 29. (False)

(24) The lesion pictured in Figure 11–1 is a complete (or classic) hydatidiform mole. Moles are common complications of gestation that occur once in every 1000 pregnancies. They represent benign tumorous proliferations of pregnancy-associated trophoblastic tissue, but they have distinct malignant potential. As shown in the micrograph, a complete mole is characterized by cystic swelling of all or most of the chorionic villi. This is accompanied by diffuse trophoblastic proliferation. Patients usually present in the fourth or fifth month of pregnancy with uterine bleeding and an abnormally large uterus for the gestational stage. **(25)** In the great majority of cases of complete hydatidiform mole, an embryo or fetus is not present. The lesions are believed to originate in most cases from fertilization of an ovum that has lost its chromosomes. **(26)** Cytogenetic studies have shown that more than 90% of classic moles have a 46,XX (normal female) karyotype **(27)** and that the entire chromosome complement comes from the sperm, a phenomenon known as androgenesis. Less commonly, empty egg fertilization by two sperm results in complete moles with 46,XY karyotypes.

(28) Although moles are benign neoplasms, they are the most common precursors of choriocarcinoma. About 1 in 40 hydatidiform moles give rise to a choriocarcinoma, whereas only about 1 in 150,000 normal pregnancies results in choriocarcinoma. (29) Serum levels of human chorionic gonadotropin are often helpful in distinguishing between a benign mole and a choriocarcinoma, because the latter usually produces higher serum levels of this hormone. Although it is the most dreaded complication of hydatidiform mole, gestational choriocarcinoma can now be cured with chemotherapy in all but the most refractory cases *(pp. 1174–1178)*.

30. (True); 31. (True); 32. (False); 33. (False); 34. (True)

Carcinoma of the prostate is the second most common form of cancer and the third leading cause of cancer deaths in males. (30) Although it can be a lethal disease, prostate cancer occurs most frequently in a clinically insignificant form that is often discovered as an incidental finding at postmortem examination or within a surgical specimen removed for other reasons. In fact, it has been estimated that about 30% of men older than 50 years harbor a stage A (confined to the prostate) prostatic carcinoma.

(31) In prostate cancer, the grade of the tumor is of particular importance in determining the prognosis, because the correlation between histologic grade and biologic behavior is very good.

(32) In contrast to benign prostatic hypertrophy, which originates from the periurethral portion of the prostate gland, almost all carcinomas arise from the peripheral zone of the gland. (33) While the cancer is still localized within the prostate, serum tumor markers, such as prostatic acid phosphatase, cannot be detected. Only when the cancer has extended beyond the prostate capsule or has metastasized or both are serum elevations of prostatic acid phosphatase detectable by either radioimmunoassay or biochemical enzymatic assay.

(34) Metastatic spread of prostate cancer occurs chiefly to bones, particularly the vertebral bodies. Metastatic lesions are characteristically osteoblastic in contrast to most other forms of metastatic carcinoma, which are osteolytic. Therefore, osteoblastic bone lesions in men with known prostate cancer are virtually diagnostic of metastatic disease *(pp. 1121–1125)*.

35. (C); 36. (B); 37. (C); 38. (B); 39. (D)

(35) Adenomyosis refers to a pathologic process within the uterus characterized by the presence of endometrial tissue deep within the myometrial wall. Although endometriosis also refers to the presence of endometrial tissue in an abnormal location, it involves extrauterine sites such as the ovaries, uterine ligaments, rectovaginal septum, or pelvic peritoneum. The two processes are biologically and clinically distinct.

(36) Adenomyosis may occur at any stage of adult life. It can be quite common among postmenopausal women and has been reported to occur in 10 to 15% of uteri examined at autopsy. In contrast, endometri-

osis is a disease of women in active reproductive life and virtually never occurs after the age of 50 years.

(37) Premenopausal women with either of these processes frequently have dysmenorrhea and other functional pain. (38) Although both disorders may produce significant discomfort, only endometriosis is associated with serious complications. In long-standing disease with tubal and ovarian involvement, repeated bleeding of the ectopic endometrium with menstrual cycles leads to progressive scarring and, eventually, sterility.

(39) Although the pathogenesis of both of these conditions is still somewhat controversial, neither of these processes is believed to be related to increased estrogen exposure. Adenomyosis represents abnormal endometrium growth in the presence of normal or low estrogen levels. Theories about the pathogenesis of endometriosis include (1) regurgitation of endometrial tissue through the fallopian tubes, (2) metaplasia of coelomic epithelium, and (3) lymphatic or vascular dissemination *(pp. 1146–1148)*.

40. (D); 41. (C); 42. (A); 43. (A); 44. (C); 45. (D); 46. (C); 47. (C); 48. (D)

Tumors of the surface epithelium of the ovary are the most common types of ovarian neoplasms, and among these, serous and mucinous tumors are the two most common variants. (40) Although the risk factors for ovarian carcinoma are much less clear than for other genital malignancies, it is at least apparent that the use of oral contraceptive steroids is not associated with ovarian carcinoma and may even decrease the risk of developing this malignancy.

(41) Both mucinous and serous carcinomas are cystic tumors in most cases and cannot be definitively differentiated from one another by gross examination. (42) One of the most important reasons to differentiate between the two tumor types is that mucinous tumors are much more commonly benign than malignant, whereas serous tumors are seldom benign. (43) Furthermore, serous tumors are far more likely than mucinous tumors to be bilateral. About 20 to 30% of benign serous tumors involve both ovaries, whereas only 55% of benign mucinous tumors are bilateral. Malignant serous tumors are bilateral in about two-thirds of cases, in striking contrast to the 20% bilaterality rate of mucinous malignancies. (44) "Borderline" tumors are lesions that by histopathologic criteria are neither clearly benign nor clearly malignant. They represent a group of intermediate-grade tumors of low malignant potential. About 15% of either mucinous or serous neoplasms are borderline tumors.

(45) Simultaneous occurrence of an endometrial carcinoma in a significant number of cases is a property associated with endometrioid carcinomas of the ovary rather than serous or mucinous neoplasms.

(46) Despite the difference in frequency of occurrence, malignant variants of both serous and mucinous tumors have certain similarities in biologic behavior, the strongest being their tendency to spread by direct

seeding throughout the peritoneal cavity. For both tumors, metastasis by lymphatic or hematogenous routes is much less common.

(47) Another feature common to both serous and mucinous tumors is the presence of psammoma bodies within the tumor or its metastases. Although characteristic, psammoma bodies are not pathognomonic of ovarian carcinoma. They may occur in any type of papillary malignancy, including those of the pancreas or thyroid (see Chapter 14, Question 8).

(48) In contrast to malignant germ cell tumors of the ovary, epithelial tumors are not associated with increased serum levels of embryonic proteins such as α-fetoprotein or gonadotrophic hormones (pp. 1158–1163).

49. (B); 50. (A); 51. (B); 52. (C)

Ovarian stromal tumors are of particular interest because of their ability to elaborate hormones. (49) Because hilus cell (pure Leydig's cell) tumors predominantly synthesize androgens, they usually cause masculinization with hirsutism, voice changes, and clitoral enlargement. (50) Granulosa cell tumors, in contrast, are predominantly estrogen producing and greatly predispose to endometrial carcinoma (see Question 2). About 10 to 15% of patients with estrogen-producing granulosa cell tumors eventually develop endometrial carcinoma.

(51) A pathognomonic histologic feature of hilus cell tumors (as well as testicular Leydig's cell neoplasms) is the rod-shaped crystalloids of Reinke, which appear in the cytoplasm of about half of these tumors.

(52) Although occasionally troublesome or even dangerous (see Question 50) because of their hormone-producing capacity, both of these tumor types tend to be benign in their biologic behavior. Granulosa cell tumors exhibit malignant behavior in 5 to 25% of cases; hilus cell tumors are almost always benign (pp. 1167–1170).

53. (C); 54. (A); 55. (B); 56. (E); 57. (D)

Benign cystic lesions are extremely common in the female genital tract. They are commonly the result of cystic dilatation of either an inflamed normal gland or a remnant of an embryologic structure. (53) Bartholin's cysts arise from inflamed vulvovaginal glands and are often associated with gonorrheal infections.

(55) Similarly, nabothian cysts originate from inflamed endocervical glands. In contrast to Bartholin's cysts, however, these lesions are not usually the result of gonococcal infection. They usually occur as a result of so-called nonspecific cervicitis, a commonplace inflammatory process thought to be caused by a variety of bacteria, including streptococci, enterococci, *Escherichia coli*, and staphylococci.

(54) Among the developmental structures that may persist as remnants and undergo cystic change are the Gartner's duct cysts of the vagina, which represent mesonephric ductal structures, and (57) hydatid cysts of Morgagni of the fallopian tube, which arise from wolffian duct remnants.

(56) Endometriosis of the ovary (see Question 38) may, with repeated bleeding, undergo cystic change. These cysts have a distinctive gross appearance characterized by a brown, hemosiderin-laden wall and turbid hemorrhagic cyst fluid. On the basis of this appearance, they have become known as chocolate cysts (pp. 1128, 1133, 1138, 1140, 1148, 1156–1157).

58. (E); 59. (A); 60. (A); 61. (D); 62. (B)

Although germ cell tumors represent only 15 to 20% of all ovarian cancers, they comprise the vast majority (about 95%) of testicular malignancies. (58) Among the malignant germ cell tumors in both sexes, the most biologically primitive (the dysgerminoma in females and the seminoma in males) are the most common (see Question 6). (59) Overall, testicular germ cell tumors are almost always malignant, and ovarian germ cell tumors are almost always benign. Benign cystic teratomas or dermoid cysts constitute about 95% of ovarian germ cell tumors. These teratomas are very well differentiated. Although they contain primarily ectodermal structures, mesodermal and endodermal elements are also encountered and are also well differentiated. (60) Occasionally, a single histologic element of an ovarian teratoma comprises the entire tumor, a phenomenon known as monodermal or specialized teratoma. One of the most interesting of these is a tumor composed entirely of mature thyroid tissue known as struma ovarii. Because these tumors may hyperfunction, they may be a rare cause of hyperthyroidism.

(61) Like fetal tissues arising from germ cells, germ cell tumors synthesize embryonic and trophoblastic polypeptides, which serve as useful tumor markers. Alpha-fetoprotein (AFP), the major serum protein of the early fetus, is synthesized by the yolk sac as well as the fetal intestine and liver. Analogously, yolk sac tumors synthesize AFP almost exclusively. Embryonal carcinoma and teratomas may both synthesize AFP, but these tumors usually produce both AFP and human chorionic gonadotropin (HCG) simultaneously. (62) At the other end of the spectrum, choriocarcinoma usually produces only HCG like its normal counterpart, the trophoblast. Frequently, especially in testicular neoplasms, mixtures of these "pure" patterns of tumor differentiation occur simultaneously and, in turn, cause mixed patterns of oncofetal antigen and hormone elaboration (pp. 1108–1115, 1164–1167).

12

The Breast

DIRECTIONS: For Questions 1 to 8, choose the ONE BEST answer to each question.

1. The most important prognostic feature in invasive breast cancer is:

A. The histologic type of the tumor
B. The grade of the tumor
C. The size (diameter) of the tumor
D. The status of the draining lymph nodes
E. The presence or absence of estrogen receptors on tumor cells

2. Poor prognosis in breast cancer is associated with:

A. The presence of the *neu* oncogene
B. The absence of estrogen receptors
C. The presence of aneuploidy
D. All of the above
E. None of the above

3. All of the following statements about intraductal carcinoma of the breast are true EXCEPT:

A. It is not usually detectable by palpation
B. It is usually detectable by mammography
C. Draining lymph nodes contain metastases in only 1% of cases
D. The risk of invasive carcinoma is increased in both breasts
E. It can often be cured by surgical excision

4. Gynecomastia is associated with all of the following EXCEPT:

A. Alcoholic cirrhosis
B. Prostatic carcinoma
C. Cimetidine ingestion
D. Leydig's cell tumor
E. Klinefelter's syndrome

5. All of the following statements about sclerosing adenosis are true EXCEPT:

A. It is a variant of fibrocystic disease
B. It typically lacks cysts
C. Florid cases resemble carcinoma clinically
D. Florid cases resemble carcinoma histologically
E. It is considered a premalignant condition

6. All of the following are risk factors for breast cancer EXCEPT:

A. Close relatives with breast cancer
B. Early menarche
C. Early menopause
D. History of endometrial carcinoma
E. Obesity

DIRECTIONS: For Questions 7 to 19, ONE or MORE of the completions given correctly finishes the incomplete statement. Choose:

A—if only *1,2, and 3* are correct
B—if only *1 and 3* are correct
C—if only *2 and 4* are correct
D—if only *4* is correct
E—if all are correct

7. Features that invariably indicate malignant transformation in cystosarcoma phyllodes (phyllodes tumor) include:

1. Ulceration of the overlying breast skin
2. Invasion of the adjacent breast tissue
3. Cellular anaplasia
4. Rapid increase in size

A. 1,2,3   B. 1,3   C. 2,4   D. 4 only   E. All

8. Microscopic features of gynecomastia include:

1. Ductal hyperplasia
2. Stromal hyalinization
3. Stromal hyperplasia
4. Lobular hyperplasia

A. 1,2,3 B. 1,3 C. 2,4 D. 4 Only E. All

9. The ducts of the normal breast are correctly described as

1. Modified eccrine glands
2. Composed of a single layer of cells
3. Increasing their mitotic activity in response to estrogens
4. Forming a network of circumferentially anastomosing channels throughout the breast

A. 1,2,3 B. 1,3 C. 2,4 D. 4 Only E. All

10. Histologic types of breast carcinoma associated with a better overall prognosis than infiltrating ductal carcinoma (the most common type) include:

1. Tubular carcinoma
2. Papillary carcinoma
3. Colloid (mucinous) carcinoma
4. Medullary carcinoma

A. 1,2,3 B. 1,3 C. 2,4 D. 4 Only E. All

11. Carcinoma of the male breast is correctly described as:

1. About 100 times less common than female breast cancer
2. Having a better overall prognosis than female breast cancer
3. Metastasizing in the same pattern as female breast cancer
4. Usually preceded by gynecomastia

A. 1,2,3 B. 1,3 C. 2,4 D. 4 Only E. All

12. Paget's disease of the breast is associated with:

1. Dermal lymphatic invasion from an underlying ductal carcinoma
2. An osteolytic-osteoblastic process in bone
3. A better prognosis than infiltrating ductal carcinoma of comparable stage
4. Occurrence in the absence of a palpable breast mass

A. 1,2,3 B. 1,3 C. 2,4 D. 4 Only E. All

13. Benign histologic lesions that are associated with an increased risk of breast carcinoma include

1. Atypical ductal hyperplasia
2. Multiple intraductal papillomas
3. Atypical lobular hyperplasia
4. Apocrine metaplasia

A. 1,2,3, B. 1,3 C. 2,4 D. 4 Only E. All

14. High level of estrogen receptors in a breast cancer is likely to be associated with*

1. A high degree of tumor cell differentiation
2. Previous exposure to estrogenic drugs
3. Therapeutic response of the tumor to tamoxifen
4. Therapeutic response of the tumor to doxorubicin (Adriamycin)

A. 1,2,3 B. 1,3 C. 2,4 D. 4 Only E. All

15. Lesions of the breast that are characteristically tender or painful include:

1. Galactocele
2. Mammary duct ectasia
3. Cystic disease
4. Infiltrating ductal carcinoma

A. 1,2,3 B. 1,3 C. 2,4 D. 4 Only E. All

16. Fibroadenoma of the breast is known to:

1. Represent both a stromal and a glandular proliferation
2. Be rare before age 30
3. Be a sharply circumscribed lesion
4. Often harbor a carcinoma

A. 1,2,3 B. 1,3 C. 2,4 D. 4 Only E. All

17. Features characteristic of fibrocystic disease include:

1. Stromal degeneration (atrophy)
2. Proliferation of small ductules
3. Acute inflammation
4. Proliferation of ductal epithelium

A. 1,2,3 B. 1,3 C. 2,4 D. 4 Only E. All

18. A 35-year-old woman notices a lump in the upper outer quadrant of her left breast; it fluctuates in size with her menstrual cycles. This clinical behavior is compatible with:

1. Fibroadenoma
2. Intraductal papilloma
3. Cystic disease
4. Infiltrating ductal carcinoma

A. 1,2,3 B. 1,3 C. 2,4 D. 4 Only E. All

19. A 50-year-old woman has a brownish discharge from the nipple but has no palpable mass in her breast. This clinical situation describes:

1. Intraductal papilloma
2. Duct ectasia
3. Paget's disease
4. Galactocele

A. 1,2,3 B. 1,3 C. 2,4 D. 4 Only E. All

DIRECTIONS: For Questions 20 to 37, the set of lettered headings is followed by a list of numbered words or phrases. For each numbered word or phrase choose:

A—if the item is associated with (A) only
B—if the item is associated with (B) only
C—if the item is associated with *both* (A) and (B)
D—if the item is associated with *neither* (A) nor (B)

For each of the characteristics listed below, choose whether it describes ductal carcinoma, lobular carcinoma, both, or neither.

    A. Ductal carcinoma
    B. Lobular carcinoma
    C. Both
    D. Neither

20. Occurs most frequently in the upper outer quadrant of the breast

21. Is commonly palpable in the in situ state

22. Commonly produces scirrhous tumors

23. Produces Paget's disease in the nipple

24. Tends to arise multicentrically in the same breast

25. Occurs bilaterally in approximately 20% of cases

26. Is commonly associated with calcifications on mammography

For each of the characteristics listed below, choose whether it describes medullary carcinoma, colloid (mucinous) carcinoma, both, or neither.

    A. Medullary carcinoma
    B. Colloid (mucinous) carcinoma
    C. Both
    D. Neither

27. Represents a variant of lobular carcinoma

28. Occurs bilaterally twice as frequently as usual ductal carcinoma

29. Typically feels soft on palpation

30. Composed of anaplastic tumor cells with a high mitotic rate

31. Characterized histologically by a lymphocytic infiltrate

32. Commonly contains numerous large foci of necrosis and hemorrhage

For each of the characteristics listed below, choose whether it describes inflammatory carcinoma of the breast, acute mastitis, both, or neither.

    A. Inflammatory carcinoma of the breast
    B. Acute mastitis
    C. Both
    D. Neither

33. The involved breast is usually red and hot

34. The process is usually unilateral

35. Skin retraction is a common clinical finding

36. The process is more common in women older than 50 years

37. Neutrophils are found in affected ducts

The Breast

1. (D) Overall, the status of the draining lymph nodes of the breast that contains malignancy is the most important prognostic factor in breast cancer once the tumor has become invasive ("infiltrating" rather than in situ carcinoma) and largely determines the survival rate. The size (transverse diameter) of the tumor and the fixation of nodes or the tumor to the skin or deeper structures are factors considered in the assessment of stage. Although the histologic type of the tumor and its grade are significant prognostic factors, neither as accurately reflects the clinical course and survival rates of breast cancer patients as the degree of nodal involvement (*p. 1200*).

2. (D) On the whole, invasive breast cancers with high levels of estrogen and/or progesterone receptors have a better prognosis than those with low levels or no receptors. The presence of amplified or activated oncogenes, particularly the *neu*oncogene, and aneuploidy (randomly increased DNA content) in breast cancers also correlates with poor prognosis. Nevertheless, none of these features as a single finding is now thought to be as strongly predictive of outcome (survival) in patients with early breast cancer as lymph node status (see Question 1) (*pp. 1193, 1201*).

3. (C) Intraductal carcinoma of the breast is, by definition, an in situ malignancy of ductal epithelium. At this stage, the malignant ductal cells have grown vertically into the duct lumen and/or horizontally along the length of the duct, but they have not yet penetrated the ductal basement membrane. They have not gained access to the lymphatics and blood vessels of the periductal stroma and cannot metastasize. Thus, draining lymph nodes are always free of tumor. At this stage, the tumor can be cured in most cases by excisional biopsy alone. Unfortunately, however, intraductal tumors are difficult if not impossible to detect by palpation. At best, they

may be felt as foci of slightly increased consistency as a result of the dilatation and solidification of the affected ducts. More often, special screening techniques such as mammography, xerography, or thermography are required to detect small and early cancers like these. Intraductal carcinoma most markedly increases the risk of invasive carcinoma in the involved breast (28% of women treated with biopsy alone develop invasive carcinoma in the same region as the original tumor), but the risk also increases for the contralateral breast (*pp. 1193–1194, 1200*).

4. (B) In men, elevated serum levels of either estrogen or prolactin may cause gynecomastia (see Question 8). Conditions that cause hyperestrogenism in males are diverse. Cirrhosis causes hepatic parenchymal destruction, which leads to decreased catabolism of estrogenic compounds. A small percentage of patients treated with cimetidine for peptic ulcer disease develop gynecomastia as a consequence of elevated serum levels of prolactin caused by the drug. Leydig's (interstitial) cell tumors of the testis are often hormonally active and may secrete a large variety of steroid hormones, including estrogens. Patients with Klinefelter's syndrome have atrophic testes and primary hypogonadism. The levels of circulating androgens in these patients are drastically reduced, and relative hyperestrogenism with gynecomastia results. Gynecomastia may even occur in puberty or in the very aged as a result of changes in the ratios of circulating androgens and estrogens. It may also develop with chronic use of marijuana or heroin and may even occur without apparent cause.

Carcinoma of the prostate does not itself cause gynecomastia. However, therapies for this disease that involve hormonal manipulations such as estrogen administration or castration may lead to the subsequent development of gynecomastia (*p. 1202*).

5. (**E**) Sclerosing adenosis is a benign condition characterized by proliferation of both intralobular connective tissue and small ductules or acini. Although sclerosing adenosis is considered a variant of fibrocystic disease, it typically lacks cysts. On the contrary, the lumina of the glandular elements are either small or lacking altogether. Sclerosing adenosis is also distinctive because it often resembles carcinoma both clinically and histologically. Like carcinoma, it often presents as a mass that is hard and poorly localized on palpation. Histologically, the proliferation of small glandular structures and nests or cords of cells within a densely fibrous stroma closely resembles infiltrating carcinoma. Sclerosing adenosis, however, is benign in its biologic behavior and is not associated with increased risk of breast carcinoma (*pp. 1185, 1188*).

6. (**C**) Although the etiology of human breast cancer is still not entirely known, epidemiologic studies have shown that certain clinical factors are associated with development of the disease and are now considered risk factors for breast carcinoma. Major categories of risk factors include (1) genetic background (race and family history), (2) endogenous hormonal factors related to reproductive history, and (3) premalignant pathologic lesions in the breast tissue, specifically epithelial hyperplasia.

Women with a strong family history of breast cancer (carcinoma developing in first-degree female relatives) are at exceptionally high risk. The younger the relatives at the time of developing cancer, the greater the risk.

In general, the longer the uninterrupted exposure to endogenous estrogens, the greater the risk of developing breast carcinoma. Nulliparity, early menarche, and late menopause, therefore, all are risk factors. Endometrial carcinoma is also known to be associated with uninterrupted estrogen stimulation (of endometrial glands). Because breast cancer and endometrial carcinoma share this risk factor, the development of endometrial carcinoma is often accompanied by the development of a breast malignancy in the same patient, and a history of endometrial carcinoma represents a risk factor for breast cancer.

Less well understood is the relationship of obesity to increased risk of breast cancer. Estrogen metabolism clearly is altered in obese women, and synthesis of estrone is increased. Some investigators have hypothesized that increased fat in the diet may augment steroid (estrogen) hormone production by providing increased amounts of precursor substrate molecules. Furthermore, it is known that adipose tissue directly contributes to increased estrogen production by converting androstenedione of adrenal origin to estrone. The local effects of this may be highly significant, because breast tissue (especially in obese women) is composed largely of fat (*pp. 1192–1193*).

7. (**C**) Despite its name, cystosarcoma phyllodes is a tumor that is rarely cystic and is not a true sarcoma. It may not even be malignant. It is more akin to a bizarre and aggressive form of fibroadenoma, which it resembles histologically. *Phyllodes* is a Greek term that refers to the leaf-like, scalloped appearance of these tumors. It is a locally expansile lesion that may grow to enormous size, causing pressure necrosis and ulceration of the overlying skin. However, ulceration, even with rupture through the capsule or fungating growth through the skin, does not necessarily indicate malignancy. Invariable indications of malignant transformation include rapid increase in size and invasion of adjacent breast tissue by the malignant stromal component. Histologic findings of stromal anaplasia, increased stromal cellularity, and high mitotic rate are indicative of malignancy, but in many instances, cellular anaplasia may occur in biologically benign tumors. Even malignant cystosarcoma phyllodes is a tumor of low virulence and remains localized for long periods of time. Although it metastasizes to distant sites in 15% of cases, this usually occurs late in the course of the disease. Simple mastectomy is usually the treatment of choice (*p. 1191*).

8. (**A**) Gynecomastia refers to enlargement of the male breast in response to hyperestrogenism or increased prolactin. The major histologic component of the normal male breast is fibrostromal tissue. The glandular component consists exclusively of major mammary ducts and secondary branches, but lobular elements are not present. As in women, breast elements in men are responsive to estrogenic stimulation and undergo hyperplasia when exposed to excessive estrogens. Microscopically, gynecomastia is characterized by proliferation of ductal epithelium (epithelial hyperplasia and stromal hyperplasia) and stromal hyalinization. Because lobules are not a component of the male breast, lobular hyperplasia is not a feature of gynecomastia (*p. 1202*).

9. (**B**) Embryologically, the breast derives from the epidermis and represents a group of modified eccrine (sweat) glands. Like eccrine ducts elsewhere in the body, the mammary ducts are lined by a double layer of epithelial cells—an inner layer of cuboidal secretory epithelial cells and an outer layer of flattened myoepithelial cells. Ductal elements are supported by a collagenized connective tissue stroma admixed with fat. Breast tissue is hormonally responsive and undergoes cyclic changes with the menses. During the first half of the cycle, estrogens stimulate proliferative activity in the epithelium of the ducts and gland buds, whereas progesterone causes stromal as well as terminal duct cell growth in the latter half of the cycle. The overall architectural organization of the mammary ducts is strictly compartmentalized into about 20 wedge-shaped lobes, each of which is drained by a separate excretory duct. Each compartment (lobe) is discrete, and the ductal channels within it do not anastomose with the ducts of adjacent lobes. This architectural arrangement is a fundamental concept in breast pathology, because lesions arising within a duct in a single lobe cannot spread to other breast segments via the ductal system and can be adequately excised with a segmental mastectomy (*pp. 1181–1182*).

10. (E) Tubular carcinoma of the breast is a form of ductal carcinoma displaying a high degree of differentiation. It behaves less aggressively than infiltrating ductal carcinoma and has a low incidence of axillary lymph node metastasis. Papillary carcinoma, colloid (mucinous) carcinoma, and medullary carcinoma are variants of ductal carcinoma that also have a relatively good prognosis because they tend to metastasize to axillary lymph nodes less frequently than the usual infiltrating ductal carcinoma. The long-term survival rates for papillary, medullary, and colloid carcinomas are about 65%, 58%, and 58%, respectively, about twice the survival rate for infiltrating ductal carcinoma (29%). The reason for this difference in behavior is unknown, however (*pp. 1195–1198, 1200*).

11. (B) Carcinoma of the male breast is a very rare entity and, compared with carcinoma of the female breast, has an incidence ratio of 1:100. When it does occur, however, carcinoma of the male breast has a worse prognosis than carcinoma of the female breast. Because men have a small amount of breast tissue, tumors can rapidly infiltrate the underlying chest wall or the overlying skin. Thus, skin involvement by fixation, ulceration, and microscopic Paget's disease is relatively much more common in males than in females. Overall, however, dissemination of breast cancer in men follows the same pattern as in women, and axillary lymph node metastases are present at the time of discovery in about 50% of cases. Although the predisposing factors for carcinoma in the male breast remain obscure, there is no evidence that gynecomastia is related to the development of carcinoma. Carcinoma does not develop with increased frequency in patients with gynecomastia, and conversely, patients with carcinoma rarely have a history of preceding or coexisting gynecomastia (*p. 1202*).

12. (D) Paget's disease of the breast is a form of ductal carcinoma arising in the major excretory ducts beneath the nipple and extending outward along the duct toward the skin surface, directly invading the nipple epidermis. The primary tumor may or may not show stromal invasion and may often appear in the absence of a palpable breast mass. Skin involvement is, however, considered a grave finding in any breast carcinoma, and patients with Paget's disease have the same prognosis as patients with usual infiltrating ductal carcinoma of similar stage (Stage III). When comparing Paget's disease arising from an in situ lesion (no penetration through the duct basement membrane or invasion of periductal stroma) with other in situ ductal carcinomas, however, Paget's disease has a distinctly worse prognosis, with a 30 to 40% incidence of metastasis at the time of surgery.

Although the eczematous appearance of the skin in Paget's disease may resemble inflammatory carcinoma of the breast clinically, the two lesions can be differentiated from one another by their histologic appearance. Inflammatory carcinoma of the breast corresponds to dermal lymphatic invasion from an underlying breast carcinoma (see Question 33), whereas Paget's disease refers to epidermal involvement. Paget's disease of the breast is not to be confused with Paget's disease of bone, a totally unrelated disorder. Paget's disease of bone is a benign disorder of unknown cause; it is characterized by an osteolytic-osteoblastic process in the bones of affected individuals (*pp. 1198, 1200, 1328*).

13. (A) Epithelial hyperplasias of either ductal or lobular origin are the two forms of benign breast disease that are associated with increased risk of development of carcinoma. The more severe and atypical the hyperplasia, the greater the risk of carcinoma is considered to be. Although intraductal papillomas are benign growths within lactiferous ducts and are usually solitary and do not give rise to papillary carcinoma, multiple intraductal papillomas behave more like epithelial hyperplasias and are associated with an increased risk of carcinoma. Apocrine metaplasia is a very common, innocuous feature of fibrocystic disease of the breast and is virtually always a benign lesion (*pp. 1187–1188, 1191*).

14. (B) The therapeutic response of a breast cancer to hormonal manipulation (hormone ablation by oophorectomy and adrenalectomy or competitive inhibition by synthetic, hormonally inactive hormone analogs) is directly proportional to the quantity of estrogen and progesterone receptors expressed by the tumor cells. Thus, quantitative analysis of estrogen and progesterone receptor protein is often performed on fresh tissue from a surgically excised tumor to determine whether recurrent or concurrent disease would be responsive to this form of adjuvant therapy. In general, the greater the differentiation of the tumor, the greater the number of estrogen receptors. Although estrogen is known to act as a promoter in breast carcinogenesis, previous exposure to exogenous estrogen is not known to influence the estrogen receptor positivity of the breast tumors developing under this influence. Although there is a high correlation between estrogen receptor positivity of a tumor and its response to antiestrogenic drugs such as tamoxifen (a synthetic estrogen analog), estrogen receptor positivity has no predictive value in the response of the tumor to nonhormonal chemotherapeutic agents such as doxorubicin (Adriamycin) (*pp. 1200–1201*).

15. (A) Pain (or tenderness to palpation) is a symptom more often associated with benign rather than malignant diseases of the breast and is characteristic of such lesions as galactocele, mammary duct ectasia, and cystic disease. Although infiltrating ductal carcinoma may present as a painful lesion in rare patients, the tumor most often comes to the patient's or physician's attention as a firm but painless mass in the breast (*pp. 1184–1186, 1189, 1200*).

16. (B) The fibroadenoma is the most common benign tumor of the female breast and is found most frequently in women younger than 30 years old. It is believed to arise from breast lobules representing a proliferation of both the stromal and glandular elements. Although it may be confused clinically with a cyst, a fibroadenoma is usually easy to differentiate clinically from carcinoma because of its sharply circumscribed borders and rubbery consistency. Although the overwhelming majority of fibroadenomas are completely benign, the epithelial element, like the epithelial elements elsewhere in the breast, may give rise to a carcinoma. This, however, is an extremely rare event (*pp. 1189–1190*).

17. (C) Fibrocystic disease of the breast is a very common condition caused by an exaggeration of the response of stromal and glandular breast elements to the cyclic hormonal cycles of menses. Stromal elements are rather unidirectional in their response, undergoing proliferative rather than degenerative changes. Stromal hyperplasia with increased collagen production (stromal sclerosis or fibrosis) may be the predominant feature in fibrocystic disease or may be accompanied by various degrees of epithelial hyperplasia. Types of hyperplastic epithelial responses that may occur in fibrocystic disease include proliferation of small ductules or acinar structures (adenosis), proliferation of ductal lining cells (intraductal hyperplasia), and cyst formation. Fibrocystic disease is not an inflammatory condition and is not characteristically associated with the presence of acute inflammation histologically unless infection has been superimposed on the process. Nonspecific chronic inflammation in the form of stromal lymphocytic infiltrates, on the other hand, is a common finding in fibrocystic disease (*pp. 1185–1188*).

18. (C) In the fluctuating hormonal environment produced by the normal menstrual cycle, cyclic variation in the size of hormonally responsive proliferative lesions of the breast such as fibroadenomas and cystic disease is common and helps to differentiate these lesions from malignancies. Intraductal papillomas are not known to fluctuate noticeably with hormonal cycles and are almost always found in a subareolar location, not in the upper outer quadrant. Malignant processes, although most common in the upper outer quadrant, tend to increase relentlessly in size without fluctuation in response to hormonal cycles (*pp. 1189–1190, 1194–1200*).

19. (A) Nipple discharge in a middle-aged woman may result from either a benign or neoplastic process involving the major excretory ducts of the breast. Intraductal papilloma of the nipple is a lesion that usually affects women of middle age and often causes nipple discharge. It is a benign neoplastic growth of the lactiferous duct epithelium and forms multiple delicate papillae. Duct ectasia, an inflammatory disorder principally involving the major excretory ducts, tends to occur in the fifth or sixth decade of life. It often causes discharge from the nipple as well as pain and induration. Paget's disease of the breast is the principal malignant process causing nipple discharge and must be differentiated from benign

conditions producing this symptom. Paget's disease represents a form of ductal carcinoma involving the major excretory ducts and the skin of the overlying nipple. In addition to an oozy, bloody discharge, the nipple often shows eczematous changes and fissuring or ulceration with surrounding inflammatory hyperemia and edema. A galactocele is a cystic dilatation of an obstructed duct occurring during lactation and does not correspond to the situation described in the question (*pp. 1184–1185, 1191, 1198*).

20. (C); 21. (D); 22. (A); 23. (A); 24. (B); 25. (B); 26. (C)
(20) Both ductal and lobular carcinomas of the breast occur with greatest frequency in the upper outer quadrant, which is the region of greatest concentration of glandular tissue in the breast. **(21)** In general, neither ductal carcinoma in situ nor lobular carcinoma in situ is palpable. It is infiltrating tumor with its sclerotic stromal response that presents clinically as a firm lump. **(22)** Infiltrating tumors of ductal origin classically induce marked stromal sclerosis. Such tumors have a hard, cartilaginous consistency on palpation and are known as scirrhous tumors. Although the great majority of scirrhous tumors are infiltrating ductal carcinomas, any given scirrhous malignancy may be of either ductal or lobular origin. Most invasive lobular carcinomas, however, are rubbery and typically are not scirrhous. **(23)** Paget's disease of the breast is produced only by ductal carcinoma that arises in a major excretory duct and extends to involve the skin of the nipple.

Lobular carcinoma is associated with two clinically important features: **(24)** a tendency to be multicentric within the same breast and **(25)** a high incidence of bilaterality (approaching 20% as compared with 10 to 12% bilaterality in ductal carcinomas). Bilaterality and multicentricity are not unique to lobular carcinoma but occur about twice as frequently with lobular carcinomas as ductal carcinoma.

(26) Because early breast cancers are often nonpalpable, special techniques such as radiologic imaging (e.g., mammography) are needed for breast cancer screening. Mammography can detect the microcalcifications that are associated with invasive breast cancer of either ductal or lobular origin. Although this technique identifies calcifications in about 60% of cancers, the finding is not diagnostic of malignancy. Nearly as many benign lesions contain calcifications as well. Thus, biopsy or cytologic studies are usually needed for definitive diagnosis (*pp. 1199–1200*).

27. (D); 28. (D); 29. (C); 30. (A); 31. (A); 32. (A)
(27) Both medullary carcinoma and colloid carcinoma of the breast arise from ductal epithelial cells and represent variants of ductal carcinomas. **(28)** The incidence of bilaterality in patients with either of these tumor types is not significantly different from that in patients with usual ductal carcinoma. **(29)** Unlike usual ductal carcinomas, medullary carcinoma and colloid carcinoma induce little stromal response. They typically feel soft on palpation and may resemble each other

clinically. (30) Histologically, however, the two variants are distinctly different. Medullary carcinomas are characterized by a high degree of anaplasia and a high mitotic rate (31) and are typically accompanied by an abundant lymphocytic infiltrate. (32) In addition, medullary carcinomas typically contain foci of hemorrhage and necrosis that are large and numerous, whereas colloid carcinomas create large, pale gray-blue gelatinous masses that are not typically associated with hemorrhage or necrosis (*pp. 1195, 1198*).

33. (C); 34. (C); 35. (C); 36. (A); 37. (B)

(33) Although inflammatory carcinoma of the breast shares some clinical features with mastitis, it is not truly an inflammatory process. Inflammatory carcinoma is actually an infiltrating ductal carcinoma of the breast with a characteristic tendency to extensively invade the lymphatics of the breast and overlying skin. Acute mastitis is a true inflammatory process caused by bacteria (usually *Staphylococcus aureus*), which gain access to the breast substance through cracks created in the nipple skin during nursing. The involved breast in both inflammatory carcinoma and acute mastitis is usually reddened, swollen, and warm to touch. (34) In both processes, the involvement is typically unilateral and (35) produces skin retraction or nipple retraction as a result of the accompanying marked edema. (36) Inflammatory carcinoma is more common in women older than 50 years (because infiltrating ductal carcinoma itself is more common in this age-group), whereas mastitis is a disease of young lactating women. (37) Histologically, the presence of numerous neutrophils within affected ducts is characteristic only of acute mastitis (*pp. 1184, 1199*).

13

The Skin

DIRECTIONS: For Questions 1 to 12, choose the ONE BEST answer to each question.

1. All of the following descriptions are characteristic of basal cell carcinoma EXCEPT:

    A. Grows slowly
    B. Rarely metastasizes
    C. Sometimes pigmented
    D. Associated with papillomavirus infection
    E. Associated with sun exposure

2. A healthy 20-year-old woman develops hives when she eats nuts. All of the following statements about this situation are true EXCEPT:

    A. The development of the skin lesions is mediated by IgE
    B. Mast cell degranulation occurs in the lesions
    C. Complement activation is important in the pathogenesis of the lesions
    D. The lesions typically regress within 24 hours
    E. Aspirin administration is contraindicated

3. All of the following statements about the excised lesion shown in Figure 13–1 are true EXCEPT:

    A. It is a very common lesion
    B. The cell of origin is a melanocyte
    C. Infiltration of the deep dermis indicates aggressive biologic behavior
    D. Mitoses are rarely found in these lesions
    E. It is unlikely to undergo malignant transformation

4. A patient notices a deeply pigmented, raised nodule with indefinite borders on the upper extremity. Although a nodular melanoma is suspected, none of the following lesions can be ruled out on clinical inspection EXCEPT:

    A. Basal cell carcinoma
    B. Seborrheic keratosis
    C. Blue nevus
    D. Dermatofibroma
    E. Lentigo simplex

5. All of the following statements about malignant melanoma are true EXCEPT:

    A. It is etiologically related to sun exposure
    B. It is typically uniformly pigmented
    C. It does not metastasize during its horizontal growth phase

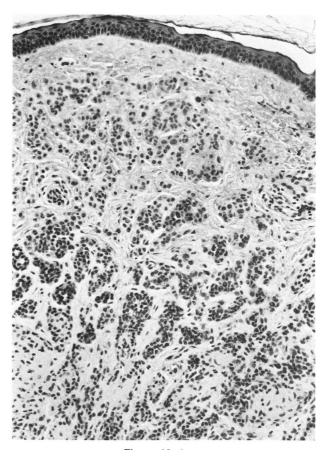

Figure 13–1

D. The probability of metastasis is directly proportional to depth of dermal infiltration
E. Increased early diagnosis has greatly improved survival rates

6. Which of the following statements about mycosis fungoides is true?

A. Lesions resemble superficial fungal infection
B. The causative agent is an atypical mycobacterium
C. Suppressor T cells with convoluted nuclei are present in the lesions
D. Hematogenous involvement is known as Sézary's syndrome
E. Munro's microabscesses are diagnostic

7. All of the following characteristics are typical of dysplastic nevi EXCEPT:

A. Variability in pigmentation
B. Occurrence almost exclusively on sun-exposed body surfaces
C. Predisposition to intralesional melanoma formation
D. Predisposition to melanoma formation in unaffected skin
E. Occurrence in individuals with the heritable melanoma syndrome

8. Which of the following would be the LEAST likely cause of thrombocytopenia-induced purpuric lesions developing in a patient with promyelocytic leukemia?

A. Hypersplenism
B. Bone marrow replacement
C. Intercurrent infection
D. Disseminated intravascular coagulation
E. Administration of drugs

9. Langerhans' cells are correctly characterized as:

A. Giant cells in tubercular granulomas
B. Pancreatic islet cells
C. Melanocyte precursors
D. Antigen-presenting dendritic cells
E. Transformed lymphocytes

10. All of the following statements regarding actinic keratosis are true EXCEPT:

A. It is a premalignant skin condition
B. It is caused by sun exposure
C. Cytologic atypia of basal cells is characteristic
D. Proliferating basal cells typically disrupt the basement membrane
E. Elastosis of the subjacent dermis is characteristic

11. Which of the following skin disorders is LEAST likely to occur in an individual with diffuse B-cell lymphoma?

A. Xanthoma
B. Acanthosis nigricans
C. Squamous cell carcinoma
D. Cutaneous necrotizing vasculitis
E. Mycosis fungoides

12. All of the following statements are true of psoriasis EXCEPT:

A. The epidermal mitotic rate is increased
B. Other organ systems are often involved
C. Lesions are sometimes precipitated by trauma
D. Epidermal microabscesses are seen histologically
E. The disorder is usually self-limited

DIRECTIONS: For Questions 13 to 23, ONE or MORE of the completions given correctly finishes the incomplete statement. Choose:
A—if only *1, 2, and 3* are correct
B—if only *1 and 3* are correct
C—if only *2 and 4* are correct
D—if only *4* is correct
E—if all are correct

13. Mitoses occur in more than one cell layer above the basal layer of the epidermis in:

1. Squamous cell carcinoma in situ
2. Lentigo
3. Psoriasis
4. Normal skin

A. 1,2,3   B. 1,3   C. 2,4   D. 4 Only   E. All

14. Benign fibrous histiocytomas:

1. Represent fibroblastic proliferations
2. Are sometimes called sclerosing hemangiomas

3. Cause hyperpigmentation of the overlying epidermis
4. Are rapidly growing, locally aggressive lesions

A. 1,2,3   B. 1,3   C. 2,4   D. 4 Only   E. All

15. Palpable purpura developing in patients treated for chronic myelogenous leukemia is caused by

1. Malignancy-associated vasculitis
2. Drug sensitivity
3. Intercurrent infection
4. Leukemic infiltration of skin

A. 1,2,3   B. 1,3   C. 2,4   D. 4 Only   E. All

16. Squamous cell carcinoma is correctly described as:

    1. The most common skin tumor with significant metastatic potential
    2. Common on the backs of the hands
    3. Appearing as leukoplakia in mucosal sites
    4. Occurring with increased frequency in immunosuppressed persons

       A. 1,2,3   B. 1,3   C. 2,4   D. 4 Only   E. All

17. A patient with new skin lesions is found to have a gastric carcinoma. Which of the following cutaneous lesions are consistent with this situation?

    1. Seborrheic keratosis
    2. Acanthosis nigricans
    3. Erythema nodosum
    4. Paget's disease

       A. 1,2,3   B. 1,3   C. 2,4   D. 4 Only   E. All

18. Dermatitis herpetiformis is accurately characterized as:

    1. Usually very pruritic
    2. Typically producing subepidermal blisters
    3. Associated with nontropical sprue
    4. Caused by herpesvirus infection

       A. 1,2,3   B. 1,3   C. 2,4   D. 4 Only   E. All

19. Cutaneous horns are produced by which of the following skin disorders?

    1. Actinic keratosis
    2. Verruca vulgaris
    3. Seborrheic keratosis
    4. Squamous cell carcinoma

       A. 1,2,3   B. 1,3   C. 2,4   D. 4 Only   E. All

20. A patient taking sulfonamides has an increased probability of developing which of the following cutaneous lesions?

    1. Erythema multiforme
    2. Erythema nodosum
    3. Urticaria
    4. Melasma

       A. 1,2,3   B. 1,3   C. 2,4   D. 4 Only   E. All

21. Glomus cells are correctly described as:

    1. Smooth muscle cells
    2. Regulating arterial blood flow in the skin
    3. Responsive to temperature changes
    4. Giving rise to extremely painful tumors

       A. 1,2,3   B. 1,3   C. 2,4   D. 4 Only   E. All

22. Xeroderma pigmentosum is associated with an increased incidence of which of the following neoplasms?

    1. Malignant melanoma
    2. Lung cancer
    3. Basal cell carcinoma
    4. Colon cancer

       A. 1,2,3   B. 1,3   C. 2,4   D. 4 Only   E. All

23. Characteristics of keratoacanthoma include:

    1. Histologic resemblance to squamous cell carcinoma
    2. Rapid growth
    3. Extension of the lesion into the dermis
    4. Spontaneous regression

       A. 1,2,3   B. 1,3   C. 2,4   D. 4 Only   E. All

24. Characteristics typical of lichen planus include:

    1. Pruritic lesions
    2. Purple lesions
    3. Self-limited (spontaneously resolving) lesions
    4. Band-like lymphoid infiltrates in the upper dermis

       A. 1,2,3   B. 1,3   C. 2,4   D. 4 Only   E. All

25. True statements about mastocytosis include:

    1. It is characterized by mast cell proliferation in the skin
    2. It is the cause of urticaria pigmentosa
    3. It is associated with dermatographism
    4. It represents metastasis from a malignant mastocytoma in the bone marrow

       A. 1,2,3   B. 1,3   C. 2,4   D. 4 Only   E All

DIRECTIONS: For Questions 26 to 40, the set of lettered headings is followed by list of numbered words or phrases. For each numbered word or phrase choose:
   A—if the item is associated with (A) only
   B—if the item is associated with (B) only
   C—if the item is associated with *both* (A) and (B)
   D—if the item is associated with *neither* (A) nor (B)

For each of the characteristics listed below, choose whether it describes Spitz nevus, nodular malignant melanoma, both, or neither.

   A. Spitz nevus
   B. Nodular malignant melanoma

   C. Both
   D. Neither

26. Lesions consist of pleomorphic proliferations of melanocytes with a high mitotic rate

27. Deep infiltration of the underlying dermis by the tumor cells is a prominent feature

28. Infiltration of the overlying epidermis by the tumor cells is a common feature

29. Lesions occur only in adults

30. Lesions typically show variegated pigmentation

For each of the following statements, choose whether it describes molluscum contagiosum, verruca vulgaris, both, or neither.

    A. Molluscum contagiosum
    B. Verruca vulgaris
    C. Both
    D. Neither

31. The lesion is caused by a virus

32. Children and young adults are most commonly affected

33. The process spares mucous membranes

34. Cytoplasmic vacuolization (koilocytosis) is a characteristic feature

35. Lesions are self-limited (regress spontaneously)

For each of the following characteristics, choose whether it describes pemphigus vulgaris, bullous pemphigoid, both, or neither.

    A. Pemphigus vulgaris
    B. Bullous pemphigoid
    C. Both
    D. Neither

36. Subepidermal blisters are characteristic

37. Acantholysis in the blistered epidermis is typical

38. Injury is mediated by autoantibodies

39. Oral involvement is common

40. Scalp and face lesions are common

1. (D) Basal cell carcinomas are common, slow-growing malignant epidermal tumors that rarely metastasize. Histologically, the tumors are composed of small, dark basaloid cells with scant cytoplasm usually growing in nests with peripheral palisading. Some tumors contain melanin pigment and may resemble nevi or melanomas on clinical examination. Like malignant melanomas and squamous cell carcinomas of the skin, basal cell carcinomas are etiologically related to actinic radiation and tend to occur on sun-exposed body sites. In contrast to mucocutaneous squamous cell carcinomas, however, these tumors are not known to be associated with human papillomavirus infection (*pp. 1288–1289*).

2. (C) Urticaria, otherwise known as hives, is a very common skin disorder characterized by focal swelling and itching (pruritic wheals). It is caused by localized mast cell degranulation and resultant dermal microvascular hyperpermeability. The pathogenesis of urticaria includes both immunologic and nonimmunologic mechanisms. In IgE-mediated immunologic urticaria (allergic type), specific antigen sensitivity to foods, pollens, or drugs produces a type I hypersensitivity immune response with mast cell degranulation and a histamine-induced increase in venular permeability. In IgE-independent urticaria, direct stimulation of mast cell degranulation can be produced in sensitive individuals by drugs such as opiates, curare, radiographic contrast agents, or certain antibiotics. In either case, resolution of the lesions typically occurs within hours.

Complement activation is not involved in the pathogenesis of either IgE-dependent or IgE-independent allergic urticaria, and vasculitis is not produced. This contrasts with immunologic urticaria resulting from type III hypersensitivity responses, which are mediated by immune complexes. Acute necrotizing vasculitis is produced as a result of immune complex deposits and complement activation in the walls of small vessels. The associated urticaria is understandably much more persistent than that produced by type I reactions, and underlying vasculitis should be suspected in individuals in whom urticarial reactions do not resolve within 24 hours.

Prostaglandins retard IgE-dependent release of mast cell granules. Agents that act as arachidonic acid metabolism inhibitors, such as aspirin, tend to potentiate or may even cause IgE-mediated urticaria by impairing prostaglandin synthesis. Therefore, aspirin would be contraindicated in the clinical situation described in the question (*pp. 173–176, 178–181, 1296*).

3. (C) The lesion pictured in Figure 13–1 is an intradermal nevocellular nevus. Nevocellular nevi are extremely common benign tumors of melanocytes; they may be either congenital or acquired. Neval cells typically are round to oval and contain uniform nuclei. They grow in nests, which may be present at the dermoepidermal junction (junctional nevus), only within the dermis (intradermal nevus), or in both places simultaneously (compound nevus). They are thought to arise at the dermoepidermal junction and migrate downward with time. Infiltration of the deep dermis, therefore, does not indicate more aggressive biologic behavior. On the contrary, neval cells tend to become more cytologically and histochemically "mature" with downward progression into the dermis. They cluster, become spindle shaped, and lose their tyrosinase activity, coming to resemble neural tissue more than melanocytes. The process of neuralization can be diagnostically helpful in distinguishing some forms of nevi from malignant melanoma. Typical intradermal nevi rarely show mitoses on histologic examination and have little malignant potential. They are usually readily distinguished from dysplastic nevi, lesions with distinct malignant potential.

Dysplastic nevi are compound (rather than intradermal) nevi with both cytologic and architectural atypia and are known to be precursors of malignant melanoma. Characteristically, however, the progression to malignancy in dysplastic nevi virtually always begins with the junctional component. Thus, mature intradermal nevi lacking a junctional component are typically considered innocuous (*pp. 1279–1282*).

4. (E) Basal cell carcinomas, seborrheic keratoses, nevocellular nevi, or dermatofibromas all can appear as nodular hyperpigmented lesions. When deeply pigmented, any of these lesions, including the darkly pigmented blue nevus (a histologic variant of a nevocellular nevus), may be confused clinically with malignant melanoma. In contrast, lentigo simplex is never nodular and is usually relatively lightly pigmented. Lentigenes are benign hyperplasias of melanocytes. They are macular lesions that are usually tan to brown and, unlike freckles, do not darken with exposure to sunlight (*pp. 1279–1281, 1283–1284, 1288–1289, 1290*).

5. (B) Malignant melanoma is a relatively common, highly aggressive neoplasm. Like most epithelial malignancies, it is related etiologically to sun exposure. Hereditary factors and the development of precursor lesions (dysplastic nevi, see Question 7) are also important in its pathogenesis. Melanomas are typically asymptomatic, but the lesions can be recognized on clinical inspection by their typical variegated pigmentation (a mixture of shades of brown, black, blue, red, gray, or even white) and irregular notched borders. Increased recognition of these features has resulted in earlier diagnosis and surgical removal of most tumors and a dramatic improvement in the survival rate for this disease (83% in the United States in 1983). The prognosis correlates closely with the tumor stage. Melanomas tend to grow horizontally within the epidermis and superficial dermis for prolonged periods of time before infiltrating vertically. During the horizontal growth phase, melanomas do not have the capacity to metastasize and can be cured with surgical resection. When the tumor develops vertical growth, it becomes nodular in appearance and acquires metastatic potential. The deeper the invasion, the greater the probability of metastasis. In fact, the probability of metastasis can be predicted by measuring (using an ocular micrometer) the depth of invasion of the malignancy in the resection specimen (*pp. 1282–1283*).

6. (D) Mycosis fungoides is a T-cell lymphoma that arises primarily in the skin but may evolve into generalized systemic disease with involvement of lymph nodes and viscera. The development of a leukemia-like picture with seeding of the blood by malignant T cells accompanied by diffuse erythroderma and cutaneous scaling is known as Sézary's syndrome.

Although the name is suggestive of fungal infection, mycosis fungoides neither clinically resembles nor has any association with mycotic infection of the skin. Although the etiology of mycosis fungoides is still poorly understood, there is evidence that at least some cases may be related to retrovirus infection. (There is certainly no association with atypical mycobacterial infection).

The early lesions of mycosis fungoides resemble eczema both clinically and histologically, but even at this stage, karyotypic abnormalities of lymphocytes in the blood and lymph nodes can be observed. Plaquelike lesions develop as the disease progresses and are characterized by an intensification of the features of the eczematous phase with the addition of Pautrier's microabscesses (collections of Sézary-Lutzner cells, see below) in the epidermis. These are not to be confused with the Munro's microabscesses of psoriasis, which are collections of neutrophils in the stratum corneum. The diagnosis of mycosis fungoides depends on the identification of tumor cells (Sézary-Lutzner cells) within the characteristic superficial dermal band-like inflammatory infiltrates and Pautrier's abscesses of the skin lesions. Sézary-Lutzner cells are CD4+ helper T cells with hyperchromatic, highly convoluted cerebriform nuclei (*pp. 1293–1294*).

7. (B) Dysplastic nevi (also known as BK moles) constitute a distinct subset of nevocellular nevi that are morphologically highly atypical and undergo malignant transformation with much higher frequency than ordinary nevi. They are considered true precursors of malignant melanoma. Unlike ordinary nevi, dysplastic nevi tend to be variably pigmented (variegated), have irregular borders, and occur on non–sun-exposed as well as sun-exposed skin sites. They are associated with an increased risk of melanoma in the clinically unaffected as well as the lesional skin. The occurrence of dysplastic nevi in the heritable melanoma syndrome (dysplastic nevus syndrome), in which the trait is autosomal dominant and associated with a susceptibility gene located on the short arm of chromosome 1, suggests that genetic factors may play a strong part in the development of these lesions. For persons with the dysplastic nevus syndrome, the actuarial probability of developing melanoma is 56% at age 59. Thus, the importance of identification and prophylactic surveillance of such individuals is obvious (*pp. 1280–1281*).

8. (A) A reduction in the platelet count is the most common cause of generalized bleeding and is most commonly manifested by petechial skin lesions. Thrombocytopenia results from any condition causing either decreased platelet production, increased platelet destruction, sequestration of platelets, or dilution of platelets (massive transfusions). The risk of developing thrombocytopenia through several of these mechanisms is increased in patients with acute leukemia. Leukemic infiltration of the bone marrow replaces normal hematopoietic elements and causes decreased production of platelets. Administration of drugs, particularly chemotherapeutic agents, further reduces normal hematopoiesis. Immunopathologic mechanisms associated with drugs or intercurrent infection may also cause increased platelet destruction. Patients with promyelogenous leukemia are especially prone to increased platelet destruction from disseminated intravascular coagulation, because the cytoplasmic granules that characterize the neoplastic promyelocytes are rich in a thromboplastin-like substance capable of activating the coagulation cascade.

Although patients with chronic myelogenous leukemia may develop massive splenomegaly leading to platelet sequestration (hypersplenism), splenomegaly is usually not a feature of the acute forms of leukemia (*pp. 691–693*).

9. (D) Langerhans cells are bone marrow-derived, antigen-presenting cells of the epidermis. They are dendritic in shape and have clear cytoplasm. Langerhans cells can be unequivocally identified in the electron microscope by their pathognomonic pentilaminar cytoplasmic granules (Birbeck granules), some of which have dilated tips and resemble tiny matchsticks or tennis rackets. Because Langerhans cells contain hydrolytic enzymes and exhibit cell surface markers (such as class II HLA antigens) characteristic of monocytes and macrophages, it is likely that they are descendants of this cell line. They interact with cutaneous T cells in the presentation of antigens, but Langerhans cells themselves are not lymphocytes. Although the terminology is sometimes confusing, Langerhans cells have nothing to do with the pancreatic islets of Langerhans or with the Langhans' giant cells of tubercular granulomata (*pp. 66, 168, 992, 1277, 1292*).

10. (D) Actinic (solar) keratosis is a premalignant condition in which progressively dysplastic epidermal changes precede the development of squamous cell carcinoma. It is caused by chronic exposure to sunlight. Although the lesions are often hyperplastic and hyperkeratotic, epidermal atrophy may also be seen. Deposition of abnormal thickened blue-gray elastic fibers in the dermis (elastosis) is also characteristic. However, the essential microscopic features of actinic keratosis is cytologic atypia of the epidermis, characteristically seen first and most prominently in the lowermost layers. The atypia may progress to involve the full thickness of the epidermis, becoming squamous cell carcinoma in situ (Bowen's disease). With penetration of the underlying basement membrane by the proliferating cells, the process evolves to invasive squamous cell carcinoma (*pp. 1286–1288*).

11. (E) Xanthomas, lesions composed of lipid-laden foamy histiocytes, may occur in normal individuals or in association with hyperlipidemic disorders (either acquired or familial), but are also known to develop in association with malignancies (especially lympho- or myeloproliferative neoplasms). Likewise, acanthosis nigricans, a lesion characterized by epidermal thickening and hyperpigmentation, has both a benign and a malignancy-associated form. It usually occurs as either a heritable trait or in association with obesity or endocri-

nopathies, but it too can be associated with an underlying malignancy.

Patients with lymphoma, perhaps as a result of endogenous or chemotherapeutic immunosuppression, are prone to develop second malignancies, especially cutaneous squamous cell carcinomas.

Numerous conditions are associated with cutaneous vasculitis: lymphomas, leukemias, carcinomas, infections, drug sensitivities, C2 deficiency, and collagen-vascular diseases.

Mycosis fungoides is itself a T-cell lymphoma originating in the skin and is not a paraphenomenon of a lymphoproliferative disorder (*pp. 295, 1284, 1288, 1291, 1293*).

12. (E) Psoriasis is a common chronic inflammatory dermatosis characterized by scaling lesions that persist for years. It may also involve organs besides the skin, such as the musculoskeletal system (e.g., psoriatic arthritis and myopathy). Psoriatic skin lesions are characterized by increased epidermal cell turnover (mitotic rate) with epidermal thickening, elongation of rete ridges, and numerous mitotic figures. The stratum granulosum is typically thinned or absent, the overlying stratum corneum is parakeratotic, and small neutrophilic abscesses are present in the superficial epidermis (spongiform pustules) and stratum corneum (Munro's microabscesses). Although association with certain HLA types suggests a genetic predisposition for the disease, lesions may be precipitated in susceptible individuals by trauma (the Koebner phenomenon) (*pp. 1300–1301*).

13. (B) Mitoses occurring in the suprabasal cell layers of the epidermis usually indicate a pathologic process. In normal skin, mitosis occurs only in the basal layer itself or at most one cell layer above. In some inflammatory processes and in cell tumors of the epidermis, mitotic figures may be found in more superficial locations. Although lentigo simplex is characterized by a benign proliferation of melanocytes in the epidermis, the proliferating cells are limited to the basal layer. Histologically, mitotic figures are seldom seen in lentigenes. The presence of mitoses high in the epidermis with superficial migration of melanocytes suggests a melanocytic malignancy rather than lentigo. As in all intraepidermal malignancies, mitotic figures may be seen at any level from the deepest to the most superficial layers in squamous cell carcinoma in situs. Psoriasis is a disease characterized by very rapid turnover of epidermal keratinocytes, and mitoses commonly occur as high as two cell layers above the basal zone but rarely higher (*pp. 1279, 1282, 1288, 1300*).

14. (A) Benign fibrous histiocytomas are intradermal tumors of fibroblasts and histiocytes. The most common form of fibrous histiocytoma in the skin is a dermatofibroma. The histologic variant containing numerous blood vessels is called a sclerosing hemangioma. These lesions have a completely benign behavior, being neither locally aggressive nor rapidly growing. The dermal lesions have poorly demarcated borders and are accompanied by hyperplasia and hyperpigmentation of the overlying epidermis, which can cause confusion with melanoma clinically. The superficial fibrous histiocytomas of the dermis are virtually always of the benign type. Malignant fibrous histiocytomas do occur; however, they are usually large and located in deeper soft tissues and bone. Malignant lesions are recognized by their pleomorphism and high mitotic rate (*pp. 1290, 1373*).

15. (E) Purpura represents hemorrhage into the skin and, when caused by inflammatory damage to vessel walls, will produce palpable induration. An important cause of palpable purpura is cutaneous necrotizing vasculitis. This disorder produces fibrinoid necrosis of venular walls with extravasation of red blood cells and serum. Neutrophils and cellular debris are present in and around the walls of the damaged vessels. The lesions are believed to be produced by an immune complex-mediated mechanism (type III hypersensitivity, p. 178) in which complement is activated.

Numerous diverse conditions are associated with this type of vasculitis. In many cases, the sources of the inciting antigens are well defined. Drugs, foreign proteins (serum sickness), viruses, and bacteria (intercurrent infections) are common examples. In other disorders, although the known association with vasculitis may be well established, the precise antigen is unknown, or multiple diverse antigens may be involved. Examples of such situations include vasculitis associated with malignancy (leukemias, lymphomas, and carcinomas), collagen-vascular disease, Henoch-Schönlein purpura, and C2 deficiency. Although it is not mediated by immunologic mechanisms, leukemic infiltration of the skin can be purpuric in character and must always be included in the differential diagnosis of palpable purpura in this setting. The histopathology of these lesions is not that of a necrotizing vasculitis but of a dense dermal infiltrate of myeloid cells, including numerous immature forms (*pp. 93, 178–181, 692*).

16. (E) Squamous cell carcinoma (SCC) is the most common skin tumor having significant potential for metastasis. Basal cell carcinoma is more common than SCC but virtually never metastasizes. Melanoma is considerably more aggressive than SCC but is less common. Epidermal SCC often arises from dysplastic premalignant lesions induced by chronic sun exposure and radiation damage (actinic keratoses), but in addition to ultraviolet irradiation, a number of other contributing factors may be important in the pathogenesis of SCC. For example, tumorigenesis is favored by immunologic suppression as a result of chemotherapy or organ transplantation. Thus, as many as 4% of iatrogenically immunosuppressed patients may develop SCC, often within relatively a short period after therapy. Sunlight itself has depressive effects on epidermal Langerhans cells and may contribute to immunosuppressive permissive conditions for SCC development in otherwise normal, immunocompetent individuals.

The backs of the hands and the face (typically chronically sun exposed) are common sites of SCC occurrence. In curious contrast to SCC, basal cell carcinomas, tumors also related to chronic sun exposure, are uncommon on the backs of the hands. On mucous membranes, SCC usually has the appearance of white patches called leukoplakia. However, because this appearance may be produced by benign conditions as well, biopsy may be needed to differentiate benign from malignant leukoplakia (*pp. 1287–1289*).

17. (A) Seborrheic keratosis, acanthosis nigricans, and erythema nodosum all are benign dermal lesions that may be associated with underlying malignancy. Seborrheic keratoses appearing suddenly in association with a gastrointestinal malignancy is known as the Leser-Trélat sign. The majority of malignancies associated with acanthosis nigricans are adenocarcinomas, most commonly of gastric origin. Erythema nodosum, although most often idiopathic or associated with infections or drugs, may also occur with visceral malignancy. In contrast to these disorders, Paget's disease is itself a malignant disease process. It presents invasion of the epidermis by adenocarcinoma cells, usually originating from a tumor in an underlying or adjacent structure. It most often refers to nipple involvement by a subjacent ductal carcinoma of breast (*pp. 1198, 1283–1284, 1299*).

18. (C) Dermatitis herpetiformis (DH) is a rare but very distinctive blistering disease having a strong association with celiac disease (gluten enteropathy or sprue). Although not all patients with celiac disease have DH, it appears that almost all patients with DH have celiac disease (often clinically latent). It is believed that the immunologic response to gluten in these individuals constitutes the underlying pathogenesis of both diseases. The lesions of DH consist of urticarial plaques and vesicles that are characteristically extremely pruritic (itchy). The vesicles of DH are frequently grouped like those seen in herpesvirus infection (hence the name of the disease), but the cause of DH is not at all related to viral infection. The blisters of DH are typically subepidermal, caused by a separation of the dermoepidermal junction beginning at the tips of the dermal papillae (between rete ridges). By immunofluorescence, granular deposits of IgA are localized in the tips of the involved papillae (*pp. 1305–1306*).

19. (A) Exuberant conical excrescences of keratin known as cutaneous horns may be the predominant clinical feature of several diverse epidermal lesions. Warts (papillomavirus lesions), actinic keratoses, seborrheic keratoses, and squamous cell carcinomas all may appear clinically as cutaneous horns and require biopsy for definitive diagnosis. Seborrheic keratosis is a common benign tumor of basaloid keratinocytes growing in cords and sheets and superficially forming horned cysts. It is usually exophytic but occasionally grows inward, extending into the dermis (inverted seborrheic keratosis) (*pp. 1284, 1286*).

20. (A) Erythema multiforme is an uncommon self-limited dermatosis that causes a cytotoxic pattern of injury in the epidermis. It is believed to represent a hypersensitivity response to certain infection or drugs. Its association with specific drugs is well established, and sulfonamides, penicillin, barbiturates, salicylates, hydantoins, and antimalarial drugs are among the primary offenders.

Erythema nodosum is a type of panniculitis (i.e., inflammation of the subcutaneous fat). Like erythema multiforme, it is also commonly associated with infections of the administration of certain drugs, especially sulfonamides.

Urticaria (hives) may develop in an individual taking antibiotics such as sulfonamides either as a result of an immunologically mediated hypersensitivity response to the drug or as a direct action of the drug on mast cells causing their degranulation.

Melasma is a mask-like zone of facial hyperpigmentation commonly occurring in pregnancy. It is thought to result from enhanced transfer of pigment from melanocytes to keratinocytes in response to hormonal changes. It may also occur with the administration of some drugs such as oral contraceptives or hydantoins but is not associated with antibiotic use (*pp. 1279, 1296, 1298–1299*).

21. (E) Glomus bodies are specialized smooth muscle cells that regulate arterial blood flow through arteriovenous shunts in the skin in response to temperature changes. Tumors of these cells commonly occur on the distal portions of the fingers and toes, where glomus bodies are most numerous. Tumors of glomus cells are characteristically exquisitely painful and bothersome but have virtually no malignant potential (*p. 589*).

22. (B) Xeroderma pigmentosum is an autosomal recessive disorder characterized by predisposition to chromosomal breakage secondary to defective excision-repair of DNA. Several distinct subsets of this disease have been defined, each with a specific enzymatic defect. The major subset lacks dimeric endonucleases. Because of the inability to repair acquired cellular mutations in the skin induced by ultraviolet irradiation, affected individuals have a markedly increased predisposition to skin cancers. All sunlight-induced epidermal malignancies (basal cell carcinomas, squamous cell carcinomas, and melanomas) occur with greatly increased frequency in individuals with xeroderma pigmentosum. However, there is no increased predisposition to major visceral malignancies such as cancers of the lung, colon, or breast. This suggests that the mutagenic effects of sunlight on the skin far exceed the effects of all other environmental mutagens on the body (*pp. 266, 274, 1287*).

23. (E) Keratoacanthomas are rapidly growing but benign tumors of keratinocytes. Their cause is unknown. These lesions may closely resemble squamous cell carcinomas both clinically and histologically. They may deeply penetrate the underlying dermis but never extend beyond the depth of adjacent hair follicles. Differentiation from squamous cell carcinoma depends on the overall symmetrical, smooth contour of the lesion and the mature, homogenous, glassy appearance of its component squamous cells. Although alarming in appearance, keratoacanthomas regress spontaneously and heal without treatment (*p. 1285*).

24. (E) Lichen planus, a chronic inflammatory dermatosis of unknown cause, is characterized by "pruritic, purple, polygonal papules." The lesions occur on both the skin and the mucous membranes. Although oral lesions may persist for years, lichen planus is a self-limited disorder, resolving spontaneously within 12 to 24 months. Histologically, the lesions typically show degeneration and necrosis of the basal keratinocytes and a band-like (lichenoid) infiltrate of lymphocytes along the dermoepidermal junction (*pp. 1301–1302*).

25. (A) Mastocytosis represents a spectrum of disease in which mast cells proliferate in the skin and sometimes in other organs as well. The most common subset of mastocytosis is called urticaria pigmentosa, a localized cutaneous from of the disease that predominantly affects children. Mastocytosis may be systemic in distribution with mast cell infiltration of many organs (e.g., bone marrow, liver, spleen, lymph nodes) in addition to skin involvement. The clinical signs of mastocytosis are related to the effects of mast cell products such as histamine and heparin. Two common signs are dermatographism (dermal edema resembling a hive resulting from localized stroking of uninvolved skin) and Darier's sign (dermal edema resulting from stroking of lesional skin). It is unclear whether mastocytosis is a true neoplasm or whether the defect results from altered mast cell maturation or proliferation in response to abnormalities of the local microenvironment. However, it does not represent metastatic disease from an underlying malignancy in the bone marrow (*pp. 1294–1295*).

26. (C); **27.** (C); **28.** (B); **29.** (D); **30.** (B)

The Spitz nevus, once called juvenile melanoma, is an uncommon nevocellular nevus that occurs predominantly in childhood but can also arise in adults. Spitz nevi are benign in their biologic behavior but are characterized by histologic features usually associated with malignancy. The neval cells typically show striking nuclear irregularities; and mitoses may be numerous, causing confusion with malignant melanoma. In addition, the lesions are often highly infiltrative and extend deep into the dermis. In contrast to most malignant melanomas, their pigmentation is usually sparse, and the nevi appear clinically as pink-tan papules or nodules.

Dermal infiltration is not an innocuous feature in nodular malignant melanoma; its extent is the most important factor in determining prognosis in this disease. Malignant melanoma can occur in any age-group, although it is most common between the ages of 40 and 60. In contrast to Spitz nevi, malignant melanomas are most often heavily but variably pigmented with shades of black, brown, blue, red, or other huses. Histologically, melanomas are composed of markedly atypical neoplastic melanocytes and show frequent mitoses. Helpful features in the diagnosis of malignant melanoma include the involvement of the overlying epidermis and the presence of atypical mitoses; these features are typically lacking in Spitz nevi (*pp. 1279–1280, 1282–1283*).

31. (C); 32. (C); 33. (D); 34. (B); 35. (D)

Molluscum contagiosum and verruca vulgaris are the two most common viral lesions of skin. Molluscum contagiosum is caused by a poxvirus, whereas verruca vulgaris is caused by papillomaviruses of the papovavirus group. Both occur most frequently in children and young adults and are characterized by epidermal hyperplasia. Both may occur on mucous membranes. Virally infected keratinocytes in both conditions exhibit characteristic histologic changes. Verrucal keratinocytes typically show marked cytoplasmic vacuolization known as koilocytosis and zones of pallor surrounding infected nuclei. Virally infected keratinocytes in molluscum contagiosum are uniquely characterized by large, homogenous eosinophilic cytoplasmic inclusions (molluscum bodies) containing replicating virions that compress the nucleus to one side of the cell. Both molluscum contagiosum and verruca vulgaris are contagious diseases, caused by direct contact, and both are self-limited, regressing spontaneously within 6 months to 2 years (*pp. 1307–1308*).

36. (B); 37. (A); 38. (C); 39. (C); 40. (A)

Pemphigus vulgaris and bullous pemphigoid are both uncommon autoimmune blistering (bullous) diseases. Pemphigus vulgaris is characterized by antibody-mediated damage to intercellular cement substances in the epidermis causing dissolution or lysis of the epithelium (acantholysis). Bullous pemphigoid, in contrast, is characterized by subepidermal blisters mediated by autoantibodies to basal lamina and hemidesmosomal antigens. Both diseases may involve mucosal as well as cutaneous surfaces, but the characteristic distribution of lesions differs in the two diseases. Pemphigus vulgaris typically involves the scalp and face as well as the axilla, groin, trunk, and points of pressure. Bullous pemphigoid lesions occur predominantly on the inner aspects of the thighs, flexor surfaces of the forearms, groin, axilla, and lower abdomen but spare the face and scalp (*pp. 1304–1305*).

The Endocrine System

DIRECTIONS: For Questions 1 to 11, choose the ONE BEST answer to each question.

1. A woman fails to lactate or menstruate after giving birth. Which of the following is the most likely cause?

A. Sheehan's syndrome
B. Chromophobe adenoma
C. Empty sella syndrome
D. Hypothalamic glioma
E. Basophilic adenoma

2. Simple goiter is associated with all of the following EXCEPT:

A. Fluorides in the water supply
B. Puberty
C. Androgenic steroid therapy
D. Dietary iodine deficiency
E. Pregnancy

3. The most common cause of the syndrome of inappropriate antidiuretic hormone secretion is:

A. Subdural hematoma
B. Radiation injury to the hypothalamus
C. Meningitis
D. Oat cell carcinoma of lung
E. Pituitary adenoma

4. A goitrogen is a substance that:

A. Mimics the action of T_3
B. Mimics the action of T_4
C. Suppresses T_3 and T_4 synthesis
D. Mimics the action of thyroid-stimulating hormone (TSH)
E. Depletes the body of iodine

5. A 30-year-old woman with infectious mononucleosis suddenly develops a painful enlarged thyroid. The most likely diagnosis is:

A. Subacute lymphocytic thyroiditis
B. Reidel's thyroiditis
C. Thyroid abscess

D. Subacute granulomatous thyroiditis
E. Hashimoto's thyroiditis

6. Thyroid enlargement is greatest in:

A. Graves' disease
B. Simple goiter
C. Hashimoto's thyroiditis
D. Multinodular goiter
E. de Quervain's thyroiditis

7. A lobe of thyroid removed from a man with thyrotoxicosis contained the 2.0-cm nodule pictured in Figure 14–1. The lesion is most likely:

A. A medullary carcinoma
B. A papillary carcinoma
C. A multinodular goiter
D. A follicular carcinoma
E. A follicular adenoma

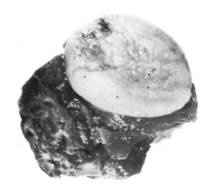

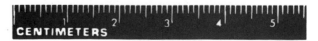

Figure 14–1

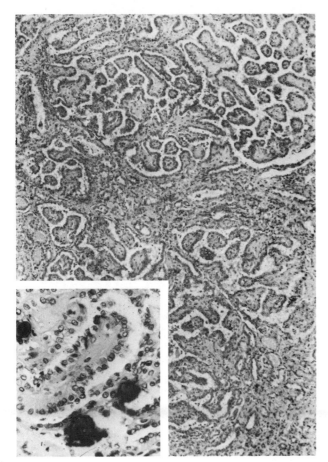

Figure 14-2

C. Preference for lymphatic rather than hematogenous spread
D. Strong association with external irradiation
E. Appearance as a "cold" nodule on thyroid scan

9. Parathyroid hormone increases serum calcium by all of the following mechanisms EXCEPT:

A. Reduces renal calcium excretion
B. Increases intestinal absorption of calcium
C. Blocks calcitonin secretion from the thyroid
D. Produces an immediate efflux of calcium from bone
E. Produces a prolonged release of calcium from bone through osteoclast activation

10. On a checkup visit to his physician, a 50-year-old man who has noticed some muscle weakness and fatigability is found to have hypercalcemia by routine laboratory tests. Statistically, it is most likely that this man has:

A. Primary parathyroid hyperplasia
B. Secondary parathyroid hyperplasia
C. A parathyroid adenoma
D. A parathyroid carcinoma
E. A nonparathyroid carcinoma

11. Hyperaldosteronism associated with an adrenal adenoma is known as:

A. Bartter's syndrome
B. Nelson's syndrome
C. Conn's syndrome
D. Cushing's syndrome
E. None of these

8. All of the following characteristics are associated with the thyroid lesion pictured in Figure 14–2 EXCEPT:

A. Aggressive biologic behavior and poor prognosis
B. Multifocality within the thyroid gland

DIRECTIONS: For Questions 12 to 17, ONE or MORE of the completions given correctly finishes the incomplete statement. Choose:
A—if only *1,2, and 3* are correct
B—if only *1 and 3* are correct
C—if only *2 and 4* are correct
D—if only *4* is correct
E—if all are correct

12. Somatostatin exerts inhibitory control over:

1. Insulin
2. Thyrotropin
3. Glucagon
4. Growth hormone

   A. 1,2,3   B. 1,3   C. 2,4   D. 4 Only   E. All

13. Which of the following characteristics describes the disease of the thyroid pictured in Figure 14–3?

1. Occurs predominantly in women
2. Is caused by a suppressor cell deficiency
3. Is characterized by TSH receptor autoantibodies
4. Is characterized by antimicrosomal antibodies

   A. 1,2,3   B. 1,3   C. 2,4   D. 4 only   E. All

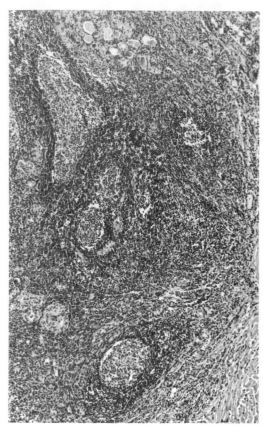

Figure 14–3

14. Features associated with medullary carcinoma of the thyroid include:

1. Neurosecretory granules
2. Amyloid stroma
3. Prostaglandin production
4. Calcitonin production

   A. 1,2,3   B. 1,3   C. 2,4   D. 4 Only   E. All

15. Most females born with 21-hydroxylase deficiency would be expected to have:

1. Clitoral hypertrophy
2. Reduced aldosterone levels
3. Elevated adrenocorticotropic hormone (ACTH) levels
4. Hypertension

   A. 1,2,3   B. 1,3   C. 2,4   D. 4 Only   E. All

16. The possible occurrence of pheochromocytoma should be expected in patients with which of the following disorders?

1. Medullary carcinoma of the thyroid
2. Pituitary adenoma
3. Parathyroid adenoma
4. Pancreatic islet cell adenoma

   A. 1,2,3   B. 1,3   C. 2,4   D. 4 Only   E. All

17. Thymomas are correctly described as:

1. Composed of neoplastic T cells
2. Often associated with myasthenia gravis
3. Responding to treatment with thymosin
4. Rarely occurring in children

   A. 1,2,3   B. 1,3   C. 2,4   D. 4 Only   E. All

DIRECTIONS: For Questions 18 to 22, you are to decide whether EACH choice is TRUE or FALSE.

For each of the following statements about Graves' disease, decide whether it is TRUE or FALSE.

18. It can be distinguished from all other forms of thyrotoxicosis by the presence of proptosis

19. It is usually caused by toxic nodular goiter

20. Virtually all patients have anti-TSH receptor antibodies

21. It has the same HLA genotype association as Hashimoto's thyroiditis

22. Localized myxedema is a characteristic clinical feature

DIRECTIONS: For Questions 23 to 51, the set of lettered headings is followed by a list of numbered words or phrases. For each numbered word or phrase choose:
    A—if the item is associated with (A) only
    B—if the item is associated with (B) only
    C—if the item is associated with *both* (A) and (B)
    D—if the item is associated with *neither* (A) nor (B)

For each of the following characteristics, choose whether it describes Cushing's syndrome, acromegaly, both, or neither.

    A. Cushing's syndrome
    B. Acromegaly
    C. Both
    D. Neither

23. Caused by basophilic adenoma of the pituitary

24. Caused by lung cancer

25. Rarely associated with visual field defects

26. Produces hyperglycemia

27. Produces hypertension

28. Produces osteoporosis

29. Produces changes in the facial appearance

For each of the characteristics listed below, choose whether it describes myxedema, Addison's disease, both, or neither.

    A. Myxedema
    B. Addison's disease
    C. Both
    D. Neither

30. In adults, the disease is most commonly caused by an autoimmune process

31. Fatigability and constipation are common symptoms

32. Hypertension is frequently produced

33. Cardiomyopathy is characteristic

34. Hyperpigmentation is characteristic

35. Mental dysfunction is common

36. Candidiasis and hypoparathyroidism are associated disorders

For each of the characteristics listed below, choose whether it describes pheochromocytoma, neuroblastoma, both, or neither.

    A. Pheochromocytoma
    B. Neuroblastoma
    C. Both
    D. Neither

37. Characteristically elaborates catecholamines

38. Primarily affects children older than 5 years

39. Is virtually always malignant

40. Carries a worse prognosis when occurring in extra-adrenal sites

41. Occasionally regresses spontaneously

For each of the statements below, choose whether it describes insulin-dependent diabetes mellitus, non–insulin-dependent diabetes mellitus, both, or neither:

    A. Insulin-dependent diabetes mellitus
    B. Non-insulin-dependent diabetes mellitus
    C. Both
    D. Neither

42. Underutilization of glucose is characteristic

43. Cellular insulin resistance is a major feature

44. Obesity is a major pathogenetic factor

45. Autoantibodies against pancreatic islet cells are characteristic

46. Strong associations with specific HLA types exist

47. Viral infection of the islet cells is causally related in some cases

48. Hyperglucagonemia is usually present

49. Most affected individuals develop retinopathy

50. Most treated individuals now enjoy a normal life expectancy

51. Ketoacidosis is a major cause of death

DIRECTIONS: Questions 52 to 69 are matching questions. For each numbered item, choose the most likely associated lettered item from those provided. Each numbered item has ONLY ONE answer. Within each group, each lettered item may be the answer to one, more than one, or none of the numbered items.

For each of the endocrine organs listed below, choose whether its embryologic origin is from Rathke's pouch, the foramen caecum, pharyngeal pouches, or none of these.

    A. Rathke's pouch
    B. Foramen caecum
    C. Pharyngeal pouches
    D. None of these

52. Thyroid gland

53. Parathyroid glands

54. Thymus gland

55. Anterior pituitary gland

56. Posterior pituitary gland

57. Pineal gland

For each of the characteristics listed below, choose whether it describes prolactin, growth hormone, corticotropin, thyrotropin, or none of these.

    A. Prolactin
    B. Growth hormone
    C. Corticotropin
    D. Thyrotropin
    E. None of these

58. A hormone produced in the hypothalamus

59. The hormone most often secreted by chromophobes

60. Cause of the most common endocrinopathy produced by pituitary tumors

61. A hormone rarely elaborated by pituitary adenomas

62. A hormone frequently secreted by pituitary carcinomas

63. The most common hormone to be affected in an isolated pituitary hormone deficiency

64. The first hormone to produce a clinically evident deficiency in panlobular pituitary destruction

For each of the characteristics listed below, choose whether it describes pituitary dwarfism, cretinism, achondroplastic dwarfism, or none of these.

    A. Pituitary dwarfism
    B. Cretinism
    C. Achondroplastic dwarfism
    D. None of these

65. Characterized by autosomal dominant inheritance

66. Produces mental retardation

67. Produces a large head and body relative to extremities

68. Associated with a broad, flat nose and large tongue

69. Cannot be prevented with treatment

The Endocrine System

ANSWERS

1. (A) Postpartum pituitary necrosis, also known as Sheehan's syndrome, is one of the three most common causes of pituitary hypofunction. Nonfunctioning (usually chromophobe) pituitary adenomas and the empty sella syndrome are the two others, but they are not related to pregnancy. It is believed that during pregnancy the pituitary enlarges to almost twice its normal size, compressing its own venous vasculature and causing relative ischemia. Thus, an episode of sudden systemic hypotension, such as that which may occur from blood loss during delivery, precipitates ischemic necrosis of the anterior lobe. The posterior pituitary, which is less vulnerable to anoxia, is spared.

Hypothalamic tumors such as gliomas can cause anterior pituitary hypofunction but do so far less commonly than the disorders mentioned above and have no known association with pregnancy (*pp. 1210–1213*).

2. (C) Simple goiter is a thyroid enlargement due to compensatory hypertrophy and hyperplasia. It diffusely involves the entire gland without producing nodularity and does not usually produce thyroid function abnormalities (i.e., affected individuals are typically euthyroid). Because the enlarged follicles are filled with colloid, simple goiter has also been called colloid goiter. In the United States, it is the most common thyroid abnormality. The disorder either arises sporadically in association with altered physiologic (e.g., hormonal) factors, occurs as a consequence of hereditary defects in iodine metabolism or hormone transport, or far more commonly occurs as an endemic disorder related to an underlying iodine deficiency or ingested goitrogen (i.e., ingested dietary substance that promotes goiter formation).

When superimposed on a minimal iodine deficiency, physiologic stimuli that normally cause an increase in thyroid size and function (e.g., puberty, pregnancy, or stress from any source) may produce goiter. Contributory physiologic mechanisms are often multiple in these circumstances. For example, estrogen-induced increases in serum levels of thyroid-binding globulin (TBG) during pregnancy or oral contraceptive steroid use increase the amount of TBG-bound T_3 and T_4 and concomitantly reduce the unbound (active) fractions. Decreased serum concentrations of free hormones, in turn, reduce feedback inhibition of the anterior pituitary, resulting in thyroid-stimulating hormone (TSH) release and thyroid stimulation. Androgenic steroids produce the opposite effect of estrogens on thyroid activity by lowering serum levels of TBG.

Lack of iodine in the diet has been a common cause of simple goiter in the past but is decreasing in prevalence with the use of iodized salt. Because iodine is the critical element in the synthesis of both T_3 and T_4, iodine deficiency leads to decreased synthesis of these hormones and a compensatory increase in TSH. Thus, the thyroid is stimulated to increase the number of follicular cells and hormone output to achieve a euthyroid state. In addition, through autoregulation within the thyroid gland itself, follicular cells become more efficient in extracting and concentrating iodine.

With chronicity, simple goiter of any cause typically progresses to produce even greater enlargement and nodular transformation of the thyroid. The condition is then called multinodular goiter. At this stage, the goiter may be either nontoxic, hyperfunctional, or (rarely) hypofunctional. The mechanisms of nodule generation are unknown (*pp. 1215–1216, 1227–1228*).

3. (D) The syndrome of inappropriate antidiuretic hormone secretion (SIADH) is a condition characterized by independent elaboration and secretion of ADH irrespective of plasma osmolarity. Under normal conditions, the posterior lobe of the pituitary is the source of ADH, but in SIADH secretion, the source of the ADH is usually a tumor. Approximately 80% of all cases are caused by bronchogenic carcinoma, especially oat cell carcinoma, which accounts for more than 80% of all cases. Other neoplasms associated with SIADH include thymoma, pancreatic carcinoma, and lymphoma. Although intracranial hemorrhage (e.g., subdural hematoma) or infection of the central nervous system (e.g., meningitis) may occasionally cause SIADH, this is relatively uncommon.

In contrast to conditions causing an overproduction of ADH, inflammatory injury or neoplastic involvement of the hypothalamohypophyseal axis (e.g., by radiation or a pituitary adenoma) usually leads to ADH deficiency and diabetes insipidus. Although mentioned earlier as an uncommon cause of increased ADH secretion, meningitis is also occasionally known to result in decreased ADH secretion and produce diabetes insipidus (*p. 1214*).

4. (C) A goitrogen is any chemical agent that suppresses the synthesis of T_3 and T_4. With the suppression of thyroid hormone synthesis, feedback inhibition to the hypothalamus and pituitary is reduced. In turn, increased amounts of TSH are released, causing hypertrophic and hyperplastic enlargement of the thyroid gland, a condition known as goiter (*pp. 1215, 1227*).

5. (D) The sudden development of an enlarged painful thyroid in association with some form of viral infection (e.g., infectious mononucleosis, mumps, or an upper respiratory tract infection) is characteristic of a self-limited inflammation of the thyroid gland known as subacute granulomatous thyroiditis or de Quervain's thyroiditis. This entity is three to six times more common in women than in men, and its peak incidence is in the second to fifth decades of life.

In contrast to de Quervain's thyroiditis, subacute lymphocytic thyroiditis (a self-limited idiopathic lymphocytic infiltration of the thyroid) and Reidel's thyroiditis (an idiopathic fibrosing reaction) are painless processes and have no association with prior viral infections. Hashimoto's thyroiditis, an autoimmune thyroiditis that may occasionally be painful and usually occurs in females, has no known association with viral illness. Whereas thyroid abscesses may occur from direct extension of a local infectious process or even by metastatic spread, this is extremely uncommon and would not be expected in the setting of a viral illness such as infectious mononucleosis (*pp. 1220–1223*).

6. (D) Multinodular goiter, the consequence of long-standing simple goiter (see Question 2), is associated with the most extreme enlargement of the thyroid gland, which may achieve weights of more than 2000 gm (normal weight = 20 to 25 gm) in this disorder. Although Graves' disease, simple goiter, Hashimoto's thyroiditis, and de Quervain's thyroiditis all produce thyroid enlargement, it is usually modest in comparison, perhaps two- to threefold greater than normal (*pp. 1214, 1222–1223, 1225, 1228*).

7. (E) A discrete, encapsulated single nodule is apparent in the otherwise normal thyroid lobe pictured in Figure 14–1. Because the patient has thyrotoxicosis, it is most likely that this nodule represents a functioning thyroid adenoma. Although most adenomas do not function and appear as "cold" nodules on thyroid scan, some are associated with hyperfunction; these accumulate radioiodine and appear as "hot" nodules. Along with Graves' disease and toxic multinodular goiter, toxic adenomas are one of the three most common causes of thyrotoxicosis. Only rarely do well-differentiated (papillary or follicular) thyroid carcinomas secrete sufficient thyroid hormone to cause clinical hyperthyroidism; moreover, in such instances, the tumor is usually widely metastatic. Medullary carcinomas of the thyroid originate from neurosecretory parafollicular cells (C cells) and not from follicular cells; thus, they do not secrete thyroid hormones. Multinodular goiter (toxic type), although a major cause of thyrotoxicosis, is characterized by multiple thyroid nodules with enlargement of the entire gland and does not correspond to a single nodule within a normal thyroid as pictured (*pp. 1229, 1230–1238*).

8. (A) A papillary carcinoma of the thyroid with characteristic psammoma bodies is pictured in the photomicrograph in Figure 14–2. Papillary adenocarcinoma is the most common form of thyroid cancer, but fortunately the great majority of these are indolent in their biologic behavior and have an excellent prognosis. Among the salient features of this tumor are its tendency to be multifocal within the thyroid gland as a result of intraglandular spread and its preference for local lymphatic rather than hematogenous metastasis. Many cases of papillary thyroid carcinoma are associated with prior exposure to ionizing radiation, which is now known to cause thyroid carcinoma in 4 to 9% of exposed individuals. Although papillary tumors are not the only radiation-associated thyroid cancers, they are the most common. Papillary carcinomas usually appear as cold nodules on thyroid scintiscans. Although a small number of papillary tumors may concentrate iodine and elaborate thyroglobulin, they are less likely to do so than well-differentiated follicular carcinomas (*pp. 1216, 1230, 1233–1236*).

9. (C) Parathyroid hormone (PTH), the most important physiologic regulator of serum calcium levels, has several modes of action. It acts to raise serum calcium by reducing renal excretion and increasing intestinal absorption of the element. It also modulates calcium stores in the bone by two separate mechanisms. It produces an immediate efflux of calcium from bone into the blood within minutes and subsequently produces a prolonged release of calcium from bone through an increase in the number and activity of osteoclasts. However, PTH has no known direct effect on the secretion of calcitonin, the calcium-lowering hormone produced by the C cells of the thyroid (*p. 1243*).

10. (E) Hypercalcemia is caused at least as frequently by nonparathyroid cancers as by all other forms of hyperparathyroidism combined. Parathyroid adenomas and primary parathyroid hyperplasia constitute 95% of cases of primary hyperparathyroidism. Secondary hyperparathyroidism is most commonly the result of renal insufficiency and, in contrast to the primary form, is characterized by hypocalcemia. Parathyroid carcinoma, although a cause of primary parathyroid hyperfunction, is quite rare (*pp. 1243–1244*).

11. (C) Conn's syndrome is caused by an adrenal adenoma producing large amounts of aldosterone. This syndrome is characterized by sodium retention and potassium wasting, which in turn cause hypertension and neuromuscular abnormalities.

Bartter's syndrome is a form of secondary hyperaldosteronism caused by overproduction of renin by the kidneys. In contrast to other forms of secondary hyperaldosteronism, the blood pressure is usually low in patients with Bartter's syndrome rather than increased.

Nelson's syndrome, in contrast, has little to do with the adrenals. It is caused by hypersecretion of adrenocorticotropic hormone (ACTH) from a pituitary tumor that cannot be eradicated and therefore necessitates removal of the end-organs. After bilateral adrenalectomy, the feedback inhibition of cortisol on the pituitary adenoma is removed, and intense hyperpigmentation related to excess production of ACTH and melanotropin ensues.

Cushing's syndrome is caused by overproduction of glucocorticoids. It may be caused by a hyperfunctioning adrenal adenoma, but it would be the result of a cortisol-producing rather than aldosterone-producing tumor (*pp. 1208, 1254–1255, 1259*).

12. (E) Somatostatin is an intriguing inhibitory hormone that is produced in the hypothalamus as well as in many other tissues throughout the body. It exerts inhibitory control over (inhibits secretion of) a number of other hormones, including insulin, glucagon, gastrin, thyrotropin (TSH), and growth hormone (GH). Thus, it has a number of physiologic roles in addition to its well-known function as a release-inhibiting factor controlling GH and TSH release from the anterior pituitary (*pp. 992, 1207*).

13. (E) Figure 14–3 shows the typical microscopic features of Hashimoto's thyroiditis. Extensive infiltration of the thyroid by lymphoid cells in all stages of transformation and differentiation with the formation of germinal centers dominates the histologic picture. Clusters of thyroid follicles persist (top center of photograph) but are atrophic. This disease, which occurs 10 times more frequently in women than in men, is an organ-specific autoimmune disorder thought to be caused by a deficiency in thyroid antigen-specific suppressor T cells. The result is an uncontrolled immunologic attack on follicular cells by cytotoxic T cells and an unregulated T helper cell participation in the formation of autoantibodies. The autoantibodies most commonly isolated from patients with Hashimoto's thyroiditis are TSH

receptor antibodies and thyroid microsomal antibodies. Some of the TSH receptor autoantibodies appear to mimic the stimulatory action of TSH, whereas others simply block the hormone receptor site (*pp. 1220–1223*).

14. (E) Medullary carcinoma of the thyroid is a neuroendocrine tumor derived from the C cells of the thyroid. Histologically, one of its most distinctive features is amyloid stroma. As in other neuroendocrine neoplasms, neurosecretory dense core granules can be identified in the cytoplasm of medullary carcinoma cells when examined by electron microscopy. Approximately 80 to 90% of these tumors elaborate the major product of their cell of origin—the calcium-lowering hormone, calcitonin. Less frequently, medullary carcinomas produce prostaglandins or histaminase, and rarely they may secrete ACTH, vasoactive intestinal polypeptide (VIP), or serotonin. Calcitonin and/or prostaglandins induce diarrhea in about 30% of patients. Medullary carcinomas are surgically curable with early diagnosis. This is often possible with surveillance in the familial forms of the disease (medullary carcinoma is part of the multiple endocrine neoplasia syndromes types IIa and IIb; see Question 16). With advanced disease, more common with the sporadic neoplasms, mean survival approaches 5 years (*pp. 1238–1240*).

15. (A) The most common cause of congenital adrenal virilism (one of at least eight distinctive clinical syndromes known collectively as congenital adrenal hyperplasia) is 21-hydroxylase deficiency. This defect impairs the synthesis of cortisol and shunts the precursors into the alternate pathway of androgen production. As a result of increased androgens, females with this syndrome are expected to show signs of virilization such as clitoral hypertrophy. Due to the block in cortisol synthesis, feedback inhibition to the pituitary is reduced and ACTH secretion is consequently increased. In about two-thirds of individuals with 21-hydroxylase deficiency, aldosterone synthesis is also impaired, and salt wasting with hyponatremia and hyperkalemia results. This contrasts with 11-hydroxylase deficiency, in which the mineralocorticoid 11-deoxycorticosterone is produced in excess, causing hypertension and hypokalemia (*pp. 1250, 1260–1261*).

16. (B) Pheochromocytoma is a neoplasm of the adrenal medulla that usually occurs sporadically but is also known to occur in several different familial syndromes. The tumor has at least four hereditary patterns, two of which are part of a multiple endocrine neoplasia syndrome. In Sipple's syndrome (multiple endocrine neoplasia type IIa), pheochromocytoma is associated with medullary carcinoma of the thyroid and parathyroid adenoma or hyperplasia. In this syndrome, which is transmitted by autosomal dominant inheritance, the pheochromocytomas are bilateral in 60 to 100% of cases. Other hereditary patterns of pheochromocytoma include (1) multiple endocrine neoplasia type IIb (MEN IIb), in which the pheochromocytoma is associated with mucosal neuromas and a marfanoid habitus; (2) a simple autosomal dominant hereditary predisposition to pheochromocytomas; (3) association with von Recklinghausen's neurofibromatosis; and (4) association with von Hippel-Lindau disease.

Pituitary adenomas and pancreatic islet cell adenomas are part of MEN I, in which they are associated with parathyroid and adrenocortical adenomas. They are not part of the constellation of endocrine adenomas associated with pheochromocytoma (*pp. 1007–1008, 1238, 1263–1264*).

17. (C) Thymomas, although rare, are the most common neoplasm of the thymus gland and one of the most common anterior mediastinal tumors. The neoplastic element of a thymoma is not the thymic lymphocyte but rather the thymic epithelial cell. In the normal gland, this cell is the source of a humoral factor known as thymosin that influences the differentiation of thymocytes (T cells). Patients with thymomas have a striking predisposition to the development of myasthenia gravis, an autoimmune disorder characterized by autoantibodies to acetylcholine receptors in skeletal muscle motor end plates (see Chapter 15, Question 3). Approximately 15 to 44% of patients with thymoma develop myasthenia gravis, and conversely, thymic abnormalities are present in most patients with myasthenia gravis (thymomas in 15 to 40%, thymic hyperplasia in most of the remaining patients). The relationship between these two diseases is still unclear.

The great majority of thymomas occur in adults; the average age of patients with thymomas is 50 years. Most of these neoplasms are benign and can be cured by surgical excision. Malignant thymomas are rare and have a poor prognosis despite surgical resection and postoperative irradiation. Thymosin, one of the humoral factors normally produced by thymic epithelial cells that induce T-cell differentiation, has been used in the treatment of some lymphoid malignancies. However, it would not be expected to have an effect on the epithelium-derived thymoma (*pp. 1269, 1270–1271, 1366–1367*).

18. (True); 19. (False); 20. (True); 21. (False); 22. (True)

Graves' disease is thyrotoxicosis caused by a hyperfunctioning diffuse hyperplastic goiter accompanied by infiltrative ophthalmopathy and sometimes infiltrative dermopathy. It is unique among the goiters. Like simple goiter, Graves' disease is diffuse rather than nodular, but simple goiter does not cause hyperfunction. Multinodular goiter may be hyperfunctioning, but as the name indicates, the thyroid enlargement is nodular rather than diffuse. In contrast to both simple and nodular goiter, Graves' disease is not caused by goitrogens or inborn errors of metabolism (see Question 6). Like Hashimoto's thyroiditis, Graves' disease is an autoimmune form of goiter, but Hashimoto's thyroiditis typically causes hypo- rather than hyperfunction.

(18) Patients with other forms of thyrotoxicosis may have eye changes such as retraction of the upper eyelid and lid lag, but only Graves' disease causes protrusion of the globe (proptosis) due to autoimmune and inflammatory processes.

(19) In addition to Graves' disease and functioning thyroid adenomas, toxic nodular goiter is one of the three major causes of thyrotoxicosis. However, as emphasized earlier, Graves' disease refers only to diffuse hyperfunctioning goiter.

(20) In Graves' disease, autoantibodies to TSH receptor antigens are produced because of a defect in antigen-specific suppressor T cells. These antibodies bind to the TSH receptors on thyroid follicular cells and mimic the actions of TSH, inducing thyroid growth and hyperfunction. With sensitive assay techniques, TSH autoantibodies can be identified in virtually all patients with Graves' disease.

(21) Although Graves' disease and Hashimoto's thyroiditis are both thyroid-specific autoimmune disorders, they have separate and distinctive genotype associations. Graves' disease is associated with the HLA-DR3 genotype, whereas Hashimoto's thyroiditis is associated with the HLA-DR5 genotype. This difference in genotypic association presumably is related to the difference in the type of TSH-receptor autoantibodies produced in each of these diseases. In Graves' disease, the autoantibodies are predominantly stimulatory, whereas in Hashimoto's thyroiditis, blocking antibodies that bind to the TSH receptor (blocking TSH binding but causing no stimulation of the receptor machinery) may play a more important role.

(22) Infiltrative dermopathy taking the form of localized skin edema over the dorsa of the legs or feet is especially characteristic of Graves' disease. However, it is present in about 10 to 15% of patients. Although ironically referred to as "localized myxedema," this change has nothing to do with true myxedema (hypothyroidism in the older child or adult) (*pp. 1217, 1224–1227*).

23. (A); 24. (A); 25. (A); 26. (C); 27. (C); 28. (C); 29. (A)

Cushing's syndrome and acromegaly are syndromes of hormonal excess caused respectively by cortisol and GH. In the case of Cushing's syndrome, overproduction of cortisol may be caused either by a functioning neoplasm in the adrenal cortex or by adrenal response to elevated plasma levels of corticotropin (ACTH). Functional pituitary adenomas are the most common cause of both Cushing's syndrome and acromegaly.

(23) Among functional pituitary adenomas, those that secrete prolactin, ACTH, or GH are the most common. Together they constitute 70% of all functional pituitary adenomas. About 60 to 70% of all cases of Cushing's syndrome are caused by basophilic pituitary adenomas. GH-secreting adenomas are even slightly more common than ACTH-secreting lesions, but they are either acidophilic or chromophobic, not basophilic.

(24) A less common cause of Cushing's syndrome (10 to 15% of cases) is ACTH production by nonendocrine cancers as a paraneoplastic phenomenon. The most common ACTH-producing tumors are bronchogenic carcinomas (particularly oat cell carcinomas), which account for about 60% of cases of "ectopic Cushing's syndrome." Although ectopic hormone production is a relatively common paraneoplastic phenomenon, acromegaly is notably absent from the list of endocrinopathies caused by nonendocrine cancers. However, acromegaly may be produced by GH-secreting endocrine neoplasms such as pancreatic endocrine tumors or carcinoid tumors.

(**25**) Any functional pituitary tumor of sufficient size can cause manifestations of a space-occupying lesion in addition to hyperpituitarism. ACTH-producing adenomas, however, are usually very small (microadenomas) though often multiple, and they rarely cause the visual disorders associated with enlarging masses in the sella turcica. Visual field defects, usually homonymous hemianopia, most commonly result from pituitary tumors, such as GH-secreting adenomas, which tend to be large and impinge on the immediately adjacent optic chiasm and optic nerve.

(**26**) Hyperglycemia and (**27**) hypertension are clinical characteristics of both Cushing's syndrome and acromegaly. In both of these conditions, glucose intolerance may be severe enough to produce overt diabetes mellitus. (**28**) Another feature common to both of these disorders is osteoporosis. (**29**) Both Cushing's syndrome and acromegaly cause characteristic changes in the facial appearance of affected individuals. In Cushing's syndrome, central obesity is characteristic, with rounding of the face (moon faces), neck, and abdomen. Acromegaly causes bone growth with striking enlargement and coarsening of the facial features, hands, and feet (*pp. 294–295, 1207–1210, 1254–1259*).

30. (C); 31. (C); 32. (D); 33. (A); 34. (B); 35. (A); 36. (B)

Myxedema and Addison's disease are endocrine deficiency syndromes caused by hypofunction of the thyroid and the adrenal cortex, respectively. Both have profound systemic effects, some of which are similar in the two diseases.

(**30**) In adults, both myxedema and Addison's disease are most commonly caused by autoimmune processes. Hashimoto's thyroiditis, the archetype of organ-specific autoimmune diseases, is the most common cause of goitrous hypothyroidism in regions having a sufficiency of iodine. Although in the past tuberculosis was the most common cause of Addison's disease, at present the disorder is usually the result of so-called idiopathic adrenalitis, a condition believed to be autoimmune in origin. In addition, as part of a polyglandular autoimmune syndrome, the two conditions may be associated with one another or with other autoimmune disorders such as pernicious anemia or diabetes mellitus.

(**31**) Certain clinical manifestations such as fatigability and constipation are common in both diseases. (**32**) Hypertension, however, is a feature of neither myxedema nor Addison's disease. On the contrary, virtually all patients with Addison's disease are hypotensive. Myxedema causes a characteristic cardiomyopathy, and systolic pressures from the enlarged, flabby heart are

greatly reduced. However, diastolic pressures are elevated because of increased peripheral vascular resistance. (**33**) Patients with full-blown myxedema usually develop congestive heart failure. The term *myxedema heart* refers to this pathologically distinctive cardiomyopathy characterized by interstitial mucopolysaccharide deposition and swelling of myofibers with loss of striations.

(**34**) Hyperpigmentation is a distinguishing feature of Addison's disease. It results from increased secretion of ACTH as a result of lowered serum cortisol levels and reduced feedback inhibition to the hypothalamus and pituitary. Increased synthesis of both ACTH and melanotropin ensues, melanocytes are stimulated, and hyperpigmentation results.

(**35**) In contrast to cortisol insufficiency, lack of thyroid hormones produces a slowing of mental as well as physical processes. Thus, myxedema causes a reduction in intellectual function that does not occur in Addison's disease.

(**36**) As mentioned earlier, both myxedema and Addison's disease may be associated with other autoimmune diseases. It has recently become evident, however, that syndromes of multiple autoimmune disorders that include Addison's disease fall into two distinct subsets. Type I is characterized by at least two of the triad of Addison's disease, hypoparathyroidism, and mucocutaneous candidiasis. Type II, also known as Schmidt's syndrome, is characterized by Addison's disease, autoimmune thyroid disease, and/or insulin-dependent diabetes mellitus without hypoparathyroidism or candidiasis (*pp. 1220–1223, 1249, 1252–1253*).

37. (C); 38. (D); 39. (B); 40. (A); 41. (B)

Pheochromocytoma and neuroblastoma constitute the two most significant disease processes of the adrenal medulla. The pheochromocytoma originates from the adrenal medullary chromaffin cell, whereas the neuroblastoma is derived from autonomic ganglion cell precursors known as neuroblasts. (**37**) Both of these tumors characteristically elaborate catecholamines, predominantly norepinephrine in both cases. (**38**) Occurrence in older children (after age 5) would be relatively unusual for either tumor type. Approximately 80% of neuroblastomas occur in children younger than 5 years, and pheochromocytoma is most common in the fourth and fifth decades. (**39**) In sharp contrast to pheochromocytomas, which are usually benign, neuroblastomas are virtually always malignant and usually metastatic by the time the diagnosis is made.

(**40**) Only about 5% of pheochromocytomas occurring in the adrenal are malignant. Thus, they have a better prognosis than their extra-adrenal counterparts, which are much more likely to be malignant. Neuroblastomas, although invariably malignant, carry a poorer prognosis when arising in the adrenal than when occurring in extra-adrenal sites.

(**41**) One of the most intriguing behavioral features of small in situ neuroblastomas found in infancy is the high frequency of spontaneous regression. Spontaneous regression has not been observed with pheochromocytomas of any sort (*pp. 1263–1267*).

42. (C); 43. (B); 44. (B); 45. (A); 46. (A); 47. (A); 48. (C); 49. (C); 50. (D); 51. (D)

Diabetes mellitus is a chronic endocrine disorder characterized by an absolute or relative deficiency of insulin. Marked derangements in the metabolism of carbohydrate, fat, and protein are the result. The disease has two major variants: insulin-dependent diabetes mellitus (IDDM), constituting about 10 to 20% of cases, and non–insulin-dependent diabetes mellitus (NIDDM), accounting for the remaining 80 to 90%.

(**42**) Although the two variants have numerous distinctive features, they have in common an inability to utilize glucose. (**43**) In contrast to IDDM, which is the result of injury to the beta cells of the pancreatic islets producing an absolute and severe lack of insulin, only a relative lack of insulin is present in NIDDM. However, NIDDM has an additional pathogenetic feature: namely, end-organ resistance to the action of insulin at the cellular level. This universal feature of NIDDM is the result of both a decrease in cellular insulin receptors and an impairment of the postreceptor effects of insulin within the cell.

(**44**) In NIDDM (but not IDDM), obesity is a major pathogenetic factor. Even in otherwise normal individuals, obesity is associated with hyperinsulinemia and insulin resistance. In obese type II diabetics, insulin levels are lower than in weight-matched nondiabetics, suggesting a relative insulin deficiency and a failure of the overstressed beta cells to maintain a state of sustained hyperinsulinism. In addition, genetic factors may contribute to accelerated age-related loss of beta cells. It is significant that approximately 80% of patients with NIDDM are considerably overweight and that weight loss in an overweight diabetic patient notably improves the metabolic derangement.

(**45**) In contrast to NIDDM, IDDM is believed to be an organ-specific (more accurately in this case, a cell-specific) autoimmune disorder. Islet cell autoantibodies can be found in as many as 90% of all newly diagnosed cases of IDDM. Some of these antibodies are known to be complement fixing and are capable of causing pancreatic islet cell membrane damage in vitro. In some patients there is also evidence for a cellular immune response in the form of sensitized T cells reactive against beta cells. Indeed, lymphocytes are a characteristic histologic finding in the pancreatic islets of young diabetics with IDDM, a phenomenon known as insulitis.

(**46**) Although there are no specific genetic markers for either form of diabetes, it is certain that diabetes mellitus is at least in part a genetic disorder. Epidemiologic studies indicate that genetic factors play a much larger role in the induction of NIDDM than in that of IDDM. For example, the concordance rate for NIDDM in identical twins is 90 to 100%, as contrasted with a 50% concordance rate in IDDM. However, IDDM shows a strong association with specific alleles in the class II histocompatibility complex (HLA-D linked), whereas it has not been possible to demonstrate a relationship between NIDDM and specific HLA types. About 80% of patients with IDDM have HLA-DR3 or HLA-DR4 alleles, whereas in the general population the prevalence of these alleles is only 30 to 50%.

(**47**) There is also ample evidence that in a few cases IDDM may be caused by a direct, severe, virus-induced injury of the pancreatic beta cells. In most cases, however, IDDM is believed to result from a combination of factors that may include viral infection but also involve HLA-linked genetic factors and immunologic factors.

(**48**) Concomitant overproduction of glucagon is another pathogenetic factor that can be demonstrated in both major forms of diabetes. Because the metabolic effects of glucagon are directly opposite to those of insulin, absolute or relative insulin deficiency is exacerbated by glucagon excess.

(**49**) Despite the major etiologic differences between IDDM and NIDDM, their major systemic pathologic manifestations are remarkably similar. One of the most common and characteristic pathologic features of diabetes, regardless of type, is retinal vascular changes known collectively as diabetic retinopathy. It has been estimated that a patient with a 25-year history of diabetes mellitus has a 90% chance of developing this complication. (**50**) Unfortunately, both major variants of diabetes also share a shortened life expectancy. On the average, life expectancy for male diabetic patients is reduced approximately 9 years and for females, approximately 7 years.

(**51**) Happily, however, ketoacidosis is no longer a major cause of death in the diabetic population. In fact, with modern methods of treatment it has become rare as a cause of mortality. Atherosclerotic complications (e.g., myocardial infarction, cerebrovascular accidents, gangrene, renal insufficiency) are the most common causes of death in both forms of long-standing diabetes (*pp. 994–1005*).

52. (B); 53. (C); 54. (C); 55. (A); 56. (D); 57. (D)

The endocrine system is composed of numerous unique and complex organs with diverse functions and embryologic origins. A knowledge of the embryologic source of each organ is useful in understanding their respective developmental pathologies. (**52**) The thyroid gland develops from a tubular invagination at the root of the tongue called the foramen caecum. The tube, called the thyroglossal duct, elongates as the thyroid migrates to its final position in front of the trachea. Vestigial remnants of the thyroglossal duct may develop into midline cystic structures later in life and require surgical removal.

(**53**) Although at least one pair is intimately associated with the thyroid gland, the parathyroid glands originate from an altogether different embryologic source—the third (lower pair) and the fourth (upper pair) pharyngeal pouches. (**54**) Because the thymus gland also originates from the third and sometimes fourth pair of pharyngeal pouches, one or two parathyroids occasionally become enclosed within the thymic capsule.

(55) The pituitary is actually a composite gland made up of an anterior, epithelium-derived portion and a neurally derived posterior portion. The anterior pituitary is derived from an evagination of the roof of the primitive oral canal called Rathke's pouch, whereas **(56)** the posterior pituitary arises from an outpouching of the floor of the third ventricle. Although in the course of normal development Rathke's pouch is detached from its origin by the growing sphenoid bone, rests of epithelial cells may occasionally be caught below the sphenoid and give rise to pharyngeal pituitary tissue.

(57) The pineal gland, a small structure located at the base of the brain, is derived from ependymal cells lining the third ventricle. Although its function is still somewhat obscure, the pineal gland is thought to play some role in maintaining diurnal awake-asleep rhythms and sexual cycles (*pp. 1206, 1214, 1241, 1242, 1268, 1272*).

58. (E); 59. (E); 60. (A); 61. (D); 62. (E); 63. (B); 64. (E)

Prolactin, GH, corticotropin, and thyrotropin all are hormones produced in the anterior pituitary. **(58)** Hypothalamic hormones include oxytocin and vasopressin, which are stored in the posterior pituitary; in addition, the hypothalamus produces releasing factors for all six of the anterior pituitary hormones and release-inhibiting factors for at least two. **(59)** The cells of the anterior pituitary have classically been divided into three separate categories according to their staining properties with acidic and basic dyes. Acidophilic cells are now known to be lactotropes or somatotropes, whereas basophilic cells are either corticotropes, thyrotropes, or gonadotropes. Chromophobic cells (about 25% of the cell population) do not appear to contain any anterior pituitary hormones by immunohistochemical methods and are thought to be sparsely granulated cells.

(60) For reasons that are poorly understood, the vast majority of functioning pituitary adenomas secrete either prolactin, GH, or corticotropin. Hyperprolactinemia is now recognized as the most common pituitary tumor-related endocrinopathy. **(61)** Tumors secreting thyrotropin, luteinizing hormone (LH), or follicle-stimulating hormone (FSH) are very uncommon; it has been estimated that pituitary tumors elaborating thyrotropin constitute less than 1% of all pituitary adenomas. **(62)** In contrast to benign pituitary tumors, which are fre-

quently secretory, pituitary carcinomas are not only exceedingly rare but only rarely elaborate hormones.

(63) Hypopituitarism usually arises from some destructive process involving the anterior pituitary and usually involves more than one hormone. Rarely, however, pituitary insufficiency may manifest itself as an isolated hormone deficiency; in such cases, it usually takes the form of a GH deficiency.

(64) More commonly, anterior pituitary destruction leads to impaired production of all the tropic hormones. Clinically, loss of the gonadotropins (LH and FSH) is usually the first to become manifest, because it quickly produces derangements of reproductive function (*pp. 1206–1211*).

65. (C); 66. (B); 67. (C); 68. (B); 69. (C)

Dwarfism is not a discrete process but rather a retardation of growth that may occur in various diverse conditions. Hypopituitarism in prepubertal children causes so-called pituitary dwarfism. Thyroid hypofunction in infants is the cause of the growth-retarding condition known as cretinism. In contrast to these two conditions, achondroplastic dwarfism is not known to be associated with an endocrinologic deficit.

(65) Achondroplasia is an autosomal dominant disorder in which the exact pathogenetic mechanisms are unknown. The disease is characterized by a failure of cartilage cell proliferation and premature closure of the growth plates of bones performed in cartilage. **(66)** Neither pituitary dwarfism nor achondroplastic dwarfism is associated with decreased intelligence. Cretinism, however, produces profound retardation of intellectual growth as well as physical growth.

(67) Achondroplastic dwarfism can be readily distinguished on the basis of its characteristic body habitus—a large head and small extremities. Head growth is not affected in this disorder, because many bones of the face and cranium are produced by membranous rather than endochondral bone formation.

(68) A broad, flat nose and a very large protuberant tongue are characteristic features of cretinism.

(69) Because pituitary dwarfism and cretinism are the result of hormone deficiencies, they can be successfully treated if recognized early enough by iatrogenic replacement of the missing hormonal elements. There is at present no known effective therapy for achondroplasia (*pp. 1211, 1219, 1319*).

The Musculoskeletal System

DIRECTIONS: For Questions 1 to 9, choose the ONE BEST answer to each question.

1. All of the following statements about osteoblasts are true EXCEPT:

A. They are multinucleate cells
B. They are precursors of osteocytes
C. They are rich in alkaline phosphatase
D. They synthesize the collagen component of the osteoid matrix
E. They control parathormone-induced osteoclastic bone resorption

2. A muscular dystrophy can usually be differentiated from denervation change on muscle by the finding of:

A. Random and irregular variation in muscle cell size
B. Dislocation and internalization of muscle cell nuclei
C. Accumulation of phagocytic macrophages around disintegrating muscle cells
D. Proliferation of endomysial and perimysial connective tissue
E. Accumulation of fat cells between muscle fibers

3. All of the following statements about myasthenia gravis are true EXCEPT:

A. Ocular muscles are usually affected first
B. Muscle weakness progresses with persistent use
C. Muscle strength is recovered after periods of rest
D. The risk of developing autoimmune thyroid disease is increased
E. Almost all patients have underlying thymomas

4. Pyogenic osteomyelitis is associated with all of the following complications EXCEPT:

A. Periostitis
B. Pott's disease
C. Sequestrum formation
D. Brodie's abscesses
E. Involucrum formation

5. A fracture that communicates with the skin surface is known as a:

A. Pathologic fracture
B. Greenstick fracture
C. Complete fracture
D. Compound fracture
E. Comminuted fracture

6. All of the following characteristics are typical of the bone disease pictured in Figure 15–1 EXCEPT:

A. Children are virtually never affected
B. Involved bones appear thickened radiologically
C. Involved bones are characteristically extremely hard
D. Serum alkaline phosphatase levels are characteristically high
E. Affected individuals are at increased risk of developing osteosarcoma

7. The disease most frequently associated with hypertrophic osteoarthropathy is:

A. Pleural mesothelioma
B. Bronchogenic carcinoma
C. Infective endocarditis
D. Congenital heart disease
E. Ulcerative colitis

8. Which of the following statements about giant cell tumors of bone is true?

A. Children most often are affected by this neoplasm
B. The giant cells in this tumor are osteoclasts
C. Lesions typically show stippled calcifications on x-ray
D. The bones about the knee are most commonly involved
E. Most lesions exhibit highly aggressive clinical behavior

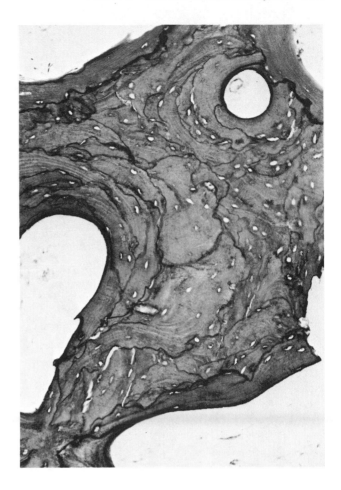

Figure 15–1

9. Pathologic features of osteoarthritis include all of the following EXCEPT:

A. Cartilage fibrillation
B. Pannus formation
C. Eburnation
D. Heberden's node formation
E. Osteophyte formation

DIRECTIONS: For Questions 10 to 13, ONE or MORE of the completions given correctly finishes the incomplete statement. Choose:

A—if only *1,2, and 3* are correct
B—if only *1 and 3* are correct
C—if only *2 and 4* are correct
D—if only *4* is correct
E—if all are correct

10. Granular cell tumors are correctly described as:

1. Arising from Schwann cell precursors
2. Occurring most commonly in the tongue
3. Inducing pseudoepitheliomatous hyperplasia in the overlying epithelium
4. Almost always benign

A. 1,2,3   B. 1,3   C. 2,4   D. 4 Only   E. All

11. Osteoporosis is a reduction in the bone mass that

1. Rarely occurs in males
2. Is caused by impaired osteoid mineralization
3. Primarily involves cortical bone
4. Predisposes to hip fractures

A. 1,2,3   B. 1,3   C. 2,4   D. 4 Only   E. All

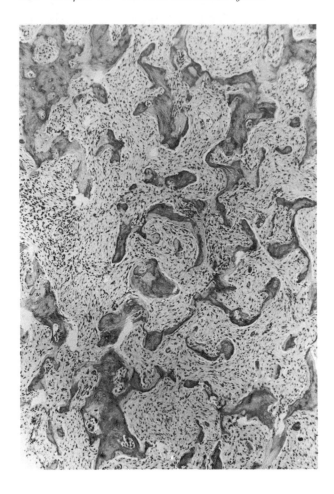

Figure 15–2

12. An asymptomatic 10-year-old boy was discovered to have a single bone involved by the lesion pictured in Figure 15–2. The patient:

1. Most likely has an underlying endocrine disorder
2. Is at increased risk of developing more of these lesions in other bones
3. Has about a 20 to 30% chance of developing an osteosarcoma

4. Most likely had this lesion in a rib

A. 1,2,3   B. 1,3   C. 2,4   D. 4 Only   E. All

13. Characteristic features of Ewing's sarcoma include:

1. Origin in epiphyses of long bones
2. Extensive invasion of adjacent soft tissues
3. High degree of cytologic pleomorphism
4. PAS-positive cytoplasmic granules

A. 1,2,3   B. 1,3   C. 2,4   D. 4 Only   E. All

DIRECTIONS: For Questions 14 to 32, you are to decide whether EACH choice is TRUE or FALSE.

For each of the following statements about normal skeletal muscle, decide whether it is TRUE or FALSE.

14. A striated muscle cell is known as a myofibril

15. Muscle cells innervated by a single motor neuron constitute a motor unit

16. Slow-twitch and fast-twitch fibers are segregated into separate muscles

17. Muscle cells undergo mitosis when regenerating

18. During regeneration, new multinucleate muscle cells form from fusion of mononuclear myotubules

For each of the following statements about rheumatoid arthritis, decide whether it is TRUE or FALSE.

19. The process tends to involve the large joints of weight-bearing areas

20. Most affected adults have rheumatoid skin nodules

21. Most affected adults have antibodies directed against IgG

22. Joint fluid in acute disease typically has normal complement levels

23. The predominant cell type found in the joint fluid in acute disease is the plasma cell

24. In the presence of hypersplenism and leg ulcers, the process is known as Felty's syndrome

25. Amyloidosis develops in more than half of cases of long-standing disease

For each of the following statements about gout, decide whether it is TRUE or FALSE.

26. Most individuals with hyperuricemia develop gout

27. An underlying disease causing excessive cell breakdown is usually present

28. Synthesis of uric acid is increased in most cases

29. Acute arthritis of the great toe is the most common presentation

30. Acute gouty arthritis is the result of urate crystal formation

31. Chronic gouty arthritis is the result of pannus formation

32. Tophi in the central nervous system are one of the most debilitating complications

DIRECTIONS: For Questions 33 to 51, the set of lettered headings is followed by a list of numbered words or phrases. For each numbered word or phrase choose:

    A—if the item is associated with (A) only
    B—if the item is associated with (B) only
    C—if the item is associated with *both* (A) and (B)
    D—if the item is associated with *neither* (A) nor (B)

For each of the characteristics listed below, choose whether it describes desmoids, nodular fasciitis, both, or neither.

    A. Desmoid
    B. Nodular fasciitis
    C. Both
    D. Neither

33. Is a true neoplasm

34. Is associated with pregnancy

35. Occurs commonly in extremities

36. Characteristically infiltrates surrounding soft tissues

37. Characteristically has a myxoid center on histologic examination

38. Tends to recur after incomplete surgical excision

39. Undergoes malignant transformation in 5 to 10% of cases

For each of the characteristics listed below, choose whether it describes osteochondromatosis, enchondromatosis, both, or neither.

    A. Osteochondromatosis
    B. Enchondromatosis

    C. Both
    D. Neither

40. Has a sex-linked mode of hereditary transmission

41. Represents multiple true neoplasms

42. Is associated with colonic polyps in Gardner's syndrome

43. Is associated with cavernous hemangioma in Maffucci's syndrome

44. Is associated with an increased risk of developing chondrosarcoma

For each of the characteristics listed below, choose whether it describes osteosarcoma, chondrosarcoma, both, or neither.

    A. Osteosarcoma
    B. Chondrosarcoma
    C. Both
    D. Neither

45. Constitutes the most common form of primary cancer of bones

46. Occurs most frequently in children and adolescents

47. Arises de novo as a primary lesion in most cases

48. Tends to arise in pelvic bones

49. Often contains both bone and cartilage

50. Rarely metastasizes to lymph nodes

51. Behaves predictably according to tumor grade

DIRECTIONS: Questions 52 to 72 are matching questions. For each numbered item, choose the most likely associated lettered item from those provided. Each numbered item has ONLY ONE answer. Within each group, each lettered item may be the answer to one, more than one, or none of the numbered items.

For each of the features listed below, choose whether it is characteristic of Duchenne type muscular dystrophy, myotonic dystrophy, congenital myopathy, all of these, or none of these.

    A. Duchenne type muscular dystrophy
    B. Myotonic dystrophy
    C. Congenital myopathy
    D. All of these
    E. None of these

52. Occurs only in males

53. Rarely associated with mental retardation

54. Incompatible with long survival

55. Characteristically involves extramuscular systems

56. Characteristically produces involvement of a single myofiber type

57. Characterized histologically by "ring fibers"

58. Caused by a myotropic virus

For each of the characteristics listed below, choose whether it describes rhabdomyosarcoma, synoviosarcoma, malignant fibrous histiocytoma, liposarcoma, or none of these.

    A. Rhabdomyosarcoma
    B. Synoviosarcoma
    C. Malignant fibrous histiocytoma
    D. Liposarcoma
    E. None of these

59. Commonly occurs in children

60. Most often has a myxoid appearance

61. Has an aggressive "alveolar" variant

62. Contains both epithelioid and spindle-shaped cells ("biphasic growth")

63. Typically produces a storiform (pinwheel) growth pattern

64. Often stains positively for lysozyme by immunohistochemistry

65. Often stains positively for keratin by immunohistochemistry

For each of the characteristics listed below, choose whether it describes osteogenesis imperfecta, osteopetrosis, achondroplasia, all of these, or none of these.

    A. Osteogenesis imperfecta
    B. Osteopetrosis
    C. Achondroplasia
    D. All of these
    E. None of these

66. Is genetically transmitted

67. Represents a defect in osteoclast function

68. Represents a defect in type I collagen synthesis

69. Represents a defect in epiphyseal cartilage growth

70. Is associated with blue sclerae

71. Is commonly complicated by multiple exostoses

72. Is commonly complicated by anemia and hepatosplenomegaly

The Musculoskeletal System

ANSWERS

1. (E) Osteoblasts are bone-forming cells that synthesize the collagenous component of the osteoid matrix. In addition, they synthesize the calcium-binding proteins required for mineralization of the osteoid that they produce. When osteoblasts become enclosed within the matrix they produce, they are then called osteocytes. Both osteoblasts and osteocytes are uninucleate and thus can be easily distinguished from osteoclasts, which are multinucleate cells. Osteoblasts are rich in alkaline phosphatase; thus, this enzyme serves as a marker for osteoblastic activity. Although the major function of the osteoblast is bone formation, osteoblasts are also thought to control bone resorption in response to parathormone via signals to osteoblasts. Without osteoblasts, parathormone-induced osteoclastic bone resorption does not occur (*p. 1315*).

2. (A) Morphologic patterns of muscle injury are limited in number and usually lack specificity for any given etiology. Therefore, specific etiologic diagnosis of muscle disease is often impossible from biopsy alone. Clinical features such as the distribution of muscle involvement and the coexistence of other organ involvement must also be considered in order to make a specific diagnosis.

Although it is true that morphologic changes on muscle biopsy are often less than pathognomonic, fairly specific changes are produced by at least some forms of muscle injury. For example, the muscular dystrophies typically produce a random and irregular variation in myofiber size. It is principally this irregular pattern of individual muscle cell involvement that differentiates muscular dystrophy from denervation—both processes that ultimately produce muscle atrophy. In contrast to the random muscle fiber muscle atrophy in the dystrophies, atrophy of fiber groups is seen in denervation. The group atrophy pattern is determined by the pattern of innervation of the affected motor nerves.

Pathologic changes such as proliferation of endomysial and perimysial connective tissue, accumulation of fat cells between myofibers, dislocation and internalization of muscle nuclei, and accumulation of phagocytic macrophages around disintegrating muscle cells are general features of muscle atrophy and do not help to differentiate muscular dystrophy from denervation atrophy (*pp. 1367–1369*).

3. (E) Myasthenia gravis (MG) is an autoimmune disorder characterized by autoantibodies to the acetylcholine receptors of postsynaptic membranes at the motor end plate. Transmission of neural impulses at the neuromuscular junction is blocked, resulting in muscle weakness. Characteristically, the first manifestation of MG is weakening of the eye muscles with diplopia and drooping of the eyelids. Trunk and limb muscles are frequently affected later in the disease. A distinctive clinical feature that sets MG apart from other muscular disorders is fatigue that increases with activity with recovery of strength after a period of rest. Individuals with MG and members of their family have an increased incidence of other autoimmune disorders including thyroid disease, rheumatoid arthritis, lupus, and pernicious anemia. The thymus appears to have a central role in the etiology of MG, but the underlying immunopathologic mechanisms are still unclear. The thymus is abnormal in nearly all patients with MG. About 15 to 40% have a thymoma, and the remainder characteristically have thymic hyperplasia. Thus, thymectomy is an important treatment modality for MG (*pp. 1366–1367*).

4. (B) Pyogenic osteomyelitis is a bacterial (or rarely fungal) infection of bone. Almost any bacterium can be responsible, but the most common organisms involved in adult disease are *Staphylococcus aureus*, *Escherichia coli*, and *Pseudomonas aeruginosa*. In neonates, *Hemophilus influenzae* and group B streptococci are common offenders. The infection most often appears to arise as a primary infection in a previously healthy individual and, in this setting, is thought to be produced by transient bacteremias from such trivial sources as injury to the intestinal mucosa, vigorous chewing of hard foods, or minor injury to the skin. Less often, the infection has a more obvious source and is the result of local trauma, metastatic seeding from a distant infection, or local spread of a contiguous soft tissue infection.

In hematogenous osteomyelitis, the inflammatory process typically begins in the marrow. With progression, it penetrates the endosteum, enters the haversian and lacunar systems of the cortex, and then invades the periosteum (periostitis). Lifting of the periosteum impairs the blood supply to the bone, and a sequestrum, a large fragment of dead bone that detaches as a free foreign body, may form as a combined result of both suppurative and ischemic injury. If endogenous reactive/reparative processes succeed in walling off the bony infection, a localized abscess may remain as a chronic nidus of infection known as a Brodie's abscess. In some cases, smoldering infection induces fibroblastic activity from the periosteum, and new bone, known as an involucrum, is formed around the inflammatory focus.

Pott's disease is tuberculous osteomyelitis of the spine. Unlike pyogenic osteomyelitis, which is typically an acute process, tuberculous osteomyelitis tends to be an insidious, chronic infection that is characteristically more destructive and resistant to control. Thus, Pott's disease commonly results in compression fractures that produce serious spinal deformities (*pp. 1320–1322*).

5. (D) Fractures of different types heal with different speeds, the repair process being affected by both the nature and the extent of the injury. A greenstick or incomplete fracture usually refers to long bone injuries in which the cortex snaps apart on one side and remains attached on the other. Complete fractures are through-and-through ruptures with total dissociation of the fractured edges. In a comminuted (means "pulverized") fracture, the bone is shattered into splinters. In a closed or simple fracture, the overlying tissue is intact, but in compound fractures, the fracture site communicates with the skin surface (*p. 1322*).

6. (C) The pathognomonic histologic feature of Paget's disease of bone (osteitis deformans), a *mosaic* pattern of bone formation, is illustrated in Figure 15–1. Paget's disease is characterized by excessive resorption of normal bone followed by excessive new bone formation in a haphazard arrangement. The newly formed osteons are demarcated by osteoid seams that form the histologic "mosaic." It is a disorder of adults of middle age or older and virtually never appears in children. Involved bones are characteristically greatly thickened, a feature readily seen on x-ray. The intense osteoblastic activity typically produces high serum alkaline phosphatase levels. In fact, the alkaline phosphatase levels in Paget's disease are generally greater than in any other bone disorder.

Although involved bones are thickened in this disease,

they are, nevertheless, extremely soft. They are composed largely of poorly mineralized osteoid matrix and vascular connective tissue and are usually light, soft, and porous. Thus, pagetic bones are prone to pathologic fractures, a common complication. The most ominous complication of Paget's disease is the development of a sarcoma in the involved bone, a consequence that occurs in about 1% of patients.

Paget's disease is an extremely common disorder of bone, but its pathogenesis is still unclear. The recent findings of intranuclear viral inclusions in osteoclasts by electron microscopy and paramyxovirus antigens by immunohistochemistry have suggested a slow-viral etiology, but virus has not yet been isolated from affected bone (*pp. 1328–1331*).

7. (B) Hypertrophic osteoarthropathy is a disorder of unknown cause characterized by periosteal inflammation at the ends of tubular bones with lifting of the periosteum, subjacent new bone formation, and arthritis of the adjacent joints. Clubbing of the digits is a common manifestation. Although it may occur in association with a wide variety of neoplastic and inflammatory disorders, the disease with which it most frequently occurs is bronchogenic carcinoma. No other single disease produces hypertrophic osteoarthropathy with as great a frequency (10% of cases) as bronchogenic carcinoma. Additional associated disorders include other intrathoracic tumors such as pleural mesothelioma, pulmonary metastases, or mediastinal Hodgkin's disease, chronic lung infection, or chronic liver disease. Clubbing alone, without distal long-bone neo-osteogenesis or arthritis, may occur with cyanotic heart disease, infective endocarditis or aortitis, inflammatory bowel disease (ulcerative colitis or Crohn's disease), or cancer of the esophagus or colon. Hypertrophic osteoarthropathy sometimes precedes clinical manifestations of an underlying disease and can call attention to it. The arthropathy is usually reversible with the surgical resection or medical correction of the underlying disorder (*p. 1333*).

8. (D) Giant cell tumors of bone encompass a spectrum of neoplasms that exhibit extremely variable biologic behavior. They are composed of mononuclear cells of mesenchymal origin and numerous multinucleate giant cells derived from the mononuclear elements. These tumors have been inappropriately known as "osteoclastomas," but the giant cells are not osteoclasts. Giant cell tumors occur most commonly in adults between the ages of 20 and 40 years and are distinctly rare in skeletally immature individuals (children). Distinctively, the lesions almost always arise in the epiphyses of long bones, most commonly around the knee. Radiographically, giant cell tumors typically appear as lytic soap-bubble lesions that notably lack stippling or calcifications.

Most giant cell tumors (70 to 75%) are composed of well-differentiated cells with few, if any, mitoses and minimal atypicality; these lesions behave clinically in a benign fashion. Only about 5 to 15% of giant cell tumors are overtly anaplastic and biologically aggressive. The remainder have an intermediate histologic appearance and a variable and unpredictable clinical course (*pp. 1343–1345*).

9. (B) Osteoarthritis (degenerative joint disease) is the most common form of arthritis. It is a destructive process, both deforming and debilitating, that may occur de novo in advanced age or at any age as a secondary consequence of congenital, structural, traumatic, metabolic, or inflammatory joint disease.

No matter what the underlying pathogenesis, the histologic changes of osteoarthritis are quite constant. Clefts appear in the surface of the articular cartilage and may extend to the underlying subchondral bone, a pathologic feature known as cartilage fibrillation. With progressive erosion of articular cartilage, focal areas of subchondral bone become denuded and sclerotic (eburnation). Bony spurs arise from the margins of the articular cartilage and may project from opposing bone, causing pain and limitation of motion. Osteophytic spurs arising from the base of the terminal phalanges are known as Heberden's nodes and are characteristic of osteoarthritis.

Pannus formation is a process characterized by intense inflammation of the synovial lining; a highly vascularized polypoid mass of inflammatory tissue arises from the synovium and often overgrows the articular surface beginning at the joint margins. Pannus formation is highly characteristic of rheumatoid arthritis but is not pathognomonic. It may also occur in other inflammatory joint disease such as that associated with psoriasis or gout. However, pannus formation is not a feature of osteoarthritis (*pp. 1346–1349, 1358*).

10. (E) Granular cell tumors are soft tissue neoplasms that are almost always benign and arise from Schwann cell precursors. In the past, because they were thought to arise from myoblastic cells, these tumors were called myoblastomas. They occur most commonly in the tongue and in the dermis or subcutis of skin on the trunk arms. It is important to recognize that granular cell tumors induce pseudoepitheliomatous hyperplasia of the overlying epithelium because this can be so exuberant as to be mistaken for a squamous cell carcinoma (*pp. 1371–1373*).

11. (D) Osteoporosis is a condition characterized by reduction in both the mineral and matrix phases of structurally normal bone. It is a ubiquitous but asymptomatic condition that affects both sexes but may be more marked in women because the rate of loss significantly increases after menopause. It is an age-related disorder associated with estrogen deficiency in women and androgen deficiency in men and probably is related to reduced physical activity and dietary calcium deficiency in both sexes. The condition is believed to be caused by accelerated bone loss along with some slowing of bone formation, the reasons for which are unclear. The bone loss is greater in trabecular than in cortical bone. Therefore, fractures of bone composed predominantly of trabecular bone such as vertebral bodies and the femoral necks are common.

Impaired osteoid mineralization is the characteristic defect in osteomalacia and rickets but is not encountered in osteoporosis (*pp. 1324–1326*).

12. (D) The bony lesion pictured in Figure 15–2 is known as fibrous dysplasia. It is characterized by haphazardly arranged trabeculae of woven bone within a background of cellular connective tissue. In about 70 to 75% of cases, the lesion is limited to a single bone and referred to as monostotic fibrous dysplasia. As in the case described in the question, the condition typically becomes manifest in childhood. The lesion is usually asymptomatic and often discovered as an incidental finding on x-ray. The rib is the most common location of monostotic fibrous dysplasia, followed by the femur, tibia, maxilla, mandible, calvarium, and humerus.

In about 30% of cases of fibrous dysplasia, multiple bones are involved. The polyostotic form of the disease usually appears at a slightly earlier age, is more likely to involve the craniofacial bones, and is less likely to involve the ribs than the monostotic form. In about 3% of cases of polyostotic fibrous dysplasia, the condition is accompanied by skin pigmentation and various endocrine disorders, including precocious sexual development (Albright's syndrome), hyperthyroidism, Cushing's syndrome, hyperparathyroidism, and others.

There is no known association between the monostotic and polyostotic forms of fibrous dysplasia; transition from the monostotic to the polyostotic form has never been reported. Therefore, a patient with a single lesion such as the one described is not at increased risk of developing multiple lesions.

Fibrous dysplasia rarely undergoes sarcomatous change. The risk of developing an osteogenic sarcoma (sometimes fibrosarcoma or chondrosarcoma) is less than 1% (*pp. 1331–1332*).

13. (C) Ewing's sarcoma is a highly malignant primary bone tumor composed of small round undifferentiated cells. It is believed to originate from a primitive neuroectodermal cell because it shares a unique and characteristic chromosomal abnormality (reciprocal translocation of long arms of chromosomes 11 and 22) with other neuroectodermal tumors and because the tumor cells can be induced to undergo neural differentiation in culture. Histologically, the tumor is composed of masses of small uniform cells with little cytologic pleomorphism. A helpful diagnostic feature of Ewing's sarcoma is the finding of characteristic PAS-positive granules in the cytoplasm of the tumor cells.

Ewing's sarcoma typically arises in the metaphyses of long tubular bones and virtually never originates in epiphyseal regions. It tends to perforate the bony cortex and penetrate adjacent soft tissues, often producing larger extraosseous than intraosseous masses. With combined surgery, chemotherapy, and radiation therapy, the 5-year survival rate for this tumor has improved from about 10% to 40 to 75% (*pp. 1342–1343*).

14. (False); 15. (True); 16. (False); 17. (False); 18. (True)
(14) Normal skeletal muscle is a marvel of structural

organization from the gross to the ultrastructural level. Each muscle is composed of numerous fascicles that represent groups of muscle cells enclosed in perimyseal connective tissue. Individual muscle cells within a fascicle are known as myofibers; each contains numerous myofibrils within its cytoplasm. Myofibrils are the contractile elements of the cell and are composed of a highly ordered array of interdigitating actin and myosin myofilaments.

(15) The functional organization of groups of muscle cells does not always correspond precisely to the architectural organization described above. Functional groupings of myofibers are known as motor units and are determined by innervation rather than by spacial contiguity or fascicular grouping. A motor unit, therefore, is composed of all myofibers innervated by a single anterior horn motor neuron.

(16) There are two functional types of muscle fibers: slow-twitch (type I) and fast-twitch (type II). The former are involved with tonic contractions (e.g., posture maintenance) and the latter with rapid phasic contractions (e.g., finger wiggling). Because it is innervation that determines myofiber type, all of the myofibers within a motor unit are of the same type. However, fiber types (and motor units) are randomly distributed in different muscles and are not separated into separate muscles as they are in other animals such as birds.

(17) Differentiated skeletal muscle cells, along with cardiac muscle and nerve cells, lack the capacity to undergo mitotic division in postnatal life. (18) Nevertheless, skeletal muscle is capable of regeneration through proliferation of myoblasts normally present between myofibers as satellite cells. Myoblasts form myotubules, which then fuse to form multinucleate myofibers (*pp. 31, 1363–1365*).

19. (False); 20. (False); 21. (True); 22. (False); 23. (False); 24. (True); 25. (False)

Rheumatoid arthritis (RA) is a chronic systemic inflammatory disease that is autoimmune in character and produces a progressive deforming arthritis as one of its primary manifestations.

(19) In contrast to osteoarthritis, which tends to involve weight-bearing joints, RA typically affects the small joints of the hands and feet in a symmetrical distribution.

(20) Rheumatoid skin nodules are a particularly distinctive but variable feature of RA and are present only in about 25% of patients.

(21) Almost all adult patients with RA have antibodies against the Fc fragment of autologous IgG. These autoantibodies, called rheumatoid factor (RF), are present only infrequently in the juvenile form of rheumatoid arthritis (Still's disease), occurring in individuals under the age of 16. (22) In the adult form of the disease, most of the RF is formed locally by the lymphoplasmacytic inflammatory infiltrate in the joints. The IgG-RF immune complexes that are formed bind and activate complement and initiate an inflammatory response. Thus, complement levels are characteristically low in the acute rheumatoid synovial effusions. (23) Neutro-

phils, attracted by the chemotactic fragments from C3 and C5, predominate in the acute phase of the disease. Neutrophils containing granular intracytoplasmic inclusions of phagocytized immune complexes are called RA cells.

(24) Felty's syndrome is one of the variant forms of rheumatoid arthritis; it refers to the combination of splenomegaly with hypersplenism and leg ulcers in association with the characteristic rheumatoid polyarthritis. Other variant forms of the disease include juvenile rheumatoid arthritis (see Question 21), ankylosing spondylitis, psoriatic arthritis, and arthritis associated with ulcerative colitis, Whipple's disease, or Sjögren's syndrome.

(25) Although RA is the second most common cause of secondary amyloidosis, only about 15 to 25% of cases of long-standing RA are complicated by this disorder. Thus, the likelihood of developing secondary amyloidosis is less for patients with RA than for those with tuberculosis or leprosy, diseases in which the prevalence of amyloidosis approaches 50% (*pp. 214, 1349–1354*).

26. (False); 27. (False); 28. (True); 29. (True); 30. (True); 31. (True); 32. (False)

Gout is a chronic disabling disease caused by the precipitation of monosodium urate crystals from supersaturated body fluids in patients with hyperuricemia. (26) Although hyperuricemia is the sine qua non of gout, it does not inevitably produce the disease. Only a fraction (about 20%) of individuals who are hyperuricemic develop gout. (27) Although gout may occur as a secondary phenomenon in any disease process causing hyperuricemia, the vast majority of cases (approximately 90%) occur in the absence of a defined metabolic defect and are referred to as primary idiopathic gout. (28) In most cases of primary gout, the hyperuricemia is primarily the result of increased uric acid synthesis rather than impaired excretion. However, a *relative* underexcretion of uric acid may coexist with the increased urate synthesis in some cases. Less frequently, underexcretion of urates is the major defect in primary gout; in about 30% of cases, no increased synthesis of uric acid can be detected. In these individuals, the hyperuricemia is believed to be renal in origin.

(29) Acute gouty arthritis of the metatarsal phalangeal joint of the great toe is the most common presentation of the disease. At least half of the initial attacks involve this joint. (30) Acute arthritis is evoked by the precipitation of urate crystals into the joint fluid. It is characterized by sudden development of swelling, redness, erythema, and excruciating pain in the involved joint; these symptoms can be mistaken for suppurative arthritis. (31) Chronic gouty arthritis is the result of multiple recurrent attacks of acute arthritis leading to inflammatory synovial pannus formation. The pannus, in turn, progressively destroys the underlying articular cartilage and ultimately causes structural deformation and disabling disease.

(32) Tophi, the pathognomonic lesions of gout, are composed of a mass of crystalline or amorphous urates surrounded by an intense inflammatory and foreign body

giant cell reaction. Because urates do not penetrate the blood-brain barrier, tophi do not develop in the central nervous system (*pp. 1355–1360*).

33. (D); 34. (A); 35. (B); 36. (C); 37. (B); 38. (A); 39. (D)

(33) Both desmoids and nodular fasciitis are considered to be forms of fibromatosis, exuberant fibrous tissue growths that are more aggressive than usual reactive proliferations but are not clearly neoplastic. Desmoids form tumorous masses that can be quite large (up to 15 cm in diameter) and may be difficult to differentiate from a sarcoma. Nodular fasciitis is somewhat of a misnomer because it does not always arise in fascia (most commonly occurs in subcutaneous tissues) and does not represent an inflammatory process. Like desmoids, nodular fasciitis is commonly mistaken clinically for a neoplasm.

(34) Some desmoids appear to be hormonally responsive lesions. Abdominal wall desmoids have a striking female predominance, generally arise during or after pregnancy, and have been found to contain estrogen receptors. Furthermore, desmoid-like masses have been produced in guinea pigs by the injection of estrogens. Extra-abdominal and intra-abdominal desmoids, however, have no sexual associations. Nodular fasciitis also occurs with equal frequency in both sexes and has no associations with pregnancy.

(35) In contrast to desmoids, which rarely arise in extremities, nodular fasciitis has a predilection for the extremities (forearm, leg, and arm). (36) Both desmoids and nodular fasciitis tend to be unifocal lesions with irregular borders that characteristically infiltrate the surrounding soft tissues. (37) Histologically, a desmoid is typically heavily collagenized in the center, whereas nodular fasciitis characteristically has a myxoid center.

(38) Both desmoid tumors and nodular fasciitis can be cured by surgical resection. However, incompletely excised desmoids tend to recur locally, whereas postoperative recurrence of nodular fasciitis, even when incompletely resected, is exceedingly rare. (39) Neither of these lesions has a propensity for neoplastic transformation. The rare reports of metastatic dissemination of a desmoid are believed to represent misdiagnosis of low-grade fibrosarcoma (*pp. 1380–1381*).

40. (D); 41. (B); 42. (A); 43. (B); 44. (C)

(40) Osteochondromatosis and enchondromatosis are syndromes characterized by multiple osteochondromas and enchondromas, respectively, lesions that are most commonly solitary and sporadic in occurrence. Osteochondromas are cartilage-capped bony projections growing from the lateral contours of endochondral bones. They are developmental aberrations rather than true neoplasms and are also known as exostoses. The syndrome of osteochondromatosis is an autosomal dominant rather than a sex-linked disorder, but it does affect males three times more often than females. (42) Multiple osteochondromas may also occur as a part of another hereditary disorder known as Gardner's syndrome, which also includes desmoid tumors, sebaceous cysts,

and adenomatous polyps of the colon. The latter pose a significantly increased risk of colonic adenocarcinoma.

(41 and 43) Enchondromas are true benign neoplasms composed of mature hyaline cartilage arising in the interior of a bone. Enchondromatosis (also known as Ollier's disease) usually develops at a younger age than osteochondromatosis and is typically discovered early in childhood, but there is no clear evidence of hereditary transmission in this disease. However, it may occur as part of a familial syndrome that also includes multiple cavernous hemangiomas known as Maffucci's syndrome.

(44) Both osteochondromatosis and enchondromatosis are associated with an increased incidence of chondrosarcoma, but the rate of malignant transformation in Ollier's disease is particularly high (30 to 50%) (*pp. 1319–1320, 1339*).

45. (A); 46. (A); 47. (C); 48. (B); 49. (C); 50. (C); 51. (B)

Malignancies arising from the cell types in bone are much less common than those arising from marrow elements (myeloma and leukemia). Although infrequent, primary bone tumors are among the most biologically aggressive neoplasms in humans. (45) Osteosarcoma is the most common cancer of bone, (46) and most commonly occur in children and adolescents. Chondrosarcoma occurs half as often as osteosarcoma but, even so, is second only to osteosarcoma in frequency. It tends to arise in middle age to later life. (47) Like chondrosarcomas, osteosarcomas arise de novo ("primary" osteosarcomas) in most cases. Less frequently, they develop in a background of preexisting bone disease ("secondary" osteosarcomas) such as Paget's disease, multiple enchondromas, multiple osteochondromas, chronic osteomyelitis, fibrous dysplasia, infarcts, or fractures of bone.

(48) Unlike osteosarcoma, which tends to arise about the knee, chondrosarcomas originate most frequently in the pelvic bones. (49) Histologically, both osteosarcomas and chondrosarcomas often contain both bony and cartilaginous elements. Their diagnosis depends on the identification of frankly malignant, anaplastic cells in association with osteoid matrix in the case of osteosarcoma or chondroid matrix in the case of chondrosarcoma. In chondrosarcomas with ossification, the bone formation occurs within cartilage, whereas in osteosarcomas, the neo-osteogenesis arises out of the background of anaplastic, osteoblastic cells. (50) It is rare for either osteosarcoma or chondrosarcoma to metastasize to lymph nodes. Hematogenous dissemination is the major mode of metastasis of both of these tumors. (51) In contrast to the experience with osteosarcoma in which there is little correlation between histologic grade and patient survival, there is an excellent correlation between the histopathology of chondrosarcomas and tumor behavior. Obviously, then, histologic grading of chondrosarcoma is of great clinical significance (*pp. 1336–1338, 1340–1342*).

52. (A); 53. (C); 54. (A); 55. (B); 56. (E); 57. (B); 58. (E)

Muscular dystrophies and congenital myopathies are inherited primary disorders of muscle fibers that produce muscle weakness, atrophy, and loss of tendon reflexes. Although the muscular dystrophies tend to have distinctive clinical features, they produce the same basic morphologic changes in the involved muscles. They typically become apparent in early childhood. Congenital myopathies, in contrast, are not clinically distinctive but produce fairly specific morphologic changes. Most congenital myopathies present as a floppy infant syndrome.

(52) Among the hereditary dystrophies and congenital myopathies, the Duchenne type and Becker's muscular dystrophies are the only two that are inherited as sex-linked conditions and occur only in males. (53) Both Duchenne type muscular dystrophy and myotonic dystrophy, the most severe and the most prevalent dystrophies, respectively, are associated with decreased intelligence. Although mild reduction in intelligence is common among individuals with Duchenne type muscular dystrophy, frank mental retardation is present only in about 30%. Most individuals with myotonic dystrophy, however, manifest frank mental retardation or even dementia. Congenital myopathies, in contrast, are rarely associated with mental retardation.

(54) Duchenne type muscular dystrophy is incompatible with long survival; it is a progressive disease that usually leads to death by age 20. Although myotonic dystrophy is also a progressive disease, muscle involvement generally proceeds far more slowly and is not totally incapacitating nor incompatible with long survival. In contrast to the muscular dystrophies, the congenital myopathies are not progressive and are compatible with a normal life span and a useful existence.

(55) Unlike the other forms of muscular dystrophy and the congenital myopathies, myotonic dystrophy characteristically involves many extramuscular systems. Thus, in addition to weakness and myotonia of the distal muscles, frontal baldness, cataracts, and testicular atrophy are major clinical features.

(56) In all forms of muscular dystrophy, there is a loss of histochemical differentiation between type I and type II myofibers, but neither fiber type is spared. Several of the congenital myopathies tend to involve one fiber type more than the other, but in no case is the damage limited to a single fiber type. (57) "Ring fibers" represent single myofibers transversely encircling other myofibers in the same bundle. They are a distinctive histologic feature of myotonic dystrophy and when present provide the opportunity to identify this form of dystrophy morphologically. (58) As stated earlier, the muscular dystrophies and congenital myopathies are hereditary disorders of muscle fibers and are not known to be related to any acquired disease such as viral infection (*pp. 1368–1370*).

59. (A); 60. (D); 61. (A); 62. (B); 63. (C); 64. (C); 65. (B)

(59 and 61) Most soft tissue sarcomas are adult tumors. Rhabdomyosarcoma is the exception, occurring most commonly in children. In contrast to other soft tissue sarcomas, rhabdomyosarcoma has an alveolar variant characterized by interlacing strands of fibrovascular stroma enclosing spaces filled with loose or solid clusters of small tumor cells. Aside from the pleomorphic variant

(a rarity), rhabdosarcomas are uncommon in adults, and 90% occur before the age of 20.

(60) Most soft tissue sarcomas manifest various histologic growth patterns. Unfortunately, many of these histologic variants overlap, making specific diagnosis of soft tissue sarcomas a challenging endeavor. The myxoid histologic variant is the most common form of liposarcoma. However, a myxoid variant is also common in malignant fibrous histiocytoma and is second only to the typical storiform-pleomorphic variant (see Question 63) in frequency.

(62) Uniquely, synoviosarcoma is characterized by a biphasic histologic pattern; it is composed of both epithelioid and spindle-shaped cells, recapitulating the derivation of cuboidal synovial lining cells from primitive mesenchymal cells.

(63) Storiform or pinwheel patterns of growth are highly characteristic of malignant fibrous histiocytoma. (64) This tumor is believed to derive from primitive mesenchymal cells capable of multidirectional differentiation. They are composed of a mixture of cells resembling fibroblasts, myofibroblasts, histiocytes, and cells with features intermediate among these types. Immunohistochemical stains for lysozyme, α_1-antitrypsin, and α_1-antichymotrypsin, enzymes that are typically present in normal histiocytes, stain most cells in these neoplasms. (65) Immunoperoxidase staining for keratin, on the other hand, is unusual for sarcomas but can often be seen in the epithelium-like components of synoviosarcomas (*pp. 1373–1377, 1378–1379*).

66. (D); 67. (B); 68. (A); 69. (C); 70. (A); 71. (E); 72. (B)

(66) Osteogenesis imperfecta, osteopetrosis, and achondroplasia are hereditary disorders of bone with varying morbidity and mortality. (67) Although there are four variants with different modes of inheritance and different clinical features, the basic defect in all forms of osteogenesis imperfecta is some biochemical abnormality in the synthesis of type I collagen. (68) In osteopetrosis, the underlying defect in both hereditary subsets is one of osteoclast function resulting in overgrowth and sclerosis of bone. (69) In achondroplasia (a form of dwarfism), a defect in epiphyseal cartilage growth results in premature ossification at the osteochondral junction and truncated growth of long bones.

(70) One of the most distinctive clinical features of all variants of osteogenesis imperfecta type IV is the appearance of the sclerae. They are translucent and look blue because of the visualization of the underlying choroid plexus.

(71) Exostoses are not associated with any of these three hereditary conditions but rather constitute a separate and unrelated hereditary condition of bone known as osteochondromatosis (see Questions 40 through 44 above).

(72) Anemia and hepatosplenomegaly are common complications of osteopetrosis. In this condition, the marked overgrowth of bone narrows the marrow cavity and in advanced cases may obliterate it altogether. In such cases, hepatosplenomegaly results from extramedullary hematopoiesis (*pp. 1318–1319*).

The Nervous System

DIRECTIONS: For Questions 1 to 7, choose the ONE BEST answer to each question.

1. All of the following conditions cause increased intracranial pressure EXCEPT:

A. Alzheimer's disease
B. Metastatic tumor
C. Cerebral infarction
D. Lead encephalopathy
E. Water intoxication

2. A disorder of the central nervous system (CNS) that is almost exclusively iatrogenic is:

A. Acute lymphocytic meningitis
B. Subcortical leukoencephalopathy
C. Subacute necrotizing encephalomyelopathy
D. Central pontine myelinolysis
E. Metachromatic leukodystrophy

3. All of the following features describe subacute sclerosing panencephalitis (SSPE) EXCEPT:

A. Occurs as a complication of rubeola infection
B. Has a long latent period
C. Has a protracted course
D. Has a high mortality rate
E. Causes primary demyelinization in the CNS

4. Which of the following statements about subacute spongiform encephalopathy (Creutzfeldt-Jakob disease) is correct?

A. The causative agent is visible only with the electron microscope
B. The affected brain is typically markedly atrophic
C. The usual mode of transmission is person to person via aerosolized droplet exposure

D. A brisk cellular immune response without granuloma formation is characteristic
E. The disease typically causes a rapidly progressive dementia

5. Which of the following statements about epidural hematoma is correct?

A. It is almost always accompanied by a skull fracture
B. The bleeding is usually of venous origin
C. The onset of symptoms is typically delayed for several hours after the vascular rupture
D. The major symptom is a fluctuating level of consciousness
E. It occasionally occurs as a result of rupture of a mycotic aneurysm

6. The most common cause of spinal cord compression is:

A. Penetrating wounds with hemorrhage into the cord
B. Spinal meningioma
C. Traumatic vertebral fracture
D. Epidural hematoma
E. Metastatic tumor

7. All of the following pathologic features are characteristic of Alzheimer's disease EXCEPT:

A. Hirano bodies
B. Senile plaques
C. Neurofibrillary tangles
D. Pick bodies
E. Granulovacuolar degeneration of neurons

DIRECTIONS: For Questions 8 to 16, ONE or MORE of the completions given correctly finishes the incomplete statement. Choose:

A—if only *1, 2, and 3* are correct
B—if only *1 and 3* are correct
C—if only *2 and 4* are correct
D—if only *4* is correct
E—if all are correct

8. Subdural empyema is associated with:

1. Bacterial meningitis
2. Skull fracture
3. Brain abscess
4. Sinusitis

    A. 1,2,3   B. 1,3   C. 2,4   D. 4 Only   E. All

9. Herpes simplex virus causes:

1. Cold sores
2. Neonatal panencephalitis
3. Keratoconjunctivitis
4. Postherpetic neuralgia

    A. 1,2,3   B. 1,3   C. 2,4   D. 4 Only   E. All

10. Berry aneurysms are correctly described as:

1. Usually atherosclerotic in origin
2. Virtually always solitary
3. Most commonly located in the basilar artery
4. The most common cause of ruptured intracranial aneurysm

    A. 1,2,3   B. 1,3   C. 2,4   D. 4 Only   E. All

11. Human immunodeficiency virus type 1 infection of the CNS causes:

1. Acute aseptic meningitis
2. Subacute encephalitis
3. Vacuolar myelopathy
4. Peripheral neuropathy

    A. 1,2,3   B. 1,3   C. 2,4   D. 4 Only   E. All

12. Carcinomatous meningitis is associated with which of the following tumors?

1. Metastatic lung cancer
2. Medulloblastomas
3. Metastatic breast cancer
4. Meningiomas

    A. 1,2,3   B. 1,3   C. 2,4   D. 4 Only   E. All

13. Meningiomas are commonly associated with:

1. Infiltrative, irregular borders
2. Penetration of the adjacent bone
3. A poor prognosis
4. Psammoma bodies

    A. 1,2,3   B. 1,3   C. 2,4   D. 4 Only   E. All

14. Typical histologic features of idiopathic parkinsonism include:

1. Neurofibrillary tangles
2. Lewy bodies
3. Severe neuronal loss in the putamen
4. Depigmentation of the substantia nigra

    A. 1,2,3   B. 1,3   C. 2,4   D. 4 Only   E. All

15. Typical features of amyotrophic lateral sclerosis include:

1. Degeneration of the upper motor neurons
2. Degeneration of the lower motor neurons
3. An inevitably fatal course
4. Infection with an enterovirus

    A. 1,2,3   B. 1,3   C. 2,4   D. 4 Only   E. All

16. Neurofibromata are correctly described as:

1. Derived from Schwann cells
2. Containing Verocay bodies
3. Often multiple
4. Eccentrically located on distal nerves

    A. 1,2,3   B. 1,3   C. 2,4   D. 4 Only   E. All

DIRECTIONS: For Questions 17 to 32, you are to decide whether EACH choice is TRUE or FALSE.

For each of the following statements about vascular disease of the CNS, choose whether it is TRUE or FALSE.

17. Neurons remain viable for only 3 to 4 minutes without blood flow

18. Ischemic encephalopathy is most commonly associated with inadequate cardiopulmonary resuscitation after cardiac arrest

19. A hemorrhagic infarct often overlaps arterial supplies

20. Cerebral hemorrhage is most often caused by hypertensive vascular disease

21. Supratentorial hemorrhage often presents clinically as intractable vomiting

22. Cerebral infarction is most commonly embolic in origin

23. Hypertensive vascular disease is associated with lacunar infarcts

24. Hypertensive encephalopathy is characterized by cortical demyelination

25. The most common cause of vascular injury in the spinal cord is hypertensive vascular disease

For each of the following statements about multiple sclerosis, choose whether it is TRUE or FALSE.

26. Most cases occur in children

27. The primary pathologic process is generalized CNS demyelinization

28. Intellectual deterioration is an early manifestation of the disease

29. The cerebrospinal fluid (CSF) typically contains increased immunoglobulins

30. Onset usually occurs shortly after a viral infection

31. Dense plaques of gliosis are a characteristic histologic feature

32. Long term corticosteroid treatment prevents progression of the disease

DIRECTIONS: For Questions 33 to 49, the set of lettered headings is followed by a list of numbered words or phrases. For each numbered word or phrase choose:
  A—if the item is associated with (A) only
  B—if the item is associated with (B) only
  C—if the item is associated with *both* (A) and (B)
  D—if the item is associated with *neither* (A) nor (B)

For each of the features listed below, choose whether it describes communicating hydrocephalus, noncommunicating hydrocephalus, both of these, or neither of these.

  A. Communicating hydrocephalus
  B. Noncommunicating hydrocephalus
  C. Both of these
  D. Neither of these

33. Often fails to produce ventricular distention

34. Associated with postmeningitic states

35. Associated with neoplasms

36. Associated with thrombosis of the dural sinuses

37. Associated with the Dandy-Walker syndrome

For each of the features listed below, choose whether it describes rabies, poliomyelitis, both of these, or neither of these.

  A. Rabies
  B. Poliomyelitis
  C. Both of these
  D. Neither of these

38. A primary infection elsewhere precedes nervous system disease

39. Diagnostic inclusions are seen in infected cells

40. The causative viral agent affects only dorsal root ganglion cells

41. Lower motor neuron paralysis is produced

42. The most common cause of death is respiratory center failure

For each of the features listed below, choose whether it describes acute disseminated encephalomyelitis, acute hemorrhagic leukoencephalopathy, both of these, or neither of these.

  A. Acute disseminated encephalomyelitis
  B. Acute necrotizing hemorrhagic leukoencephalitis
  C. Both of these
  D. Neither of these

43. The disorder is a common disease of white matter in children

44. Development of the disease is usually preceded by a nonspecific respiratory infection

45. Lymphocytes from patients with the disease are sensitized to myelin basic protein

46. Circulating antibodies to myelin basic protein are a characteristic feature

47. Recovery without neurologic impairment is the rule

48. On gross examination, the brain is usually normal

49. Vasculitis is characteristically present on histologic examination

DIRECTIONS: Questions 50 to 81 are matching questions. For each numbered item, choose the most likely associated lettered item from those provided. Each numbered item has ONLY ONE answer. Within each group, each lettered item may be the answer to one, more than one, or none of the numbered items.

For each of the characteristics of CNS cells listed below, choose whether it describes astrocytes, oligodendrocytes, ependymal cells, all of these, or none of these.

    A. Astrocyte
    B. Oligodendrocyte
    C. Ependymal cells
    D. All of these
    E. None of these

50. Defined as a neuroglial cell

51. Functions as a macrophage

52. Forms glial scars after CNS injury

53. Provides physical (structural) support for neurons

54. Maintains CNS myelin

55. Produces CSF

56. Resorbs CSF

For each of the features listed below, choose whether it describes meningococcal meningitis, mumps meningitis, tuberculous meningitis, all of these, or none of these.

    A. Meningococcal meningitis
    B. Mumps meningitis
    C. Tuberculous meningitis
    D. All of these
    E. None of these

57. The CSF sugar content is usually normal

58. The CSF protein content is usually elevated

59. Neutrophils are characteristically found in the CSF

60. Photophobia and stiff neck are not commonly present

61. Obliterative endarteritis of subarachnoid vessels is an associated complication

For each of the features listed below, choose whether it is characteristic of astrocytoma, oligodendroglioma, ependymoma, or none of these

    A. Astrocytoma
    B. Oligodendroglioma
    C. Ependymoma
    D. None of these

62. The most common brain tumor in children

63. The most common brain tumor in adults

64. The most common type of intraspinal glioma

65. Gives rise to glioblastoma multiforme

66. Characteristically tends to calcify markedly

67. Forms tumor cell rosettes as a typical histologic feature

68. Forms tumor cell pseudorosettes as a typical histologic feature

69. Typically metastasizes to bone

70. Frequently responds dramatically to chemotherapy

For each of the features listed below, choose whether it describes metachromatic leukodystrophy, Krabbe's disease (globoid cell leukodystrophy), adrenoleukodystrophy, or none of these

    A. Metachromatic leukodystrophy
    B. Krabbe's disease (globoid cell leukodystrophy)
    C. Adrenoleukodystrophy
    D. None of these

71. Usually becomes clinically manifest after age 10

72. Produced by a deficiency of cerebroside sulfatase

73. Produced by a deficiency of galactocerebroside β-galactosidase

74. Characterized histologically by multinucleate histiocytic cells in the white matter

75. Characterized histologically by diagnostic inclusion bodies in Schwann cells

For each of the causes of peripheral neuropathies listed below, decide whether it is usually associated with a pattern of ascending motor paralysis, symmetrical polyneuropathy, asymmetric polyneuropathy, or none of these.

    A. Ascending motor paralysis
    B. Symmetrical polyneuropathy

    C. Asymmetric polyneuropathy
    D. None of these

76. Diabetic neuropathy

77. Alcoholic neuropathy

78. Landry-Guillain-Barré syndrome

79. Diphtheritic neuropathy

80. Polyarteritis nodosa neuropathy

81. Lead neuropathy

1. (A) Increased intracranial pressure is the end result of myriad pathologic conditions that expand the volume of the intracranial contents beyond the limits set by its bony confines. Processes that are characterized by cellular swelling, interstitial edema, space-occupying lesions (e.g., tumors, hematomas dilated ventricles) or a combination of these lead to increased intracranial pressure. Metastatic tumor, in addition to being a space-occupying mass, also causes local damage to capillary endothelial cells and/or induces new capillary formation. Damaged capillaries that have lost their permeability barrier function or new capillaries that have not yet acquired it leak fluid into the intercellular space, a process known as vasogenic cerebral edema. Similar mechanisms of vascular injury producing vasogenic edema occur in association with infarction, lead encephalopathy, abscesses, and contusions. Water intoxication leads to cytotoxic edema by producing an acute hypoosmolar state in the plasma with a resultant shift of water into the cerebral cells to maintain osmotic equilibrium.

Alzheimer's disease, a degenerative disease of the cerebral cortex (see Question 7), is not associated with increased intracranial pressure. On the contrary, brain volume is reduced as a result of severe atrophy. The compensatory enlargement of the ventricular system is known as hydrocephalus ex vacuo. It should not be confused with obstructive or communicating hydrocephalus in which expansion of the ventricles is caused by increased cerebrospinal fluid (CSF) volume and intracranial pressure is increased (*pp. 1389–1390, 1427*).

2. (D) Central pontine myelinolysis is an iatrogenic disease characterized by demyelination in the midportion of the pons. Although small foci of involvement may be asymptomatic, large lesions produce a flaccid quadriplegia. The disorder is produced by rapid rises in serum sodium concentrations most frequently associated with intravenous administration of sodium-containing solutions.

Acute lymphocytic meningitis is caused by viral infection (e.g., mumps, ECHO viruses, coxsackievirus, Epstein-Barr virus, herpesvirus) of the meninges.

Subcortical leukoencephalopathy (Binswanger's disease) is a diffuse loss of deep hemispheric white matter associated with hypertension and atherosclerotic cerebrovascular disease. The extensive demyelination produces dementia.

Subacute necrotizing encephalomyelopathy (Leigh syndrome) is an autosomal recessive inborn error of metabolism resulting in mitochondrial defects such as cytochrome oxidase C deficiency. It produces bilateral symmetrical necrosis in the thalamus, midbrain, pons, medulla, and spinal cord.

Metachromatic leukodystrophy is a genetic autosomal recessive disorder of sphingomyelin metabolism that produces demyelination in both the central and peripheral nervous systems and has no iatrogenic component (*pp. 1393, 1408, 1434–1435, 1436, 1437*).

3. (E) Subacute sclerosing panencephalitis (SSPE) is a slow viral infection of the CNS. It is caused by the measles virus and therefore usually follows either active infection or immunization against rubeola. The disease has a long latent period and a protracted course that usually leads to death. Pathologically, the disease is characterized by inclusion bodies in neurons and oligodendroglia, extensive neuronal loss, and perivascular mononuclear cell infiltrates. Most of the injury in SSPE is sustained by the neurons, and primary demyelination is not a feature. Rather, primary demyelination is the characteristic feature of progressive multifocal leukoencephalopathy, a viral infection of oligodendrocytes (*pp. 1399–1400*).

4. (E) Subacute spongiform encephalopathy (Creutzfeldt-Jakob disease, transmissible agent dementia) is a rapidly progressive dementia caused by a poorly defined transmissible agent that has not been visualized by any method, including electron microscopic examination. The agent is resistant to ionizing radiation, ultraviolet light, and formalin. Unfortunately, the mode of transmission is unknown at present, although the disease does not appear to be highly contagious. Documented cases of person-to-person transmission have occurred via a parenteral route. The disease is characterized pathologically by neuronal loss and marked gliosis in the absence of inflammation. Intracytoplasmic membrane-bound vacuoles in neuronal and glial processes that appear grossly as spongiform change are pathognomonic. Clinically, a rapidly progressive dementia is the rule, and death usually ensues after an average survival of 7 months (*p. 1401*).

5. (A) An epidural hematoma results from bleeding into the potential space between the skull and the dura mater. Unlike subdural hematomas, which often result from blunt trauma without skull fractures, epidural hematomas almost always occur in association with an overlying skull fracture. Because the bleeding is usually of arterial origin, the rise in intracranial pressure and the onset of symptoms are typically rapid, usually developing within minutes to a few hours of the trauma. Typically, the patient momentarily recovers consciousness from the initial trauma before descending into a progressively deepening coma. Delayed onset of symptoms and a fluctuating level of consciousness are suggestive instead of a subdural hematoma. Epidural hematomas are almost always due to trauma; other causes are distinctly uncommon. Although they are rarely a cause of intracranial hemorrhage, ruptured mycotic aneurysms usually produce subarachnoid hemorrhage rather than epidural hematoma (*pp. 1406, 1409–1411*).

6. (E) Mechanical injury to the spinal cord occurs by two mechanisms: penetration and/or compression injuries. Compression injuries produce contusions of the cord. They are most frequently caused by metastatic tumor causing pathologic fractures in the spinal canal and within the vertebral bodies. Although penetrating wounds usually produce lacerations of the spinal cord, an element of compression may be introduced when concomitant hemorrhage into the cord parenchyma occurs (hematomyelia) (*p. 1412*).

7. (D) Alzheimer's disease is a degenerative disease of the cerebral cortex; it ultimately leads to dementia. Although the pathogenesis of the disease is unknown, genetic studies have shown that the defect is located on chromosome 21 in familial Alzheimer's disease. Alzheimer's disease is associated with several distinctive (although not pathognomonic) histopathologic changes in the cerebral cortex: Hirano bodies, senile plaques, neurofibrillary tangles, amyloid angiopathy, and granulovacuolar degeneration of neurons. Hirano bodies,

glassy eosinophilic inclusions composed principally of actin filaments, are seen in proximal dendrites. Senile (neuritic) plaques are dilated, tortuous, presynaptic axon terminals that may develop a central amyloid core. Neurofibrillary tangles, neurofilaments in the cytoplasm of neurons that typically encircle the nucleus and denote neuronal degeneration, are most notably, but not exclusively, associated with Alzheimer's disease. Vascular amyloid deposition (amyloid angiopathy) is found almost invariably in the intracortical and small subarachnoid blood vessels. Granulovacuolar degeneration of neurons refers to the formation of small intraneuronal cytoplasmic vacuoles, each of which contains an argyrophilic granule of unknown composition. This form of neuronal degeneration is particularly characteristic of Alzheimer's disease.

Pick bodies are cytoplasmic inclusions of neurofilaments, endoplasmic reticulum, and paired helical filaments (also found in the neurofibrillary tangles of Alzheimer's disease) in neurons of the atrophic frontal and temporal lobes of patients with Pick's disease. Like Alzheimer's disease, Pick's disease is a degenerative disease of the cerebral cortex. It produces profound dementia but typically involves only the frontal and temporal lobes. Unlike Alzheimer's disease, it conspicuously spares the posterior two-thirds of the superior temporal gyrus and only rarely affects either the parietal or occipital lobes (*pp. 1427–1429*).

8. (D) A subdural empyema is an infection (most frequently bacterial) of the skull bones or air sinuses that has penetrated into the subdural space. Thus, most patients with a subdural empyema also have sinusitis and fever. The process usually remains localized, and the underlying arachnoid mater and subarachnoid space are uninvolved. Injury to the brain may occur by indirect means such as secondary thrombophlebitis of central veins crossing the subdural space with venous infarction of the brain or by direct compression via a mass effect from the collection of subdural pus, but brain abscesses are not produced (*p. 1393*).

9. (C) Herpes simplex virus (HSV I) infections take many forms in humans. In addition to causing skin or mucosal vesicles known as cold sores or fever blisters, severe vesicular eruptions of the eye (keratoconjunctivitis) and a generalized vesiculating involvement of the skin (Kaposi's varicelliform eruption), HSV I produces both a neonatal and an adult from of encephalitis. In contrast to the adult form, which typically involves the inferior and medial regions of the temporal lobes and the orbital gyri of the frontal lobes, the neonatal form affects the entire brain. Postherpetic neuralgia, however, is a product of latent herpes zoster infection and refers to lingering pain after a case of shingles (see Question 40) (*pp. 320, 1397*).

10. (D) Berry aneurysms are developmental (often called congenital but not present at birth) arterial defects that are the most common cause (95%) of aneurysmal rupture in the CNS. They occur most commonly at the junction of the anterior cerebral and anterior communicating arteries (40%), the major bifurcation of the middle cerebral artery in the sylvian fissure (43%), and the junction of the internal carotid and posterior communicating arteries (20%). Only 4% are located in the basilar artery circulation. Although they are often solitary, more than one aneurysm is found in up to 30% of cases (*pp. 1406–1407*).

11. (E) The human immunodeficiency virus type I (HIV-1) directly infects the CNS and is associated with at least four different neuropathologic syndromes: (1) acute aseptic meningitis or, less commonly, acute encephalitis, (2) subacute encephalitis, (3) vacuolar myelopathy, and (4) peripheral neuropathy. In addition, of course, HIV-1 infection also significantly increases the risk of opportunistic CNS infections, especially from agents such as cytomegalovirus, varicella-zoster, herpes simplex, *Cryptococcus neoformans*, and *Toxoplasma gondi* (*pp. 1398–1399*).

12. (A) Carcinomatous meningitis refers to metastatic spread of tumor (not necessarily limited to true carcinoma, despite the term) via the CSF to the meningeal surfaces of the brain, spinal cord, and nerve roots. Among primary brain tumors, this mode of dissemination is most often associated with medulloblastomas, although some astrocytomas and pineal tumors grow in this pattern as well. Tumors metastatic to the brain may also spread in this manner, and the two that do so most frequently are lung and breast cancers.

Meningiomas (see Question 13) always grow as a localized mass adherent to the dura that is either bosselated (bumpy) or plaque-like. It does not cause carcinomatous meningitis (*pp. 1413, 1419, 1420, 1422*).

13. (C) Meningiomas are primary tumors of the specialized arachnoid cap cells of the meninges. They are most frequently slow-growing, well-circumscribed, benign tumors associated with a good prognosis. Only rarely do the anaplastic and papillary variants of this tumor behave in a malignant fashion and invade the brain or even metastasize. Hyperostosis of the bone overlying a meningioma is common and can be seen on radiologic studies. A common histologic characteristic of meningiomas, especially the transitional variant (the variant with histologic characteristics intermediate between the syncytial and fibroblastic variants), is the presence of psammoma bodies. These concentrically laminated spheroids of calcium salts give the tumor a gritty texture on gross examination and may appear as stippling on x-ray examination (*p. 1420*).

14. (C) Parkinsonism is a progressive disturbance of motor function characterized by damage to the striatonigral dopaminergic system. It typically results in expressionless facies, stooped posture, slowness of voluntary movement, festinating (short rapid steps) gait, rigidity, and a characteristic pill-rolling tremor. It is seen in a number of different conditions besides idiopathic Parkinson's disease, including drug/toxin injuries, postencephalitic parkinsonism, striatonigral degeneration, Shy-Drager syndrome, and progressive nuclear palsy, all of which affect the striatonigral dopaminergic system. Idiopathic Parkinson's disease (also called paralysis agitans) is the principal disease causing this syndrome. It occurs in individuals older than 50 years but is not known to be hereditary. Histologically, the disease is characterized by the presence of Lewy bodies, eosinophilic intracytoplasmic inclusion bodies, in the neurons of the substantia nigra and locus ceruleus. In addition, the melanin-containing neurons in these regions of the brain are typically depigmented.

Neurofibrillary tangles are seen in the affected neurons of postencephalitic parkinsonism (not Lewy bodies). They are not associated with idiopathic parkinsonism, however. Neuronal loss in the putamen and caudate is a characteristic of striatonigral degeneration, another degenerative disease of the basal ganglia that is clinically similar to idiopathic parkinsonism but pathologically different. In striatonigral degeneration, neither Lewy bodies (as seen in Parkinson's disease) nor neurofibrillary tangles (as seen in Alzheimer's and other degenerative diseases) are present. Diagnostic differentiation of striatonigral degeneration from Parkinson's disease is important because only the latter is responsive to levodopa treatment (*pp. 1430–1431*).

15. (A) Amyotrophic lateral sclerosis (ALS) complex (also called motor neuron disease) is a group of degenerative diseases of the pyramidal motor system with four clinical variants. The most common is amyotrophic lateral sclerosis, in which degeneration occurs in both the upper motor neurons (in the motor cortex) and lower motor neurons (in the cranial motor nuclei and anterior horns of the spinal cord). The disease has an invariably fatal outcome after a variable 2- to 6-year course.

Unlike poliomyelitis, a disease of lower motor neurons caused by an enterovirus, ALS is not known to be associated with a viral agent. The pathogenesis is unknown at present, and investigations of possible immunologic, viral, and metabolic causes have failed to demonstrate etiologic significance. Interestingly, a rare form of ALS complex (occurring in Chamorro Indians on the island of Guam) is thought to be related to toxin (flour made from seeds of the false sago palm *Cycas circinalis*) exposure (*pp. 1432–1433*).

16. (B) Neurofibromas are peripheral nerve tumors derived from Schwann cells. They are often multiple and are composed of interlacing bands of delicate spindle cells with slender, wavy nuclei. In neurofibromas, nerve fibers are found scattered throughout the tumor mass, which appears as a bulbous expansion of the entire nerve fascicle. In contrast to schwannomas, which are located eccentrically on the side of the nerve and can be surgically excised, neurofibromas cannot be resected without removing the involved nerve. Verocay bodies, a characteristic histologic feature of schwannomas, consist of palisaded nuclei in areas of high cellularity (known as Antoni A tissue, Antoni B areas being hypocellular) (*pp. 1445–1446*).

17. (True); 18. (True); 19. (False); 20. (True); 21. (False); 22. (False); 23. (True); 24. (False); 25. (False)

As a group, vascular disorders are the most common cause (about 50% of cases) of neurologic problems encountered in general hospitals. **(17)** The separate contributions of hypoxia and reduced blood flow to neurologic dysfunction are important to differentiate. Pure hypoxia (deprivation of oxygen) with maintenance of normal blood flow, as might occur on exposure to reduced atmospheric pressures, is tolerable to neurons for much longer periods of time than ischemia (reduced or interrupted blood flow). This is because cessation of blood flow is accompanied by buildup of metabolic products and pH changes that do not occur with anoxia alone. Severe hypoxia, however, is typically quickly followed by hypotension and cardiac arrest, making ischemia the final common pathway of anoxia of any cause. Of all the cells of the CNS, neurons are the most sensitive to ischemia. Evidence from experimental studies suggests that neurons can tolerate pure hypoxia for as long as 25 minutes, whereas ischemia produces permanent neuronal damage after about 4 minutes.

(18) Encephalopathic changes induced by ischemia are most commonly the result of less than effective cardiopulmonary resuscitation following cardiac arrest.

(19) Prolonged ischemia from a localized vascular obstruction, either from thrombus, embolus, or external compression, produces cerebral infarction in the distribution of the affected vessel. The infarction does not overlap arterial territories. Thus, a hemorrhagic infarct can often be differentiated from a cerebral hemorrhage that does not necessarily cause a pattern of involvement corresponding to a given vascular distribution (i.e., bleeding into tumors, amyloid angiopathy, and so on).

(20) Cerebral hemorrhage (bleeding into the brain substance) is most commonly caused by hypertensive vascular disease. In this disorder, bleeding is thought to occur from rupture of microaneurysms (Charcot-Buchard aneurysms) that form at bifurcations of intraparenchymal arteries, most commonly in the putamen (55%).

(21) Supratentorial cerebral hemorrhages tend to present as hemiplegias, whereas hemorrhage in the posterior fossa (e.g., a cerebellar hematoma) is associated with intractable vomiting, eye movement disorders, and ataxia.

(22) Although emboli are the most common cause of cerebral infarction in the distribution of the middle cerebral artery, the most common cause of cerebral infarction overall is large vessel thrombosis, usually atherosclerotic in origin.

(23) Lacunar infarcts are small infarcts in the deep portions of the brain (especially the thalamus, putamen, and internal capsule); they are characteristic of hypertensive vascular disease. Owing to their small size and variable location, lacunar infarcts can produce various ischemic syndromes or may even be asymptomatic. A pure motor hemiparesis and a pure sensory deficit are two of the recognized lacunar syndromes. They can occur from a small infarct in the internal capsule where the major tracts are compressed into a small volume.

(24) Hypertensive vascular disease is also associated with a syndrome of diffuse loss of deep hemispheric white matter with demyelination and gliosis known as subcortical leukoencephalopathy or Binswanger's disease. Both lacunae and subcortical demyelination are associated with chronic stable hypertension. Hypertensive encephalopathy, in contrast, is associated with acute malignant hypertension (e.g., eclampsia, acute nephritis), causing vascular necrosis, cerebral edema, and petechial hemorrhages.

(25) Unlike the brain, the spinal cord most often sustains vascular injury from disruption of the spinal arteries secondary to dissecting aortic aneurysms (*pp. 1403–1409*).

26. (False); 27. (True); 28. (False); 29. (True); 30. (False); 31. (False); 32. (False)

(26 and 27) The etiology of multiple sclerosis (MS) is incompletely understood. The disease causes diffuse primary demyelination in the CNS. Although it may occur in children, it usually affects adults between 20 and 40 years of age and is rare before puberty or after age 55. **(28)** The disease typically begins with paresthesias, diplopia, or cerebellar incoordination, but intellectual deterioration is not an early manifestation. **(29)** The CSF typically contains an increased immunoglobulin content, and immunoelectrophoretic analysis demonstrates oligoclonal bands that are not present in the serum. In contrast to subacute sclerosing panencephalitis (SSPE; see Question 3), in which the elevated CSF immunoglobulins are known to be directed against a specific antigen (measles virus), the antigenic targets of the CSF immunoglobulins in MS are yet unknown. Apparently, however, they are not directed against myelin. **(30)** In further contrast to SSPE, which typically occurs after a case of measles, MS is not associated with a preceding viral infection. **(31)** The characteristic brain and spinal cord plaques that occur in MS are not produced by gliosis. Rather, they consist of multiple small foci of demyelination and perivascular inflammation that have coalesced to form macroscopically visible lesions. **(32)** Although clinical trials have shown that high levels of immunosuppression can temporarily arrest the progression of MS in children, there is at present no truly effective treatment for this disease. During relapses, however, patients are often treated with adrenocorticotropic hormone or other immunosuppressive agents with some temporary benefit (*pp. 1422–1425*).

33. (D); 34. (C); 35. (B); 36. (A); 37. (B)

Distention of the ventricles by an increased volume of CSF is known as hydrocephalus. Although hydrocephalus can be caused by overproduction of fluid, decreased absorption of CSF is the most common cause.

Decreased CSF absorption may, in turn, result either from decreased transfer of CSF to the venous system by the arachnoid villi (communicating hydrocephalus) or from decreased flow through the CSF pathway to the villi as a result of obstruction (noncommunicating hydrocephalus). (33) Both types produce ventricular distention. (34) Either type may occur in a postmeningitis state, depending on the nature and extent of the injury and the location of the subsequent fibrosis. (In general, acute pyogenic meningitis of any type may cause adhesions between the meninges and the brain.) Severe pneumococcal meningitis may lead to communicating hydrocephalus from arachnoid fibrosis induced by large quantities of pneumococcal capsular polysaccharides in the subarachnoid space. Basal adhesive arachnoiditis obliterating the subarachnoid space around the brain stem may occlude the foramina of Magendie and Luschka, producing noncommunicating hydrocephalus.

(35) Obstructive (noncommunicating) hydrocephalus is characteristically seen in association with neoplasms that invade or compress the foramina in the CSF pathway. (36) Thrombosis of the dural sinuses interfere with transport of CSF into the venous system and typically produces communicating hydrocephalus. (37) The Dandy-Walker syndrome is a congenital malformation of the cerebellum in which the cerebellar vermis fails to develop. Consequently, occlusion or obliteration of the foramina of Magendie and Luschka occurs and noncommunicating hydrocephalus is produced (*pp. 1390–1391, 1441*).

38. (B); 39. (A); 40. (D); 41. (B); 42. (A)
Both rabies and poliomyelitis are viral diseases of the CNS that end in paralysis. (38) As typically occurs with most viral diseases of the CNS, poliomyelitis is preceded by a primary infection elsewhere, in this case in the gastrointestinal tract. Rabies is a noteworthy exception to this rule because the virus is inoculated directly into the peripheral nerves and ascends promptly to the brain. (39) Although other forms of viral encephalitis may be associated with inclusion bodies (e.g., intranuclear inclusions of cytomegalovirus or HSV-1, the only *diagnostic* inclusion is the Negri body of rabies. It is an eosinophilic cytoplasmic inclusion, usually round, oval, or bullet shaped and often multiple.

(40) Although rabies virus does affect the dorsal root ganglia, it also typically involves the neurons of Ammon's horn in the temporal lobe as well as the Purkinje cells of the cerebellum and the spinal cord. The principal target of poliovirus is the anterior horn cell of the spinal cord, although the posterior horn may be affected in very fulminant cases. (The viral agent that shows specific and exclusive tropism for the dorsal root ganglion cells is herpes zoster. After acute infection by herpes zoster (chickenpox), the virus remains latent for long periods of time within the dorsal root ganglia. Recrudescence of the viral infection, commonly called shingles, may occur with immunosuppression or advancing age.

(41) Rabies characteristically produces a severe encephalitis with flaccid paralysis in the late stage of the disease. In contrast, poliomyelitis, with its specifically targeted injury, characteristically causes a lower motor neuron paralysis. (42) Although the most common cause of death in both these diseases is respiratory failure, it occurs on the basis of respiratory center failure in rabies and from paralysis of the respiratory muscles in polio (*pp. 1397–1398*).

43. (D); 44. (B); 45. (C); 46. (D); 47. (D); 48. (A); 49. (B)
Acute disseminated encephalomyelitis and acute necrotizing hemorrhagic leukoencephalitis are two disorders with impossibly long names that fall into the category of perivenous encephalomyelitis. They are characterized by perivenular demyelination and a pronounced mononuclear inflammatory infiltrate. (43) Although they may occur in either children or adults, both of these diseases are extremely rare. (44) In contrast to acute disseminated encephalomyelitis, which typically occurs after a well-defined viral infection such as measles, mumps, or chickenpox, acute hemorrhagic leukoencephalitis is usually preceded only by a nonspecific respiratory tract infection. (45) Both diseases, however, are believed to be autoimmune in origin, because lymphocytes from patients with these diseases are sensitized to myelin basic protein. (46) In both diseases, the autoimmune response appears to be largely cellular rather than humoral, because antibodies to myelin proteins are not found.

(47) Unfortunately, both diseases have an extremely poor prognosis. About half of the patients with acute disseminated encephalomyelitis die in the acute phase of the disease, and those who survive usually have severe neurologic impairment. Acute necrotizing hemorrhagic leukoencephalitis is typically a rapidly fatal disorder with only rare survivors. (48) The pathologic findings in these diseases reflect their differing severity. In acute disseminated encephalomyelitis, the brain usually appears normal on gross examination, whereas in acute necrotizing hemorrhagic leukoencephalitis, the brain is soft, sometimes liquefied, and flecked with tiny hemorrhages. (49) On histologic examination, necrotizing vasculitis is seen in acute necrotizing hemorrhagic leukoencephalitis and corresponds to the hemorrhagic areas seen grossly. Although perivascular inflammation is seen in acute disseminated encephalomyelitis, vasculitis does not occur (*pp. 1425–1426*).

50. (D); 51. (E); 52. (A); 53. (A); 54. (B); 55. (E); 56. (E)
Although the neuron is the basic parenchymal element of the CNS, numerous specialized supportive and protective interstitial cells are necessary for normal neuronal functioning. (50) These supportive elements, called neuroglial cells, consist of astrocytes, oligodendrocytes, ependymal cells, and microglial cells. (51) It is the microglial cells (not presented as a choice in the question) that represent the CNS component of the monocyte-macrophage system. When activated, these cells resemble macrophages in both their cytoplasmic histochemical profiles and their phagocytic activity.

(**52 and 53**) Astrocytes form an extensive cellular plexus that serves as the structural framework for the all-important neurons. They are also thought to provide biochemical support and insulation to neighboring neurons. After injury, astrocytes are responsible for the CNS equivalent of scar formation, a process known as gliosis. In contrast to fibrosis, gliosis does not lead to the production of collagen. Rather, defects are filled by glial fibers, which are actually cellular processes of astrocytes containing abundant intermediate filaments made up of vimentin and glial fibrillary acidic protein.

(**54**) Oligodendrocytes, so called because they have fewer and shorter dendrites than astrocytes, are responsible for the production and maintenance of CNS myelin. In contrast to the Schwann cell, the myelin forming cell of the peripheral nervous system, each oligodendrocyte contributes segments of myelin sheaths to *multiple* axons. In demyelinating diseases of the CNS, oligodendrocytes sustain most of the injury.

(**55 and 56**) Although ependymal cells line the ventricles of the brain, they are not responsible for the production of the CSF contained within, nor are they responsible for its resorption. The cells of the choroid plexus produce CSF, which, after traversing the ventricles and entering the subarachnoid space, is resorbed by the cells of the arachnoid villi (*pp. 1387–1388*).

57. (B); 58. (D); 59. (A); 60. (C); 61. (C)

Meningitis refers to inflammation limited to the leptomeninges in the subarachnoid space and is most often caused by infection. The nature of the inflammatory process is largely determined by the causal organism. Acute pyogenic meningitis is usually bacterial in origin; meningococcal meningitis is a common example. Acute lymphocytic meningitis, usually virally induced, is exemplified by mumps meningitis. Chronic meningitis, a more slowly evolving process, is associated with infection by bacteria or fungi; tuberculous meningitis is a prototypic example. (**57**) Only in acute lymphocytic meningitis is the glucose content of the CSF almost invariably normal. Pyogenic meningitis causes a strikingly reduced CSF glucose content, whereas chronic meningitis is associated with a variably reduced glucose content. (**58**) In contrast, all forms of meningitis usually produce elevations in the protein content of the CSF. These vary only in magnitude.

(**59**) Large numbers of neutrophils in the CSF are characteristic of acute pyogenic meningitis such as that of meningococcal origin. In mumps meningitis, the CSF pleocytosis consists mainly of lymphocytes, and in tuberculous meningitis, it is composed largely of mononuclear cells. (**60**) Only the acute forms of meningitis, either pyogenic or lymphocytic, are associated clinically with signs of meningeal irritation: a stiff neck, headache, photophobia, irritability, and clouding of consciousness. Chronic meningitis presents with more generalized neurologic symptoms including headache, malaise, mental confusion, and vomiting rather than a stiff neck. (**61**) Obliterative endarteritis is a complication of chronic meningitis caused by the continuing inflammatory reaction around the vessels of the subarachnoid space. Because infarctions in the underlying brain may result, obliterative endarteritis is one of the most feared complications of this type of meningitis (*pp. 1392–1393*).

62. (A); 63. (D); 64. (C); 65. (A); 66. (B); 67. (C); 68. (C); 69. (D); 70. (D)

Astrocytomas, oligodendrogliomas, and ependymomas all are neuroglial tumors, but each has distinctive characteristics. (**62**) Astrocytomas are the most common type of primary brain tumor in children. In contrast to adult astrocytomas, most of which occur in the cerebral hemispheres, most astrocytomas in children occur in the cerebellum. (**63**) The most common primary brain tumor in adults is glioblastoma multiforme, constituting 25 to 30% of cases. (**65**) The astrocytoma is the tumor type that gives rise to glioblastoma multiforme, the most anaplastic of all the gliomas. Although they may arise de novo, most glioblastomas develop in preexisting astrocytomas by progressive dedifferentiation.

(**64**) In the spinal cord, the most common type of glial tumor is the ependymoma. Ependymomas constitute about 63% of intraspinal gliomas but only 5 to 6% of all intracranial gliomas. (**67 and 68**) Histologic features that are particularly characteristic of ependymomas are rosette and pseudorosette formation. A rosette is a small circle of tumor cells arranged around a central space that may contain neuroglial fibers. The tumor cells in pseudorosettes, on the other hand, are arranged around a blood vessel.

(**66**) Among the neuroglial tumors, oligodendrogliomas are distinctive in their tendency to calcify. This pathologic feature is actually a diagnostic aid, since oligodendrogliomas characteristically appear stippled with calcifications on x-ray examination and computed tomographic scan.

(**69 and 70**) Extraneural metastases from any primary intracranial tumor are distinctly uncommon, and when they occur, they are most likely to be from a glioblastoma or medulloblastoma. Another characteristic shared by all neuroglial tumors is their resistance to chemotherapy. Depending on the feasibility of surgical resection, excision and radiotherapy have thus far provided the most successful therapeutic approaches to neuroglial tumors (*pp. 1414–1417*).

71. (D); 72. (A); 73. (B); 74. (B); 75. (C)

The leukodystrophies are diseases of the white matter resulting from biochemical defects in the pathway of myelin metabolism. (**71**) All of these diseases become manifest in early childhood as symmetrical, global disorders of myelinization. (**72**) Metachromatic leukodystrophy is an autosomal recessive disorder of sphingomyelin metabolism produced by a deficiency of arylsulfatase A (cerebroside sulfatase). It usually presents as a progressive motor impairment with mental deterioration and can be diagnosed by measuring urinary arylsulfatase A. (**73 and 74**) Another autosomal recessive disorder, Krabbe's disease, results from a deficiency of galactocerebroside β-galactosidase and the accumulation of galactocerebroside. This disease usually begins within the first 6 months of life and leads to death within a year. In addition to demyelination, a characteristic histologic feature is the presence of multinuclear histocytic cells called globoid cells. (75) Adrenoleukodystrophy is a familial X-linked recessive disease leading to the accumulation of long-chain fatty acid esters of cholesterol, most likely the result of a defect in peroxisome function. It produces symmetrical demyelination in the cerebral hemispheres and adrenal failure and has a diagnostic ultrastructural feature. By electron microscopy, specific cytoplasmic inclusions composed of dense, long, thin leaflets enclosing an electron-lucent space are seen in the cerebral macrophages, adrenocortical cells, testicular Leydig's cells, and Schwann cells of patients with this disease (*pp. 1437–1438*).

76. (C); 77. (B); 78. (A); 79. (A); 80. (C); 81. (B)

Peripheral neuropathies develop whenever axonal degeneration, demyelination, or a combination of these occurs in the peripheral nervous system. They may occur in association with a large number of diseases and produce varied clinical syndromes, depending on the size and the type (sensory, motor, or autonomic) of the axons principally involved. Most major causes of peripheral neuropathy tend to produce a specific pattern of injury and corresponding clinical syndrome with variable predictability.

(76, 77, 80, 81) Diseases that produce focal patchy lesions rather than generalized diffuse injury tend to produce asymmetric neuropathy. They affect single individual nerves and produce a mononeuritis or, if more than one nerve is affected, a mononeuritis multiplex. Processes that are associated with diffuse injury, however, tend to produce symmetrical polyneuropathies. Polyarteritis nodosa, diabetes, and sarcoidosis are examples of processes that are typically focal and cause neuropathies that are usually asymmetric. Both alcohol and lead have diffuse systemic toxic effects and are associated with symmetrical sensorimotor polyneuropathies.

(78 and 79) Diseases that cause acute demyelination without significant axonal injury and an acute ascending motor paralysis include the Landry-Guillain-Barré syndrome (acute idiopathic polyneuritis) and diphtheria. The cause of the acute demyelination in the Landry-Guillain-Barré syndrome is yet unknown, although immunologic mechanisms have been implicated. Diphtheritic peripheral neuritis is the direct result of the action of diphtheria toxin on the peripheral nerve. In diphtheria, demyelination is limited to the dorsal root ganglia and the adjacent motor and sensory roots, because there is a naturally occurring defect in the blood barrier at these points, allowing penetration of the toxin (*pp. 1442–1445*).